Emergency

Care and Transportation
of the Sick and Injured

AAOS
AMERICAN ACADEMY OF ORTHOPAEDIC SURGEONS

STUDENT WORKBOOK

JONES & BARTLETT
LEARNING

World Headquarters
Jones & Bartlett Learning
25 Mall Road
Burlington, MA 01803
978-443-5000
info@jblearning.com
www.jblearning.com
www.psglearning.com

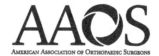

Substantial discounts on bulk quantities of Jones & Bartlett Learning publications are available to corporations, professional associations, and other qualified organizations. For details and specific discount information, contact the special sales department at Jones & Bartlett Learning via the below contact information or send an email to specialsales@jblearning.com.

Production Credits
President, Professional Education: Timothy McClinton
VP, Product Development: Christine Emerton
Director of Product Management: Jonathan Epstein
Product Manager: Carly Mahoney
Content Strategist: Barbara Scotese
Content Coordinator: Paula-Yuan Gregory
Marketing Director: Brian Rooney
VP, Manufacturing and Inventory Control: Therese Connell
Composition: S4Carlisle Publishing Services

Project Management: S4Carlisle Publishing Services
Cover Design: Scott Moden
Rights Specialist: Rebecca Damon
Project Manager: Lori Mortimer
Project Specialist: Angela Montoya
Senior Media Development Editor: Troy Liston
Cover Image: © Jones & Bartlett Learning
Printing and Binding: Sheridan

Editorial Credits
Author: Wm. Travis Engel, DO, MSc, Paramedic, FP-C, CCP-C

ISBN: 978-1-284-29242-8

6048

Printed in the United States of America
27 26 25 24   10 9 8 7 6 5

Contents

CHAPTER

1

EMS Systems

General Knowledge

Matching

Match each of the items in the left column to the appropriate definition in the right column.

_____	**1.** ALS	**A.**	An EMS professional with extensive training in ALS skills, such as intubation
_____	**2.** BLS	**B.**	A proactive process of development that capitalizes on strengths and addresses challenges
_____	**3.** EMT	**C.**	A system that assists dispatchers with unit selection
_____	**4.** AEMT	**D.**	A physician who authorizes the EMT to provide care in the field
_____	**5.** Paramedic	**E.**	The responsibility of the medical director to ensure that appropriate care is delivered by an EMT
_____	**6.** Medical control	**F.**	Legislation that protects a patient's private health information
_____	**7.** CQI	**G.**	An EMS professional trained in some ALS interventions
_____	**8.** EMS	**H.**	Advanced procedures, such as intravenous (IV) therapy, advanced airway management, and the administration of certain emergency medications
_____	**9.** MIH	**I.**	A designated location in which the EMS agency is responsible for providing prehospital care
_____	**10.** EMD	**J.**	Legislation that protects disabled individuals from discrimination
_____	**11.** Primary service area	**K.**	Physician direction to an EMS team
_____	**12.** Medical director	**L.**	Providing health care within the community rather than in an office
_____	**13.** Americans with Disabilities Act	**M.**	An EMS professional trained in BLS interventions
_____	**14.** Quality control	**N.**	Basic lifesaving interventions, such as CPR
_____	**15.** HIPAA	**O.**	A system to provide prehospital care to the sick and injured

Multiple-Choice

Read each item carefully and then select the one best response.

_____ **1.** What year was the white paper *Accidental Death and Disability: The Neglected Disease of Modern Society* published?
- **A.** 1966
- **B.** 1970
- **C.** 1984
- **D.** 1992

_____ **2.** Which of the following is true of medical control?

    A. It is determined by the dispatcher.

    B. It may consist of written or "standing" orders.

    C. It requires online radio or phone consultations.

    D. It affects only ALS providers.

_____ **3.** What is the purpose of providing mobile integrated health care (MIH)?

    A. To allow paramedics to function beyond the scope of practice

    B. To allow EMS agencies to respond to emergencies faster

    C. To educate the community on public health issues

    D. To facilitate improved access to health care at an affordable price

_____ **4.** What is the major goal of continuous quality improvement (CQI)?

    A. To perform quarterly audits of the EMS system

    B. To verify that EMTs have received BLS/CPR training

    C. To ensure that the public receives the highest standard of care

    D. To verify that the proper information is received in the billing department

_____ **5.** Which of the following involves federal legislation concerning patient confidentiality?

    A. HIPAA

    B. NAACS

    C. EMTALA

    D. FLCPC

Questions 6–10 are derived from the following scenario: After stocking the ambulance this morning, you and your partner go out for breakfast. While entering the restaurant, you see an older gentleman clutch his chest and collapse to the floor. When you get to him, he has no pulse and is not breathing.

_____ **6.** Which of the following authorizes you, as an EMT, to provide emergency care to this patient?

    A. The city council

    B. The EMS agency

    C. The medical director

    D. The fire chief

_____ **7.** In order to treat this patient, what will you need to follow?

    A. Emergency medical dispatch

    B. Continuous quality improvement (CQI)

    C. Protocols

    D. Quality control

_____ **8.** What level of training would allow you to perform cardiac monitoring and endotracheal intubation of this patient?

    A. EMR

    B. EMT

    C. AEMT

    D. Paramedic

_____ **9.** While you checked the patient's airway, breathing, and circulation, your partner considered the benefits of requesting a(n) _____ ambulance to assist with patient care.

    A. ALS

    B. CQI

    C. PSA

    D. EMD

_____ **10.** While you performed CPR on this patient, your partner retrieved the _____, which will deliver an appropriate electrical shock.

A. EMD

B. AED

C. PSA

D. GPS

True/False

If you believe the statement to be more true than false, write the letter "T" in the space provided. If you believe the statement to be more false than true, write the letter "F."

_____ **1.** EMT personnel are the highest-qualified members of the prehospital care team.

_____ **2.** The EMT scope of practice includes the use of an automated external defibrillator (AED).

_____ **3.** Personnel trained as EMRs can include law enforcement officers, firefighters, and ski patrollers.

_____ **4.** A professional appearance and manner by the EMT will help build the patient's confidence and ease the patient's anxiety.

_____ **5.** Patient care should be focused on procedures that have proven useful in improving outcomes.

_____ **6.** As a health care professional and an extension of physician care, you are not bound by patient confidentiality.

_____ **7.** Most EMS training programs must adhere to national standards established by the accrediting organizations.

_____ **8.** The medical director is responsible for authorizing and regulating all emergency medical services within the state.

_____ **9.** Advanced EMTs typically go through 1,000 to 1,300 hours of training.

_____ **10.** The development of the field medic and rapid helicopter evacuation took place during the Korean War.

Fill-in-the-Blank

Read each item carefully and then complete the statement by filling in the missing words.

1. _____ _____ _____ is a circular system of continuous internal and external reviews and audits of all aspects of an EMS system.

2. Each EMS system has a physician _____ _____, who authorizes the EMTs in the service to provide medical care in the field.

3. One of the most dramatic developments in prehospital emergency care is the use of a(n) _____ _____ defibrillator.

4. The primary _____ area is the main area in which an EMS agency operates.

5. A 9-1-1 dispatch center is called a public safety _____ _____, or PSAP.

Critical Thinking

Short-Answer

Complete this section with short written answers using the space provided.

1. Describe the EMT's role in the EMS system.

_____

_____

_____

2. What role has the US Department of Transportation played in the development of EMS?

_____

_____

_____

3. List five of the roles and/or responsibilities of being an EMT.

_____

_____

_____

4. Describe the two basic types of medical direction that help the EMT provide care.

_____

_____

_____

Ambulance Calls

The following case scenarios provide an opportunity to explore the concerns associated with patient management and to enhance critical-thinking skills. Read each scenario and answer each question to the best of your ability.

1. You are dispatched to a two-car motor vehicle collision. On arrival, you see minimal damage to both vehicles because they were traveling less than 25 mph (40 kph) when the collision occurred. You and your partner interview and examine all of the patients and find no apparent injuries. Dispatch contacts you and asks if you need an ALS crew to respond to your location.

Explain how you would respond and why.

_____

_____

_____

2. You and your partner are both EMTs and are dispatched to a private residence in response to a report of a hanging. You arrive to find a distraught man in the front yard, who quickly explains that he found his teenage daughter in the garage hanging by the neck from an extension cord. You enter the garage and find the patient unresponsive and not breathing, but with a weak pulse. Using EMT airway skills, neither of you is able to successfully open the patient's airway enough to provide ventilations.

What should you do?

_____

_____

_____

CHAPTER

2 Workforce Safety and Wellness

General Knowledge

Matching

Match each of the items in the left column to the appropriate definition in the right column.

_____	**1.** Communicable disease	**A.**	Examples include gloves, gowns, and face shields
_____	**2.** PPE	**B.**	The process of alarm, reaction, and recovery
_____	**3.** OSHA	**C.**	The regulatory compliance agency that develops and publishes guidelines that reduce hazards in the workplace
_____	**4.** Posttraumatic stress disorder	**D.**	An illness that can be spread from one person to another
_____	**5.** General adaptation syndrome	**E.**	A microorganism that is capable of causing disease in a susceptible host
_____	**6.** Pathogen	**F.**	May develop after experiencing a psychologically distressing event
_____	**7.** Transmission	**G.**	Encompasses reporting, documentation, and treatment
_____	**8.** Postexposure management	**H.**	Includes an unwelcome sexual advance or advances
_____	**9.** *Emergency Response Guidebook*	**I.**	The use of objects to limit a person's visibility of you
_____	**10.** Indirect contact	**J.**	Contact with blood, body fluids, tissues, or airborne particles
_____	**11.** Exposure	**K.**	The presence of infectious organisms in or on objects or a patient's body
_____	**12.** Infection control	**L.**	A resource detailing common hazards and proper responses
_____	**13.** Sexual harassment	**M.**	The way in which an infectious agent is spread
_____	**14.** Contamination	**N.**	Procedures to reduce transmission of infection among patients and health care personnel
_____	**15.** Concealment	**O.**	The spread of infection through an inanimate object

Multiple-Choice

Read each item carefully and then select the one best response.

_____ **1.** If you are in the first unit to arrive at the scene of a motor vehicle collision, you should:

   A. immediately extricate patients from vehicles

   B. disregard downed power lines

   C. place cones or other warning devices on the roadway to warn oncoming traffic

   D. park off of the roadway to leave room for the fire engine

_____ **2.** The stage of the grieving process where an attempt is made to secure a prize for good behavior or promise to change one's lifestyle is known as:

   A. denial

   B. acceptance

   C. bargaining

   D. depression

_____ 3. The stage of the grieving process that involves a refusal to accept diagnosis or care is known as:
  A. denial
  B. acceptance
  C. bargaining
  D. depression

_____ 4. When tools are being used during extrication, you should:
  A. protect your eyes from ultraviolet light
  B. wear eyeglasses with side shields
  C. consider wearing body armor for added protection
  D. wear a face shield or goggles

_____ 5. Which of the following is a fatigue management recommendation made by the US Department of Transportation?
  A. Napping should be discouraged while at work.
  B. Shifts should not exceed 24 hours in duration.
  C. The consumption of caffeine at work should be banned.
  D. EMS providers should get a minimum of 11 hours of sleep per night.

_____ 6. When providing support for a grieving person, it is okay to say:
  A. "I'm sorry."
  B. "Give it time."
  C. "I know how you feel."
  D. "You have to keep on going."

_____ 7. What is the first thing you should do if exposed to a patient's blood or bodily fluids?
  A. Activate your department's infection control plan.
  B. Turn over patient care to another EMS provider.
  C. Wash the exposed area with soap and water.
  D. Seek immediate medical attention.

_____ 8. _____ is a sign of compassion fatigue.
  A. Choosing to work extra shifts
  B. Excessive positivity while at work
  C. Aggression toward patients
  D. Increased empathy for patients

_____ 9. Examples of events likely to cause eustress include all of the following EXCEPT:
  A. receiving a promotion
  B. divorce or separation from a partner
  C. beginning an exercise regimen
  D. the birth of a child

_____ 10. What should you do if you suspect that your patient has tuberculosis?
  A. Place a surgical mask on yourself and the patient.
  B. Place a particulate air respirator on the patient and a surgical mask on yourself.
  C. Place a particulate air respirator on the patient.
  D. Place a particulate air respirator on yourself and a surgical mask on the patient.

_____ 11. Drug and alcohol use in the workplace causes:
  A. decreased stress for coworkers
  B. increased accidents
  C. increased decision-making ability
  D. increased physical ability

_____ **12.** Regardless of how stressful the situation is, you must focus on several factors. Which of the following factors is your top priority?
- **A.** Personal safety
- **B.** Patient care
- **C.** Scene safety
- **D.** Safety of bystanders

_____ **13.** When acknowledging the death of a child, reactions vary, but _____ is common.
- **A.** happiness
- **B.** disbelief
- **C.** apprehension
- **D.** psychosis

_____ **14.** Which of the following is NOT a way that an infectious disease is transmitted?
- **A.** Vector-borne
- **B.** Airborne
- **C.** Cyberborne
- **D.** Foodborne

_____ **15.** Which item of PPE should be the last to be removed?
- **A.** Gloves
- **B.** Masks
- **C.** Gowns
- **D.** Eye shields

_____ **16.** Which of the following is NOT considered a common hazard in a fire?
- **A.** Smoke
- **B.** Building collapse
- **C.** Toxic gases
- **D.** Bystanders

_____ **17.** _____ _____ occur(s) when insignificant stressors accumulate into a larger, stress-related problem.
- **A.** Negative stress
- **B.** Cumulative stress
- **C.** Psychological stress
- **D.** Severe stressors

_____ **18.** Events that can trigger critical incident stress include:
- **A.** mass-casualty incidents
- **B.** serious damage to your personal vehicle while off-duty
- **C.** death or serious injury of a patient's friend
- **D.** loss of equipment at the scene

_____ **19.** Consumption of _____ _____ may result in lower overall energy levels.
- **A.** simple sugars
- **B.** complex carbohydrates
- **C.** polyunsaturated fats
- **D.** lean meats

_____ **20.** The safest, most reliable sources for long-term energy production are:
- **A.** sugars
- **B.** carbohydrates
- **C.** fats
- **D.** proteins

_____ **21.** A CISM meeting is an opportunity to discuss:
   A. feelings about the incident
   B. the operational critique
   C. who is to blame for the errors
   D. opportunities for improvement

_____ **22.** Which of the following is NOT included on the CDC list of recommended immunizations for health care workers?
   A. Meningitis vaccine
   B. Hepatitis B vaccine
   C. Influenza vaccine
   D. Varicella vaccine

_____ **23.** Hazardous materials in vehicles and buildings should be clearly identified using:
   A. manifests
   B. MSDS sheets
   C. placards
   D. beacons

_____ **24.** Which of the following is true regarding cultural diversity on the job?
   A. Coworkers should never discuss race, religion, or politics.
   B. The broad range of life experiences brought by coworkers can increase the strength of the team.
   C. Teams are stronger when coworkers of similar cultural beliefs work exclusively with each other.
   D. Patients should only be treated by EMS personnel of the same race and gender when possible.

True/False

If you believe the statement to be more true than false, write the letter "T" in the space provided. If you believe the statement to be more false than true, write the letter "F."

_____ **1.** Recapping the needle from a syringe is the best way to dispose of it safely.

_____ **2.** Gloves, eye protection, and masks are the main components of PPE.

_____ **3.** Denial is usually the first step in the grieving process.

_____ **4.** Bodily fluids are generally not considered infectious substances.

_____ **5.** Most EMTs never suffer from stress.

_____ **6.** Physical conditioning and nutrition are two factors that the EMT can control in helping to reduce stress.

_____ **7.** The likelihood of you becoming infected during routine patient care is high.

_____ **8.** Construction-type helmets are not well suited for rescue situations.

_____ **9.** The religious customs and needs of the patient must be respected.

_____ **10.** Diversity is an ineffective way to strengthen a public safety workforce.

Fill-in-the-Blank

Read each item carefully and then complete the statement by filling in the missing word(s).

1. _____ is a specific type of stress that produces negative responses.

2. _____ _____ involves the contamination of food or water with an organism that can cause disease.

3. A(n) _____ _____ is a medical condition caused by the growth and spread of small, harmful organisms within the body.

4. Your safety is the most important consideration at a(n) _____ materials incident.

5. Proper _____ is the simplest, yet most effective, way to control disease transmission.

6. _____ involves the tactical use of an impenetrable barrier for protection.

7. The _____ of a human being is one of the most _____ events for another human being to accept.

8. The term _____ _____ refers to the tactics that have been shown to alleviate or eliminate stress reactions.

9. Good, productive _____ is as important as eating well and exercise in the maintenance of good health.

10. _____ _____ is important in case blood splatters toward your eyes.

Critical Thinking

Multiple-Choice

Read each critical-thinking item carefully and then select the one best response.

Questions 1–5 are derived from the following scenario: A 12-year-old boy told his grandmother that he was going to collect the day's mail, located on the opposite side of the street, for her. As he was returning with the mail, he was struck by a vehicle and was found lying lifeless in the middle of the street.

_____ 1. Which of the following would be appropriate to say to the grandmother?
   A. "Don't worry. I'm sure he'll be fine."
   B. "What were you thinking? You will be reported!"
   C. "We're placing him on a backboard to protect his back, and we'll take him to the Columbus Community Hospital. Do you know who his doctor is?"
   D. It's best not to spend time talking to the grandmother.

_____ 2. As an EMT, you know that these types of calls are coming. All of the following are ways to meet such stressful situations EXCEPT:
   A. eat a balanced diet
   B. go for walks or other forms of exercise
   C. cut down on caffeine and sugars
   D. increase overtime hours

_____ 3. You or your partner may develop _____ after experiencing this call.
   A. critical incident stress management
   B. posttraumatic stress disorder
   C. critical stress debriefing
   D. an acute stress reaction

_____ 4. What is NOT a sign of cumulative stress that you or your partner might exhibit after a stressful event has occurred?
   A. Irritability toward coworkers, family, and friends
   B. Loss of interest in work
   C. Guilt
   D. Feelings of relief

_____ 5. When should you begin protecting yourself with standard precautions on this call?
   A. As soon as you are dispatched
   B. As soon as you arrive
   C. After you assess the victim and know what you need
   D. After speaking with the grandmother

Short-Answer

Complete this section with short written answers using the space provided.

1. Describe the basic concept of standard precautions.

_____

_____

_____

2. List the five stages of the grieving process.

_____

_____

_____

3. List five warning signs of cumulative stress.

_____

_____

_____

4. List five strategies for managing stress.

_____

_____

_____

5. List the CDC-recommended immunizations for health care workers.

_____

_____

_____

6. List the three layers of clothing recommended for cold weather.

_____

_____

_____

7. List three physiological manifestations of positive and/or negative forms of stress.

_____

_____

_____

8. What are five of the common hazards associated with a fire scene?

_____

_____

_____

Ambulance Calls

The following case scenarios provide an opportunity to explore the concerns associated with patient management and to enhance critical-thinking skills. Read each scenario and answer each question to the best of your ability.

1. In the process of working a motor vehicle collision, your arm is gashed open, and you are exposed to the blood of a patient who tells you that he is HIV positive. You have no water supply with which to wash. Your patient is stable, and you are able to control his bleeding with direct pressure.

How would you best manage this situation?

_____

_____

_____

2. You are dispatched to a large apartment complex for a person in respiratory distress. You find the elderly patient living in a dark, messy apartment with many family members, both adults and children, and you know that numerous cases of tuberculosis have been reported in this particular complex.

With regard to infection control, how would you best manage this situation?

_____

_____

_____

Fill in the Patient Care Report

Read the incident scenario and then complete the following patient care report (PCR).

You and your partner are posted in the parking lot of a convenience store on McBride Avenue just west of Highway 9, cleaning and organizing the back of the ambulance, when emergency tones burst from the radio. "Truck Three, emergency traffic," the dispatcher says.

"Go ahead for Truck Three," you respond.

"Truck Three, priority one call to 7-9-7-9 Fisher Boulevard for a possible overdose. Show your time en route to be oh-nine-twelve."

You copy the assignment, activate the lights and siren, and roll off toward the address, about 14 minutes away.

As you pull up to the address, a towering, gray concrete block housing eight stories of single-room apartments, you are met by a police officer.

"So the mom calls us because she and her daughter were in the middle of a domestic issue," the officer says as he leads you through the lobby to the elevator. "By the time we got here, the 16-year-old girl had locked herself in the bathroom. I got in there and found her unconscious on the floor with a rig next to her."

"Rig?" your new partner whispers in your ear while you are waiting for the elevator to rumble to the sixth floor.

"Syringe," you say quietly as the officer steps off of the elevator and waves you to an open door.

The clock on the kitchenette microwave reads 9:29 as you enter the small, dimly lit apartment to the sounds of a woman wailing in the bathroom. Two police officers quickly move the distraught mother out of the tiny bathroom so that you can get to the unresponsive girl.

"Let's get her out into the living room," you say, using the extremity lift to move the 48-kg (106-lb) patient into the wider floor of the living room. "And watch out for that needle next to her arm; there's no cap on it."

In the living room, you determine that the girl is breathing slowly but adequately and find that she has a slow pulse. You decide to get a full set of vital signs while your partner questions the mother about the girl's history and current drug use. At 0934, the patient's blood pressure is 116/76 mm Hg; her pulse is 56 beats/min; breathing is 8 breaths/min, but with good tidal volume; and she has a pulse oximetry reading of 96%. As you are placing a nonrebreathing mask on the unresponsive girl with 15 L/min of supplemental oxygen, your partner kneels next to you and looks at his notepad.

"She attempted suicide 2 years ago by taking an overdose of aspirin and has been struggling over the past year with a heroin addiction."

"Okay," you say. "Let's get her out to the stretcher and get going."

At 0947, your partner closes you into the back of the ambulance with the patient and climbs into the cab while you obtain a second set of vital signs: blood pressure 114/74 mm Hg, pulse 48 beats/min, respirations 8 breaths/min, and SpO$_2$ 95%. Five minutes later, you arrive at the ambulance bay of the local hospital and quickly move the patient inside. You transfer her care to the emergency department staff after giving a full report to the receiving nurse. After cleaning and preparing the ambulance, you and your partner are clear at 1005.

Fill-in-the-Patient Care Report

EMS Patient Care Report (PCR)			
Date:	Incident No.:	Nature of Call:	Location:
Dispatched:	En Route:	At Scene:	Transport:	At Hospital:	In Service:

Patient Information	
Age: Sex: Weight (in kg [lb]):	Allergies: Medications: Past Medical History: Chief Complaint:

Vital Signs				
Time:	BP:	Pulse:	Respirations:	SpO$_2$:
Time:	BP:	Pulse:	Respirations:	SpO$_2$:
Time:	BP:	Pulse:	Respirations:	SpO$_2$:

EMS Treatment (circle all that apply)				
Oxygen @ ___ L/min via (circle one): NC NRM BVM	Assisted Ventilation	Airway Adjunct	CPR
Defibrillation	Bleeding Control	Bandaging	Splinting	Other:

Narrative

Skills

Skill Drills

Test your knowledge of this skill by filling in the correct words in the photo captions.

Skill Drill 2-1: Proper Glove-Removal Technique

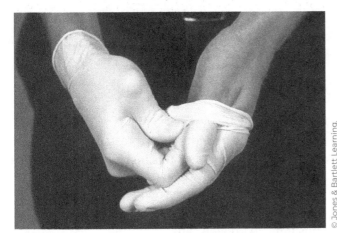

1. Partially remove the first glove by pinching at the _____. Be careful to touch only the _____ of the glove.

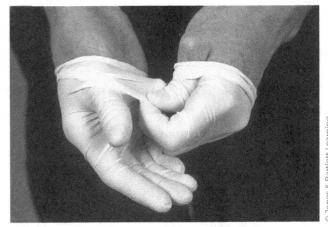

2. Remove the _____ glove by pinching the _____ with your partially gloved hand.

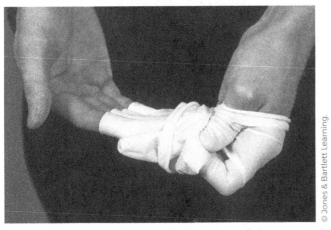

3. Pull the second glove inside out toward the _____.

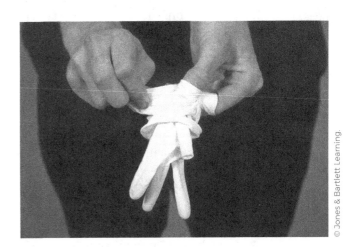

4. Grasp both gloves with your _____ hand, touching only the clean _____ surfaces.

CHAPTER

3 Medical, Legal, and Ethical Issues

General Knowledge

Matching

Match each of the items in the left column to the appropriate definition in the right column.

_____	**1.** Assault	**A.**	Being able to make rational decisions
_____	**2.** Abandonment	**B.**	The specific authorization to provide care expressed by the patient
_____	**3.** Advance directive	**C.**	Confining a person who presents a significant risk to themselves or others
_____	**4.** Battery	**D.**	The granted permission to provide treatment or care
_____	**5.** Certification	**E.**	Touching without consent
_____	**6.** Competent	**F.**	The legal responsibility to provide care
_____	**7.** Consent	**G.**	A written documentation that specifies treatment
_____	**8.** Duty to act	**H.**	Unlawfully placing a patient in fear of bodily harm
_____	**9.** Ethics	**I.**	A unilateral termination of care
_____	**10.** Expressed consent	**J.**	The failure to provide the standard of care
_____	**11.** Forcible restraint	**K.**	The manner in which you must act or behave as an EMT
_____	**12.** Implied consent	**L.**	A process that recognizes that a person has met set standards
_____	**13.** Medicolegal	**M.**	The legal assumption that treatment was desired
_____	**14.** Negligence	**N.**	Relating to law or forensic medicine
_____	**15.** Standard of care	**O.**	The philosophy of right and wrong

Multiple Choice

Read each item carefully and then select the one best response.

_____ **1.** The care that an EMT is able to provide is most commonly defined as a:
  A. duty to act
  B. competency
  C. scope of practice
  D. certification

_____ **2.** How the EMT is required to act or behave is called:
  A. the standard of care
  B. competency
  C. the scope of practice
  D. certification

_____ 3. The process by which an individual, an institution, or a program is evaluated and recognized as meeting the minimum required standards to provide safe and ethical care is called:
   A. the standard of care
   B. competency
   C. the scope of practice
   D. certification

_____ 4. Negligence is based on the EMT's duty to act, breach of duty, causation, and:
   A. expressed consent
   B. termination of care
   C. mode of transport
   D. real or perceived damages

_____ 5. While treating a patient with a suspected head injury, he becomes verbally abusive and tells you to "leave me alone." If you stop treating him, you may be guilty of:
   A. neglect
   B. battery
   C. abandonment
   D. slander

_____ 6. Good Samaritan laws generally are designed to offer protection to people who render care in good faith. They do not offer protection from:
   A. properly performed CPR
   B. acts of gross negligence
   C. improvising splinting materials
   D. providing supportive BLS to a DNR patient

_____ 7. Which of the following is generally NOT considered confidential?
   A. Assessment findings
   B. Treatment provided
   C. A patient's medical history
   D. Billing information released to third parties

_____ 8. An important safeguard against legal implication is:
   A. responding to every call with lights and siren
   B. checking ambulance equipment once a month
   C. transporting every patient to an emergency department
   D. writing a complete and accurate run report

_____ 9. Your responsibility to provide patient care is called:
   A. scope of practice
   B. duty to act
   C. DNR
   D. standard of care

_____ 10. Which of the following is NOT considered a presumptive sign of death?
   A. Absence of pupil reactivity
   B. Profound cyanosis
   C. Dependent lividity
   D. Absence of chest rise and fall

_____ 11. Definitive or conclusive signs of death that are obvious and clear to even nonmedical people include all of the following EXCEPT:
   A. profound cyanosis
   B. dependent lividity
   C. rigor mortis
   D. putrefaction

_____ **12.** Medical examiners' cases include all of the following EXCEPT:

    A. violent death

    B. suicide

    C. suspicion of a criminal act

    D. a physician's written orders for a DNR

_____ **13.** HIPAA is the acronym for the Health Insurance Portability and Accountability Act of 1996. This act:

    A. makes ambulance services accountable for transporting patients in a safe manner

    B. protects the privacy of health care information and safeguards patient confidentiality

    C. allows health insurers to transfer an insurance policy to another carrier if a patient does not pay his or her premium

    D. enables emergency personnel to transfer a patient to a lower level of care when resources are scarce

True/False

If you believe the statement to be more true than false, write the letter "T" in the space provided. If you believe the statement to be more false than true, write the letter "F."

_____ **1.** Failure to provide care to a patient once you have been called to the scene is considered negligence.

_____ **2.** For expressed consent to be valid, the patient must be a minor.

_____ **3.** If a patient is unconscious and a true emergency exists, the doctrine of implied consent applies.

_____ **4.** EMTs can legally restrain patients against their will if they pose a threat to themselves or others.

_____ **5.** DNR orders give you permission not to attempt resuscitation at your discretion.

_____ **6.** A durable power of attorney for health care is a designated person who is authorized to make medical decisions on behalf of the patient.

_____ **7.** EMT textbooks are often used in court to establish standards of care.

_____ **8.** EMTs are not typically responsible for reporting suspected child abuse.

_____ **9.** When at a crime scene, you must be careful not to disturb the scene any more than absolutely necessary.

_____ **10.** Punitive damages are intended to compensate the plaintiff for the actual injuries sustained.

Fill-in-the-Blank

Read each item carefully and then complete the statement by filling in the missing words.

1. The _____ _____ _____ outlines the care you are able to provide.

2. The _____ _____ _____ is the manner in which the EMT must act when treating patients.

3. The legal responsibility to provide care is called the _____ _____ _____.

4. The determination of _____ is based on duty, breach of duty, damages, and cause.

5. Abandonment is _____ of care without transferring that care to a medical professional who is competent to continue providing care.

6. _____ consent is given directly by an informed patient, whereas _____ consent is assumed in the unconscious patient.

7. Unlawfully placing a person in fear of immediate harm is _____, whereas _____ is unlawfully touching a person without his or her consent.

8. A(n) _____ _____ is a written document that specifies authorized treatment in case a patient becomes unable to make decisions. A written document that authorizes the EMT not to attempt resuscitation efforts is a(n) _____ _____.

9. Mentally competent patients have the right to _____ _____.

10. Incidents involving child abuse, animal bites, childbirth, and assault have _____ _____ requirements in many states.

Critical Thinking

Multiple Choice

Read the scenarios carefully and select the best responses to the questions.

At 0200, a 17-year-old boy, accompanied by his 19-year-old girlfriend, had driven to the bar to give his father (who had been drinking large amounts of alcohol) a ride home. On the way back, they were involved in a motor vehicle collision. The boy has a large laceration with profuse bleeding on his forehead. His girlfriend is unconscious on the front passenger floor. The father is standing outside the vehicle, appearing heavily intoxicated, and is refusing care.

_____ 1. Should the father be allowed to refuse care?
   A. Yes. Consent is required before care can be started.
   B. No. He is under the influence of drugs/alcohol and is therefore mentally incompetent.
   C. Yes. Consent is implied.
   D. No. You would be guilty of abandonment.

_____ 2. Why is it permissible for you to begin treatment on the girlfriend?
   A. Consent is implied.
   B. Consent has been expressed.
   C. Consent was informed.
   D. Consent is not needed.

_____ 3. As you progress in your care for the patients, the father becomes unconscious. Can you begin/continue care for him now?
   A. Yes. Consent is now implied.
   B. No. He made his wishes known before he fell unconscious.
   C. No. He just needs to sleep it off.
   D. Yes. Unconsciousness indicates informed consent.

_____ 4. With the son being a minor, what is the best way to gain consent to begin care when his father has an altered mental status or is unconscious?
   A. Due to his father being intoxicated, he is emancipated and can provide consent.
   B. Call his grandparents for consent.
   C. It is a true emergency, so consent is implied.
   D. You are covered under the Good Samaritan laws.

You respond to a single-vehicle crash on the highway west of town. On arrival, you find a 33-year-old man with an open forearm fracture who has self-extricated from his pickup truck, which is down the roadside embankment. He does not appear to have suffered any other injuries, is fully coherent, and refuses all medical care.

_____ 5. You attempt to convince the patient to go to the hospital by explaining his injuries. In an effort to obtain consent to treat this patient, what else could you do to convince him?

  A. Summon law enforcement and threaten the patient that he'll be placed into protective custody.

  B. Clearly explain the consequences of not accepting medical treatment.

  C. Proceed with treatment; consent is not required because the patient is not being rational.

  D. Allow the patient to leave the scene without a signed refusal form.

_____ 6. If you and your partner were out past the end of your scheduled shift and driving the ambulance back to base to go home when you came upon this accident, would you have a legal duty to act?

  A. No. If you were not specifically dispatched to the crash, you do not have an obligation to assist.

  B. Yes. As a trained and licensed EMT, you must assist with every medical emergency that you encounter.

  C. No. Because it is past the end of your scheduled shift, you can decide whether you want to stop and help.

  D. Yes. As a trained EMT still on-duty for an EMS system, you would have a legal and ethical obligation to stop and assist.

Short Answer

Complete this section with short written answers using the space provided.

1. In many states, certain conditions allow an emancipated minor to be treated as an adult for the purpose of consenting to medical treatment. Give three examples of emancipated minors.

_____

_____

_____

2. When does your responsibility as an EMT for patient care end?

_____

_____

3. There will be some instances when you will not be able to persuade the patient, guardian, or parent of a minor child or mentally incompetent patient to proceed with treatment. List the steps you should take to protect all parties involved.

_____

_____

_____

4. List the two rules of thumb that courts consider regarding reports and records.

_____

_____

_____

5. List the four elements that must be present for the legal doctrine of negligence to apply.

_____

_____

_____

Ambulance Calls

The following case scenarios provide an opportunity to explore the concerns associated with patient management and to enhance critical-thinking skills. Read each scenario and answer each question to the best of your ability.

1. You are dispatched to a girl complaining of abdominal pain. You arrive to find the 17-year-old girl crying and holding her abdomen. She tells you that she fell down the stairs and that she is pregnant. She is not sure how long she's been pregnant, but she is experiencing cramping and spotting. She asks you not to tell anyone and says that if you tell her parents, then she will refuse transport to the hospital.

   What do you do?

_____

_____

_____

2. You are off-duty when you see a child injured while riding his bike. You examine him and find abrasions on both knees but no other injuries. He needs help getting to his house up the street. He tells you that his mother is not home, but his grandfather is (although he is bedridden). Looking through the window, you see the house is full of clothing, garbage, and papers.

   What do you do?

_____

_____

_____

3. It is late at night when the police summon you to a motor vehicle collision. On arrival, the officer directs you to the back of his patrol car. Sitting on the seat is your patient, snoring loudly with blood covering his face. The officer states that the patient was involved in a drunk-driving accident in which he hit his head on the rearview mirror. The patient initially refused care at the scene. You were called because his wound continues to bleed. Assessment reveals a sleeping 56-year-old man with a deep, gaping wound over the right eye with moderate bleeding. During assessment, the patient wakes suddenly and pushes you away. He tells you to leave him alone.

   What actions are necessary in the management of this situation?

_____

_____

_____

Fill-in-the-Patient Care Report

Read the incident scenario and then complete the following patient care report (PCR).

It is 2115, and you are just walking out of a grocery store with a small bag of apples when the dispatch tones blare from your portable radio.

"Truck Two," the dispatcher's voice blasts from the small speaker. "Emergency call."

You pick up the pace to the ambulance, where your partner is fastening his seat belt, answering on the portable as you go. "Dispatch, go for Truck Two."

"Truck Two, I need you to head over to the intersection of Grand and Hopper for a motorcycle versus automobile." You repeat back the information, jump into the passenger seat, and pull your seat belt into position as your partner activates the lights and siren and pulls out onto the deserted street.

At 7 minutes after dispatch, you arrive at the intersection and see a small blue car with a shattered windshield sitting diagonally in the middle of the intersection. On the opposite side of the road, there is a damaged and smoking motorcycle on its side; a person is lying motionless on the pavement nearby.

The driver of the car, who is standing on the side of the road and talking on his cell phone, shouts that he is not injured, so you proceed to the woman on the ground. She appears to be approximately 24 years old; is unresponsive to pain; has bleeding from a long forehead laceration; and has inadequate, snoring respirations.

At 9 minutes after dispatch, you have your partner manually immobilize the patient's head and neck while you insert an oropharyngeal airway and begin assisting her respirations with a bag-mask device and 15 L/min of supplemental oxygen.

At 10 minutes after dispatch, a fire truck arrives on scene, and one of the firefighters obtains the patient's vitals while the others prepare the cervical collar and long backboard.

Two minutes later, the firefighter reports the patient's vitals: blood pressure, systolic 90, diastolic 54; pulse of 100 beats/min, weak and irregular; respirations of 12 breaths/min with adequate assisted tidal volume; pale, cool, and diaphoretic skin; and a pulse oximetry reading of 94%.

About 5 minutes after obtaining vitals, the patient is appropriately secured to the backboard and loaded into the ambulance for the short trip to the local university trauma center.

During the 6-minute transport to the trauma center ambulance entrance, you must continue assisting the patient's respirations and cannot repeat the vitals.

It takes a total of 14 minutes to move the patient from your gurney to the bed in the trauma bay, provide a verbal report to the nurse, and prepare the ambulance for your next call.

Fill-in-the-Patient Care Report

EMS Patient Care Report (PCR)					
Date:	Incident No.:	Nature of Call:		Location:	
Dispatched:	En Route:	At Scene:	Transport:	At Hospital:	In Service:
Patient Information					
Age: Sex: Weight (in kg [lb]):		Allergies: Medications: Past Medical History: Chief Complaint:			
Vital Signs					
Time:	BP:	Pulse: weak/irregular	Respirations:		SpO_2:
Time:	BP:	Pulse:	Respirations:		SpO_2:
Time:	BP:	Pulse:	Respirations:		SpO_2:
EMS Treatment (circle all that apply)					
Oxygen @ ___ L/min via (circle one): NC NRM BVM		Assisted Ventilation	Airway Adjunct		CPR
Defibrillation	Bleeding Control	Bandaging	Splinting		Other:
Narrative					

CHAPTER

4 Communications and Documentation

General Knowledge

Matching

Match each of the items in the left column to the appropriate definition in the right column.

_____	**1.** Base station	**A.**	A special line or frequency used exclusively for point-to-point contact
_____	**2.** Mobile radio	**B.**	A trusting relationship built with your patient
_____	**3.** Portable radio	**C.**	Utilizes an interconnected series of repeater stations for communication
_____	**4.** Repeater	**D.**	An assigned frequency used to carry voice and/or data communications
_____	**5.** Telemetry	**E.**	Radio receiver that searches across several frequencies until the message is completed
_____	**6.** UHF	**F.**	VHF and UHF channels designated exclusively for EMS use
_____	**7.** VHF	**G.**	A vehicle-mounted device that operates at a lower power than a base station
_____	**8.** Cellular telephone	**H.**	A process in which electronic signals are converted into coded, audible signals
_____	**9.** Dedicated line	**I.**	Radio frequencies between 30 and 300 MHz
_____	**10.** MED channels	**J.**	Hand-carried or handheld devices that operate at 1 to 5 watts
_____	**11.** Scanner	**K.**	A special base station radio that receives messages and signals on one frequency and then automatically retransmits them on a second frequency
_____	**12.** Channel	**L.**	Radio frequencies between 300 and 3,000 MHz
_____	**13.** Rapport	**M.**	Radio hardware containing a transmitter and receiver that is located in a fixed location

Multiple Choice

Read each item carefully and then select the one best response.

_____ **1.** Which of the following is an example of a closed-ended question?

    A. What seems to be bothering you today?

    B. Has this ever happened before?

    C. What were you doing over the past few hours?

    D. Can you describe the pain for me?

_____ **2.** The transmission range of a(n) _____ _____ is more limited than that of mobile or base station radios.

    A. portable radio

    B. 800-MHz radio

    C. cellular phone

    D. UHF radio

      3. Which of the following is TRUE when communicating with a child?

          A. Children are easily fooled by lies and deception.

          B. Avoid eye contact when speaking to a child.

          C. Children are rarely frightened by EMS providers.

          D. Calming the parents will often aid in calming the child.

      4. What is your first step when initiating communication with a non–English-speaking patient?

          A. Find out how much English the patient can speak.

          B. Speak louder to see if the patient can understand you.

          C. Skip over obtaining a medical history and go to the secondary assessment.

          D. Wait on the scene for a translator to arrive.

      5. Digital signals are also used in some kinds of paging and tone-alerting systems because they transmit _____ and allow for more choices and flexibility.

          A. numerically

          B. faster

          C. alphanumerically

          D. encoded messages

      6. The transfer of care officially occurs during:

          A. the documentation of the incident

          B. the radio report to the hospital while en route

          C. your oral report at the hospital

          D. the restocking of the unit

      7. Which of the following is FALSE with regard to simplex mode?

          A. When one party transmits, the other must wait to reply.

          B. You must push a button to talk.

          C. It is called a "pair of frequencies."

          D. Radio transmissions can occur in either direction but not simultaneously in both.

      8. Which of the following is NOT an FCC principal EMS-related responsibility?

          A. Monitoring radio operations

          B. Establishing limitations for transmitter power output

          C. Allocating specific radio frequencies for use by EMS providers

          D. Ensuring that all radios contain lithium batteries

      9. Information given to the responding unit(s) should include all of the following EXCEPT:

          A. the number of patients

          B. a list of all patient medications

          C. the exact location of the incident

          D. responses by other public safety agencies

    10. Which of the following is a reason to contact medical control?

          A. Notify the hospital of the patient's diet preference

          B. Direct orders needed to administer certain treatments

          C. Advise the hospital of the patient's primary care physician

          D. Discuss how to troubleshoot malfunctioning equipment

    11. The patient report commonly includes all of the following EXCEPT:

          A. a list of the patient's childhood illnesses

          B. the patient's age and sex

          C. a brief history of the patient's current problem

          D. your estimated time of arrival

_____ **12.** In most areas, medical control is provided by the _____ who work at the receiving hospital.
   A. nurses
   B. physicians
   C. interns
   D. staff

_____ **13.** Which of the following is NOT helpful when attempting to effectively communicate with a hearing-impaired patient?
   A. Having paper and a pen available
   B. Learning some simple phrases in sign language
   C. Shouting
   D. Speaking distinctly and at a normal pace

_____ **14.** In regard to therapeutic communication techniques, what does the term _reflection_ mean?
   A. Asking the patient to explain what he or she meant by an answer
   B. Being sensitive to the patient's feelings and thoughts
   C. Providing factual information to support a conversation
   D. Restating a patient's statement made to you to confirm your understanding

_____ **15.** When delivering a patient report, be sure that you report all patient information in a(n) _____ manner.
   A. objective
   B. accelerated
   C. sarcastic
   D. condescending

_____ **16.** Medical control guides the treatment of patients in the system through all of the following EXCEPT:
   A. hands-on care
   B. protocols
   C. direct orders
   D. post-call review

_____ **17.** When is using a closed-ended question appropriate?
   A. When patients are unable to provide long answers
   B. When you are trying to obtain the details of an event
   C. When asking about past medical history
   D. When patients are trying to explain their pain

_____ **18.** When you encounter a patient who is angry, you should:
   A. threaten the patient
   B. assume an aggressive posture
   C. stare down the patient
   D. speak calmly and slowly

_____ **19.** Which of the following is NOT included in the patient care report (PCR) narrative?
   A. Time of events
   B. Opinions about the patient
   C. Assessment findings
   D. Care provided

_____ **20.** If you make an error when documenting in a patient's record, you should:
   A. erase the error, then correct it
   B. cover it with correction fluid, then write over the top
   C. draw a single horizontal line through the error and initial it
   D. highlight the error with a marker, then write the correction next to it

_____ **21.** When caring for a visually impaired patient, you should:
  A. use sign language
  B. touch the patient only when necessary to render care
  C. try to avoid sudden movements
  D. never walk him or her to the ambulance

_____ **22.** Instances in which you may be required to file special reports with appropriate authorities include all of the following EXCEPT:
  A. gunshot wounds
  B. dog bites
  C. suspected physical, sexual, or substance abuse
  D. diabetic emergencies

True/False

If you believe the statement to be more true than false, write the letter "T" in the space provided. If you believe the statement to be more false than true, write the letter "F."

_____ **1.** The two-way radio is at least two units: a transmitter and a receiver.

_____ **2.** One of the most fundamental aspects of what EMTs do is to ask questions.

_____ **3.** Ethnocentrism occurs when you consider your own cultural values to be equal to those of others.

_____ **4.** Speaking louder to a non–English-speaking patient will increase his or her ability to understand you.

_____ **5.** If a patient refuses care and transport, you do not need to complete a PCR.

_____ **6.** Falsifying information on the PCR may result in suspension and/or revocation of your certification or license.

_____ **7.** EMS systems that use repeaters are unable to get good signals from portable radios.

_____ **8.** Children can easily see through lies or deception.

_____ **9.** When speaking on the radio, speak in plain English and avoid code words.

_____ **10.** Your PCR will reflect on you professionally and can be used as evidence in court.

Fill-in-the-Blank

Read each item carefully and then complete the statement by filling in the missing words.

1. The _____ section of the PCR is arguably the most important portion.

2. A two-way radio consists of two units: a(n) _____ and a(n) _____.

3. A(n) _____ _____, also known as a "hot line," is always open or under the control of the individuals at each end.

4. _____ is anything that dampens or obscures the true meaning of a message.

5. Refusal of care is a common source of _____ in EMS.

6. _____ are commonly used in EMS operations to alert on- and off-duty personnel.

7. When the first call to 9-1-1 comes in, the dispatcher must try to judge its relative _____ to begin the appropriate EMS response using emergency medical dispatch protocols.

8. The principal reason for radio communication is to facilitate communication between you and _____ _____.

9. A(n) _____ is an assigned frequency or frequencies used to carry voice and/or data communications.

10. _____-_____ _____ are important to use when patients are unable to provide long or complete answers to questions.

11. To ensure complete understanding, once you receive an order from medical control, you must _____ the order back, word for word, and then receive confirmation.

12. By their very nature, _____ _____ do not require direct communication with medical control.

13. The _____, pace, and _____ of the language will tell you about the mood of the person communicating.

14. Children can easily see through lies or deception, so you must always be _____ with them.

15. If the patient does not speak any English, in an emergency, you can use a family member or friend to act as a(n) _____.

16. It is _____ _____ to use military time in EMS documentation.

17. _____ adult patients have the right to refuse treatment.

Multiple Choice

Read each critical-thinking item carefully and then select the one best response.

Questions 1–5 are derived from the following scenario: You have just finished an ambulance run where a 45-year-old man had driven his SUV into a utility pole. The driver was found slumped over the steering wheel, unconscious. A large electrical wire was lying across the hood of the vehicle. After securing scene safety, you were able to approach the patient and complete a primary assessment, in which you found a 6-inch (15.4-cm) laceration across his forehead. The patient regained responsiveness, was alert and oriented, and refused care.

_____ 1. Should an EMT document this call, even though the patient refused care?
   A. No. You only need to document when you have actually provided care.
   B. No. This was not a billable run.
   C. Yes. Documentation is needed regardless.
   D. Both A and B.

_____ 2. Which of the following would NOT be important to document?
   A. That the scene needed to be made safe
   B. That ensuring scene safety delayed care
   C. That you completed a primary assessment
   D. What you and your partner were doing prior to receiving the call

_____ 3. While writing the report, you made an error. How should this be corrected?
   A. Draw a single line through it.
   B. Erase the mistake.
   C. Cover up the mistake with correction fluid.
   D. Completely cross out the error by repeatedly drawing multiple lines through it.

_____ **4.** What is NOT a consequence of falsifying a report?
  A. It may result in the suspension and/or revocation of your license.
  B. It gives other health care providers a false impression of assessment/findings.
  C. It results in poor patient care.
  D. It results in good patient care.

_____ **5.** If the patient refuses to sign the refusal form:
  A. Sign it yourself and state: "Patient refused to sign."
  B. You cannot let the man leave the scene until he either goes with you or signs the form.
  C. Have a credible witness sign the form, testifying that he or she witnessed the patient's refusal of care.
  D. If the patient refuses care, you don't have to document it.

Short Answer

Complete this section with short written answers using the space provided.

1. List the five principal FCC responsibilities related to EMS.

_____

_____

_____

2. What are the 10 Golden Rules that will help calm a patient and establish a therapeutic rapport?

_____

_____

_____

3. List the six functions of a PCR.

_____

_____

_____

4. Describe the two types of PCRs generally in use in EMS systems.

_____

_____

_____

Ambulance Calls

The following case scenarios provide an opportunity to explore the concerns associated with patient management and to enhance critical-thinking skills. Read each scenario and answer each question to the best of your ability.

1. You are in the dispatch office filling in for the EMS dispatcher, who needed to use the restroom. The phone rings, and you answer it to hear a hysterical woman screaming about a child falling into an old well. The only information she is providing is that he is 5 years old and is not making any noise. The address is on the computer display.

   How would you best manage this situation, and what additional help would you call for?

   _____

   _____

   _____

2. You respond to an "unknown medical problem" in an area commonly populated by Hispanic Americans. You arrive to find several individuals speaking to a middle-aged man. They seem to be concerned about him and motion you toward the patient. You attempt to gain information about the situation, but your patient does not speak English, and you do not speak Spanish. The patient has no outward appearance of any problems.

   How would you best manage this situation?

   _____

   _____

   _____

3. You are dispatched to the parking lot of a grocery store for a "confused child." You arrive to find a young boy who is developmentally disabled. He cannot communicate who he is or where he lives. He is frightened but appears otherwise unharmed.

   How would you best manage this situation?

   _____

   _____

   _____

Fill-in-the-Patient Care Report

Read the incident scenario and then complete the following PCR.

You watch the digital clock on the dashboard change to 1711 and flip through the stack of PCRs that you have accumulated during the past 10 hours of your busy shift, ensuring that they are all complete. Ten minutes later, the dispatcher contacts you on the radio and requests that you and your partner respond to 18553 Old Redwood Highway for a dirt bike accident.

Six minutes later, your partner pulls off the main road and into a sprawling green field dotted with motocross riders in multicolored pads and helmets. One small group of riders off in the distance begins jumping up and down, waving their arms. The ambulance moves slowly across the smooth, solid ground, and a minute later, you arrive at the group's location. You see a rider lying on the ground with blood covering his lower left leg.

"He ripped his foot off," a teenage girl with long blonde hair shouts as you step out of the truck. "Please help him quick!"

You kneel next to the 19-year-old injured man as your partner gets the equipment from the back of the ambulance. The young man is pounding his fist on the ground and yelling in pain, holding his injured leg tightly with one gloved hand. The foot of his left leg is hanging limply, almost completely severed from the ankle and bleeding profusely.

You immediately apply pressure to the end of the patient's leg with a trauma dressing as three firefighters arrive. You direct two of the firefighters to remove the patient's helmet while you immobilize his spine. Your partner and the third firefighter prepare the cervical collar and long backboard.

Once the patient is immobilized on the backboard and your partner has initiated high-flow oxygen therapy with a nonrebreathing mask, you bandage the dressings in place (after noting that the bleeding has almost completely stopped) and direct the loading of the 73-kg (161-lb) patient into the ambulance. You make a mental note that you had been on the scene for only 8 minutes.

You obtain a complete set of vital signs just as your partner is pulling away from the grass and back onto the road. You find the following: blood pressure is 104/66 mm Hg; heart rate is 102 beats/min; respirations are 18 breaths/min and unlabored; skin is pale, cool, and moist; and oxygen saturation is 97%. You immediately cover the patient with a blanket to preserve his body temperature.

After contacting the receiving trauma center with a verbal report and ETA, you repeat the vital signs about 5 minutes after the first set. You find his blood pressure is at 110/72 mm Hg, heart rate is 90 beats/min, respirations are 14 breaths/min and still unlabored, color is returning to his skin, and the pulse oximeter is showing 99%. Just as you finish obtaining the vitals, your partner opens the back doors, and you deliver the patient to the waiting team in the trauma bay.

Twenty minutes later, after providing an appropriate report to the charge nurse, turning over care of the patient, and properly cleaning and disinfecting the ambulance, you call yourselves back in service and head back to the post.

Fill-in-the-Patient Care Report

EMS Patient Care Report (PCR)					
Date:	Incident No.:		Nature of Call:		Location:
Dispatched:	En Route:	At Scene:	Transport:	At Hospital:	In Service:
Patient Information					
Age: Sex: Weight (in kg [lb]):			Allergies: Medications: Past Medical History: Chief Complaint:		
Vital Signs					
Time:	BP:		Pulse:	Respirations:	SpO$_2$:
Time:	BP:		Pulse:	Respirations:	SpO$_2$:
Time:	BP:		Pulse:	Respirations:	SpO$_2$:
EMS Treatment (circle all that apply)					
Oxygen @ ____ L/min via (circle one): NC NRM BVM		Assisted Ventilation	Airway Adjunct		CPR
Defibrillation	Bleeding Control	Bandaging	Splinting		Other:
Narrative					

Medical Terminology

General Knowledge

Matching

Match each of the items in the left column to the appropriate definition in the right column.

_____	**1.** Prefix	**A.**	Bottom of the foot
_____	**2.** Suffix	**B.**	Motion away from the midline
_____	**3.** Superior	**C.**	Belly side of the body
_____	**4.** Distal	**D.**	Occurs before the root word
_____	**5.** Ventral	**E.**	Bending of a joint
_____	**6.** Plantar	**F.**	Occurs after the root word
_____	**7.** Abduction	**G.**	Farther from the trunk
_____	**8.** Supine	**H.**	Back surface of the body
_____	**9.** Flexion	**I.**	Lying face up
_____	**10.** Posterior	**J.**	Nearer to the head

Match each of the prefixes in the left column to the appropriate definition in the right column.

_____	**11.** Tachy-	**A.**	Four
_____	**12.** Post-	**B.**	Over, excessive, high
_____	**13.** Quad-	**C.**	Rapid, fast
_____	**14.** Bi-	**D.**	Before
_____	**15.** Brady-	**E.**	Two
_____	**16.** Pre-	**F.**	Slow
_____	**17.** Hyper-	**G.**	After, behind

Match each of the suffixes in the left column to the appropriate definition in the right column.

_____	**18.** –megaly	**A.**	Disease
_____	**19.** –oma	**B.**	Surgical removal of
_____	**20.** –ectomy	**C.**	Tumor
_____	**21.** –algia	**D.**	Inflammation
_____	**22.** –logist	**E.**	Pertaining to pain
_____	**23.** –pathy	**F.**	Enlargement
_____	**24.** –itis	**G.**	Specialist

Multiple Choice

Read each item carefully and then select the one best response.

_____ 1. A patient was involved in a motor vehicle crash. He has abrasions to both arms. What word is used to describe this?

A. Medial

B. Bilateral

C. Lateral

D. Ventral

_____ 2. While assessing a patient, you note a slow pulse. How would you describe this?

A. Tachycardia

B. Brachiocardia

C. Retrocardia

D. Bradycardia

_____ 3. You are reviewing a patient care report (PCR) and notice the abbreviation DOE. What does this mean?

A. Dead on extrication

B. Director of EMS

C. Dyspnea on exertion

D. Diabetes of elderly

_____ 4. You are transporting a 72-year-old female from a hospital to an extended care facility. When reviewing her chart, you note she underwent a pleurocentesis. What does this mean?

A. Removal of lung tissue

B. Draining fluid from the chest

C. Surgical opening of the chest

D. Examination of the lung with a scope

_____ 5. You arrive at the scene of a motorcycle crash. You find the patient lying prone on the ground. What does this mean?

A. The patient is lying face down

B. The patient is lying face up

C. The patient is sitting up at 45°

D. The patient is sitting up at 90°

_____ 6. While obtaining a history on a patient, she informs you that she has a carcinoma of the liver. What does this mean?

A. Enlargement of the liver

B. Inflammation of the liver

C. Cancerous tumor of the liver

D. Noncancerous tumor of the liver

_____ 7. You are preparing a patient for transport. A nurse informs you the patient has a history of AMI. What does this mean?

A. Acute marrow inflammation

B. Acute myocardial infarction

C. Acute musculoskeletal infection

D. Acute myocardial ischemia

_____ 8. Just prior to transporting a patient from a hospital to an extended care facility, the medical control physician informs you the patient is to remain NPO. What does this mean?

A. No pulmonary oxygen

B. Noting by parenteral route

C. No pulmonary obstructions

D. Nothing by mouth

_____ **9.** You are examining a patient who experienced a TIA. What does this mean?
     A. Transient ischemic attack
     B. Total ischemic attack
     C. Transient intestinal atrophy
     D. Tissue inhibiting attack

_____ **10.** You are caring for a 6-year-old child with a recent diagnosis of pharyngitis. What does this mean?
     A. Pain in the throat
     B. Disease of the throat
     C. Inflammation of the throat
     D. Paralysis of the throat

True/False

If you believe the statement to be more true than false, write the letter "T" in the space provided. If you believe the statement to be more false than true, the letter "F."

_____ **1.** Not all medical terms will have a prefix.

_____ **2.** The ankle is proximal to the knee.

_____ **3.** The abbreviation CRNA means Certified Registered Nurse Anesthetist.

_____ **4.** The suffix "-megaly" means enlargement.

_____ **5.** The word root occurs before the prefix.

_____ **6.** When a term has more than one word root, a combining vowel must be placed between the two roots.

_____ **7.** Singular words that end in "a" change to "es" when plural.

_____ **8.** The wrist is proximal to the elbow.

_____ **9.** The abbreviation for deep vein thrombosis is DVT.

_____ **10.** The suffix "-plegia" refers to plastic surgery.

Fill-in-the-Blank

Read each item carefully and then complete the statement by filling in the missing words.

1. _____ means closer to or on the skin.

2. The _____ part of the body, or any body part, is the portion nearer to the head.

3. The bottom of the foot is referred to as the _____ surface.

4. The way to describe the sections of the abdominal cavity is by _____.

5. _____ is motion toward the midline.

6. The parts that lie closer to the midline are called _____ (inner) structures.

7. A patient who is sitting upright is said to be in the _____ _____.

8. When trying to define a term, begin with the _____ and work backward.

9. The body is in the _____ position when lying face down.

10. _____ take the place of words to shorten notes or documentation.

Labeling

Label the following diagrams with the correct terms.

1. Directional Terms

A. _____

B. _____

C. _____

D. _____

E. (side of the patient) _____

F. _____

G. _____

H. _____

I. (side of the patient) _____

J. (toward the head) _____

K. (toward the feet) _____

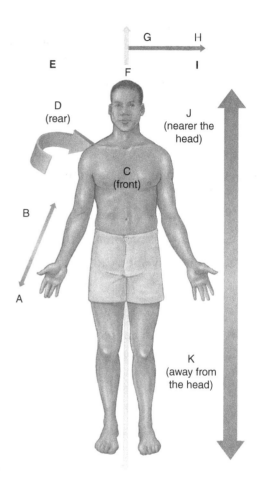

© Jones & Bartlett Learning.

2. Movement Terms

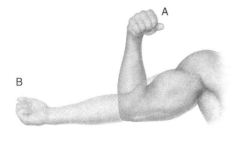

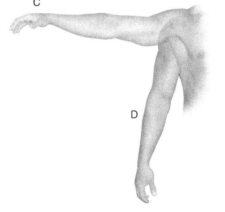

© Jones & Bartlett Learning.

A. _____

B. _____

C. _____

D. _____

Critical Thinking

Multiple Choice

Read each critical-thinking item carefully and then select the one best response.

_____ 1. You respond to the home of a 38-year-old female who complains of nausea and vomiting. The patient informs you she has been ill for the past 3 days with nausea and vomiting and states that she cannot "keep anything down." When questioned how many times she's vomited in the past 24 hours, she tells you at least 30 times. When giving a radio report to the receiving hospital, what term would you use to describe the patient's condition?

    A. Hypergastritis

    B. Hypernausea

    C. Hyperemesis

    D. Hypervomitus

_____ 2. You are examining a 28-year-old male who was stabbed following an altercation in a local bar. He has a stab wound to the right upper quadrant of the abdomen. You also notice a scar to the right lower quadrant. When you question the patient about the scar, he tells you his appendix was removed 3 years ago. What term can be used to describe which side the wound and the scar are located on in relation to the abdomen?

    A. Contralateral

    B. Ipsilateral

    C. Bilateral

    D. Retrolateral

_____ 3. A 52-year-old male called for EMS because he is experiencing a headache. The patient tells you this is "the worse headache of my life." On examination, you note the patient has photophobia. What does this term mean?

    A. Fear of cameras

    B. Fear of photographs

    C. Fear of x-rays

    D. Fear of light

_____ 4. You are called to the home of a 60-year-old female with chest pain. The patient provides you with a paper listing her medical history. Most of the items on the list are abbreviated. The list includes HTN, IDDM, GERD, CAD, MRSA, and PVD. Which abbreviation on that list describes a condition involving the gastrointestinal tract?

    A. IDDM

    B. MRSA

    C. GERD

    D. PVD

Short Answer

Complete this section with short written answers using the space provided.

1. List the four movement terms and their definitions.

_____

_____

_____

2. What are the five rules to use when converting terms from singular to plural?

_____

_____

_____

3. What are the four components that comprise a medical term?

_____

_____

_____

4. A combining vowel shown with the word root is called a combining form. List five of the most common combining forms found in EMS.

_____

_____

_____

Fill-in-the-Patient Care Report

Read the incident scenario and then complete the following PCR using medical terminology and abbreviations learned in this chapter.

You and your partner stop for something to eat at a local fast-food restaurant. While eating your lunch, you look at your watch and notice it's exactly noon. You are amazed that you're actually eating lunch on time. In that instant, you are dispatched to 152 East Bramble Street for a male with chest pain. As you clean up from lunch, your partner acknowledges the call and marks your unit en route at 1202. The dispatcher tells you this is a 53-year-old male with a history of diabetes and hypertension who experienced chest pain while mowing his lawn.

You arrive on scene at 1210 and are greeting by the patient's wife. She tells you the patient was mowing the lawn and then experienced a sudden onset of central chest pain that radiated to his jaw. He informed his wife of his symptoms, and she immediately called for EMS. You enter the patient's home and find him sitting on the couch. He appears short of breath and is holding his left hand to his chest. You introduce yourself to the patient and ask what's bothering him. He complains of chest pain and shortness of breath. As your partner places the patient on high-flow oxygen at 15 L/min via nonrebreathing mask, you request ALS and continue to get additional information from the patient and his wife. The patient tells you he has a history of hypertension, noninsulin-dependent diabetes, gastroesophageal reflux disease, and surgery to remove his appendix. His medications include metformin, lisinopril, and omeprazole. He denies any allergies.

Your partner obtains vital signs at 1215 and tells you the following results: pulse 82/regular, respirations 16, blood pressure 148/92, SpO_2 98% on oxygen. You perform a secondary assessment and note the patient's lungs are clear in all fields, and his abdomen is nontender. In addition, he has equal pulses in all of his extremities.

Following your assessment, you package the patient in a semi-Fowler's position on the litter and transport him to the local hospital at 1220. You are only 2 minutes from the local hospital and cancel ALS due to your quick travel time. The unit arrives at the hospital at 1223. The patient reports that he is feeling better since he was placed on oxygen. You transfer care to the emergency department staff and provide the nurse with a verbal report as your partner restocks the unit for the next call. You call dispatch and mark your unit back in service at 1235.

Fill-in-the-Patient Care Report

EMS Patient Care Report (PCR)					
Date:	Incident No.:		Nature of Call:		Location:
Dispatched:	En Route:	At Scene:	Transport:	At Hospital:	In Service:
Patient Information					
Age: Sex: Weight (in kg [lb]):			Allergies: Medications: Past Medical History: Chief Complaint:		
Vital Signs					
Time:	BP:		Pulse:	Respirations:	SpO_2:
Time:	BP:		Pulse:	Respirations:	SpO_2:
Time:	BP:		Pulse:	Respirations:	SpO_2:
EMS Treatment (circle all that apply)					
Oxygen @ ___ L/min via (circle one): NC NRM BVM		Assisted Ventilation	Airway Adjunct		CPR
Defibrillation	Bleeding Control	Bandaging	Splinting		Other:
Narrative					

CHAPTER

6 The Human Body

General Knowledge

Matching

Match each of the items in the left column to the appropriate definition in the right column.

_____ **1.** Capillary vessels

_____ **2.** Anatomic position

_____ **3.** Midsagittal plane

_____ **4.** Flexion

_____ **5.** Tidal volume

_____ **6.** Hypoxic drive

_____ **7.** Epidermis

_____ **8.** Peristalsis

_____ **9.** Pathophysiology

_____ **10.** Ligament

_____ **11.** Symphysis

_____ **12.** Diffusion

_____ **13.** Residual volume

_____ **14.** Dead space

_____ **15.** Stoke volume

A. The outermost layer of skin

B. Fibrous tissue that connects bones to bones

C. The amount of air moved in and out of the lungs in a single breath

D. A study of how normal physiology is affected by disease

E. Standing, facing forward, palms facing forward

F. A wave-like contraction of smooth muscle

G. Allow contact between the blood and the cells of the tissues

H. Does not participate in gas exchange

I. A joint that has grown together to form a stable connection, allowing only slight motion

J. An imaginary vertical line dividing the body into equal left and right halves

K. Air that remains in the lungs after exhalation

L. The volume of blood pumped with each contraction

M. A backup system to control respirations

N. The movement from higher concentration to lower concentration

O. The bending of a joint

For each of the bones listed in the left column, indicate whether it is an upper extremity bone (A) or a lower extremity bone (B).

_____ **16.** Talus

_____ **17.** Patella

_____ **18.** Clavicle

_____ **19.** Fibula

_____ **20.** Calcaneus

_____ **21.** Ulna

_____ **22.** Humerus

A. Upper extremity bone

B. Lower extremity bone

For each of the muscle characteristics described in the left column, select the type of muscle from the right column.

_____ **23.** Attaches to the bone

_____ **24.** Found in the walls of the gastrointestinal tract

_____ **25.** Forms the major muscle mass of the body

_____ **26.** Under the direct control of the brain

_____ **27.** Found only in the heart

_____ **28.** Cannot function on anaerobic metabolism

_____ **29.** Responsible for all bodily movement

_____ **30.** Can generate its own electrical impulses

A. Skeletal

B. Smooth

C. Cardiac

For each of the parts of the nervous system in the left column, select the phrase in the right column with which it is associated.

_____ **31.** Spinal cord

_____ **32.** Central nervous system

_____ **33.** Sensory nerves

_____ **34.** Motor nerves

_____ **35.** Brain

_____ **36.** Peripheral nervous system

A. Exits the brain through an opening at the base of the skull

B. Transmit electrical impulses to the muscles, causing them to contract

C. Brain and spinal cord

D. Links the central nervous system to various organs in the body

E. Carry sensations of taste and touch to the brain

F. Controls all functions of the body

Multiple Choice

Read each item carefully and then select the one best response.

_____ **1.** Which of the following would be considered an underlying cause of shock?

    A. Increased blood volume

    B. Increased pumping ability of the heart

    C. Loss of blood vessel control

    D. Decrease in anaerobic metabolism

_____ **2.** In the female, what structure carries the ovum to the uterus?

    A. Ovary

    B. Fallopian tube

    C. Vas deferens

    D. Seminal vesicles

_____ **3.** The leaf-shaped flap of tissue that prevents food and liquid from entering the trachea is called the:

    A. uvula

    B. epiglottis

    C. laryngopharynx

    D. cricothyroid membrane

_____ **4.** Which of the following systems is responsible for releasing chemicals that regulate body activities?
   A. Nervous
   B. Endocrine
   C. Cardiovascular
   D. Skeletal

_____ **5.** Which of the following vessels does NOT carry blood to the heart?
   A. Inferior vena cava
   B. Superior vena cava
   C. Pulmonary vein
   D. Pulmonary artery

_____ **6.** The_____ is connected to the intestine by the bile ducts.
   A. Stomach
   B. Spleen
   C. Appendix
   D. Liver

_____ **7.** Which of the following is NOT a function of the urinary system?
   A. Fluid control
   B. Hormone regulation
   C. pH balancing
   D. Waste filtration

_____ **8.** What organ secretes enzymes that are used to digest fats, starches, and protein?
   A. Liver
   B. Gallbladder
   C. Pancreas
   D. Spleen

True/False

If you believe the statement to be more true than false, write the letter "T" in the space provided. If you believe the statement to be more false than true, write the letter "F."

_____ **1.** The aorta is the only artery that supplies the groin and lower extremities with blood.

_____ **2.** The knee is a ball-and-socket joint.

_____ **3.** The phalanges are the bones of the fingers and toes.

_____ **4.** The right atrium receives blood from the pulmonary veins.

_____ **5.** There are 10 ribs located in the thorax.

_____ **6.** Exhaled air contains 21% oxygen.

_____ **7.** The spleen is a solid organ that is commonly injured in abdominal blunt-trauma injuries.

Fill-in-the-Blank

Read each item carefully and then complete the statement by filling in the missing words.

1. There is/are _____ cervical vertebrae.

2. The lower jawbone is the _____.

3. There is a total of _____ lobes in the right and left lungs.

4. There are _____ pairs of ribs in the thorax.

5. The spinal column has _____ vertebrae.

6. The ankle is formed by the _____,_____, and _____.

7. The cerebrum, which is the largest part of the brain, is composed of four lobes: _____,_____, _____, and _____.

8. The _____ space is the space between the cells.

9. The movement of air between the lungs and the environment is called _____.

10. How much air is being effectively moved during ventilation and how much blood is gaining access to the alveoli is called the _____ ratio.

Labeling

Label the following diagrams with the correct terms.

1. The Skull

A. _____

B. _____

C. _____

D. _____

E. _____

F. _____

G. _____

H. _____

I. _____

J. _____

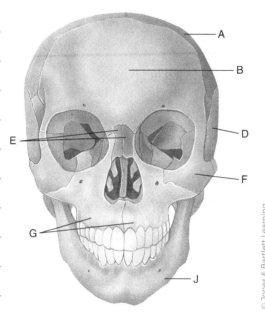

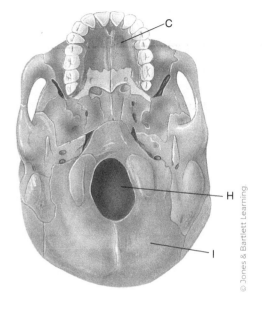

2. The Spinal Column

A. _____

B. _____

C. _____

D. _____

E. _____

F. _____

G. _____

H. _____

I. _____

J. _____

K. _____

L. _____

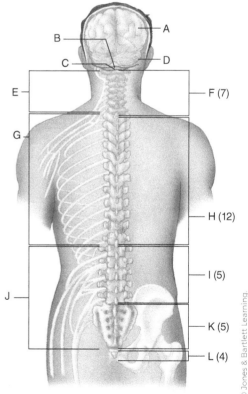

3. The Thorax

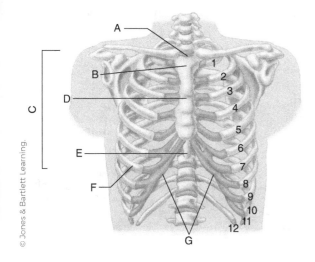

A. _____

B. _____

C. _____

D. _____

E. _____

F. _____

G. _____

4. The Shoulder Girdle

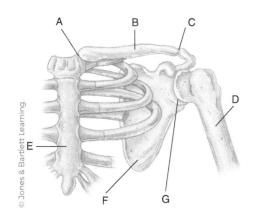

A. _____

B. _____

C. _____

D. _____

E. _____

F. _____

G. _____

5. The Wrist and Hand

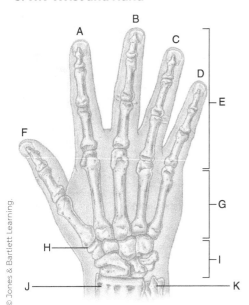

A. _____

B. _____

C. _____

D. _____

E. _____

F. _____

G. _____

H. _____

I. _____

J. _____

K. _____

6. The Pelvis

A. _____

B. _____

C. _____

D. _____

E. _____

F. _____

G. _____

H. _____

I. _____

J. _____

K. _____

L. _____

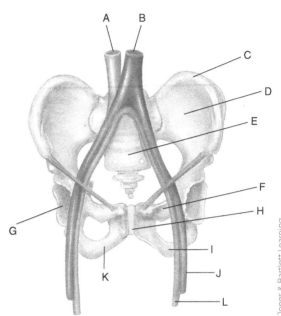

7. The Lower Extremity

A. _____

B. _____

C. _____

D. _____

E. _____

F. _____

G. _____

H. _____

I. _____

J. _____

K. _____

L. _____

M. _____

N. _____

O. _____

P. _____

Q. _____

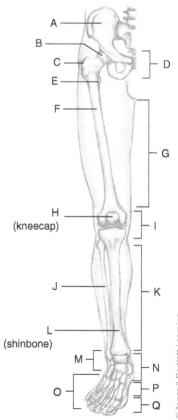

8. The Foot

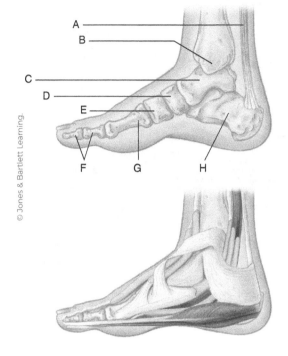

A. _____

B. _____

C. _____

D. _____

E. _____

F. _____

G. _____

H. _____

9. The Respiratory System

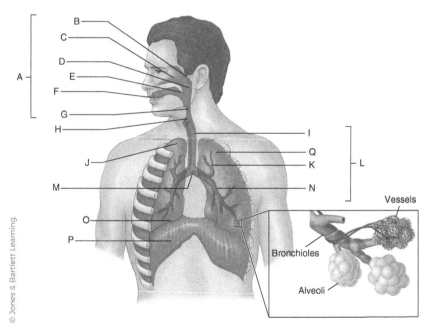

Vessels

Bronchioles

Alveoli

A. _____

B. _____

C. _____

D. _____

E. _____

F. _____

G. _____

H. _____

I. _____

J. _____

K. _____

L. _____

M. _____

N. _____

O. _____

P. _____

Q. _____

10. The Circulatory System

A. _____

B. _____

C. _____

D. _____

E. _____

F. _____

G. _____

H. _____

I. _____

J. _____

K. _____

L. _____

M. _____

UPPER BODY

A

C

B

CO$_2$ O$_2$ D

Superior vena cava

Pulmonary arteries bring oxygen-poor blood from the heart to the lungs.

E

F

G

RIGHT LUNG

CO$_2$

CO$_2$ H

LEFT LUNG

O$_2$

O$_2$

I

J

K

L

M

F

Inferior vena cava

Pulmonary veins bring oxygen-rich blood from the lungs to the heart.

B

CO$_2$ O$_2$

Tissue cells

LOWER BODY

11. Central and Peripheral Pulses

A. _____

B. _____

C. _____

D. _____

E. _____

F. _____

G. _____

H. _____

I. _____

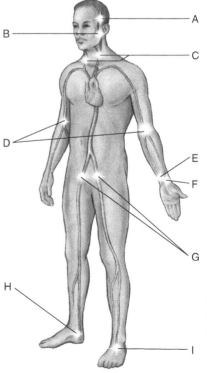

A

B

C

D

E

F

G

H

I

12. The Brain

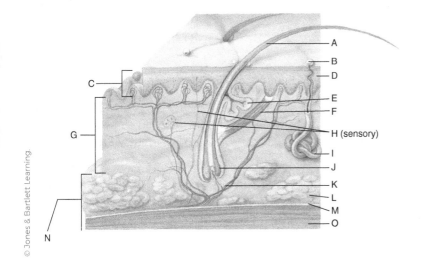

A. _____

B. _____

C. _____

13. Anatomy of the Skin

A. _____

B. _____

C. _____

D. _____

E. _____

F. _____

G. _____

H. _____

I. _____

J. _____

K. _____

L. _____

M. _____

N. _____

O. _____

14. The Male Reproductive System

A. _____

B. _____

C. _____

D. _____

E. _____

F. _____

G. _____

H. _____

I. _____

J. _____

K. _____

L. _____

M. _____

FRONT VIEW   SIDE VIEW

A B C D H I J K L E F G M

© Jones & Bartlett Learning.

15. The Female Reproductive System

A. _____

B. _____

C. _____

D. _____

E. _____

FRONT VIEW   SIDE VIEW

A B C D E

© Jones & Bartlett Learning.

Critical Thinking

Multiple Choice

Read each critical-thinking item carefully and then select the one best response.

Questions 1–5 are derived from the following scenario: Kory, a 16-year-old boy, attempted to jump down a flight of stairs on his skateboard but landed facedown on his chest and stomach, where he stayed until found. He was not wearing a helmet, and he hit the pavement with his head. Two bones were protruding from his right ankle.

_____ 1. Which of the following bones are most likely fractured?
   A. Ulna/Radius
   B. Acromion/Humerus
   C. Tibia/Fibula
   D. Patella/Fibula

_____ 2. What part of his spinal column do you want to keep immobilized so as not to move any of its seven vertebrae?
   A. Cervical
   B. Thoracic
   C. Sacrum
   D. Coccyx

_____ 3. If Kory were to develop pain in his right upper quadrant, what organ may be causing the pain?
   A. Liver
   B. Stomach
   C. Spleen
   D. Appendix

_____ 4. If Kory were to go into shock from his injuries, what type of shock will he most likely experience?
   A. Cardiogenic
   B. Obstructive
   C. Hypovolemic
   D. Septic

_____ 5. Which of the following pulses is located near Kory's leg injury?
   A. Brachial
   B. Dorsalis pedis
   C. Ulnar
   D. Superficial temporal

Short Answer

Complete this section with short written answers using the space provided.

1. List the five components of blood and each of their functions.

_____

_____

_____

2. List the five sections of the spinal column and indicate the number of vertebrae in each.

_____

_____

_____

3. What organs are in each of the quadrants of the abdomen?

RUQ: _____

LUQ: _____

RLQ: _____

LLQ: _____

4. List in order the structures that blood flows through when circulating through the heart and lungs.

1. _____

2. _____

3. _____

4. _____

5. _____

6. _____

7. _____

8. _____

9. _____

Ambulance Calls

The following case scenarios provide an opportunity to explore the concerns associated with patient management and to enhance critical-thinking skills. Read each scenario and answer each question to the best of your ability.

1. You are dispatched to the scene of a bar fight. A 34-year-old man has been stabbed in the right upper quadrant of the abdomen with a knife.

What organs might be affected by this wound?

_____

_____

_____

2. You are dispatched to a one-vehicle motor vehicle crash, car versus telephone pole. You arrive to find an unrestrained driver who is complaining of chest pain. You notice the steering wheel is deformed.

Based on this information, what anatomic structures are potentially injured?

_____

_____

_____

3. You are dispatched to a local BMX bike track just down the road from the fire station. You arrive to find a 14-year-old boy walking toward you, holding his left arm in place. He tells you that as he was turning a corner on the track, he fell off his bike and landed on his shoulder.

What anatomic structures are potentially injured?

_____

_____

_____

Fill-in-the-Patient Care Report

Read the incident scenario and then complete the following patient care report (PCR).

You note that it has been far too quiet this evening as you and your partner sit overlooking the west end of the city. An approaching car's headlights briefly illuminate the cab of the ambulance before swinging around a curve, dropping you back into darkness again. The radio buzzes, and you both snap to attention.

"Six-nineteen from central, I've got a priority-one call. Please proceed to the intersection of Alpha Street and 15th Avenue for an assault. Police reporting the scene as secure. I'm showing you assigned at 2312."

Your partner acknowledges the call as you pull out of the parking lot and begin the 17-minute cross-town trip to the scene location. On arrival, you are directed to a 38-year-old, 115-pound (52-kg) woman who is lying on the sidewalk, arms wrapped tightly around her torso.

"There was a fight over at Hank's bar," the police officer squatting next to the patient tells you. "Linda here was attacked by several other ladies and assaulted pretty severely in the street."

You kneel next to the moaning woman and explain that you are there to help her. After confirming a patent airway, you ask the police officer to hold the patient's head in a neutral, in-line position while you initiate high-flow oxygen therapy via a nonrebreathing mask set at 15 L/min. You and your partner then apply a cervical collar, secure the patient to a long backboard, and load her into the ambulance. You look at your watch and see that it has been 29 minutes since the initial dispatch.

Your partner jumps into the back of the ambulance with the patient while you slide into the cab, notify dispatch of your departure from the scene, and pull away, heading toward the university trauma center 13 minutes south on 15th Avenue. Your partner finds darkening bruises on the patient's upper arms, the left side of her chest, and down the front of both legs. Her stomach is distended and rigid, causing her to wince and cover her torso with her hands when touched.

By the time you pull to a stop in the hospital's ambulance bay, your partner has obtained two sets of vital signs— the first, 2 minutes following departure from the scene, and the other 6 minutes later. The results were, in order: blood pressure, 108/56 mm Hg and 104/54 mm Hg; pulse, 96 beats/min and 104 beats/min; respirations, 16 breaths/min (good tidal volume but labored) and 18 breaths/min (adequate tidal volume and labored); and pulse oximetry 96% and 95%. The patient also seemed to be growing more anxious during the transport and was treated for shock with blankets and proper positioning.

You and your partner quickly transfer the patient to the open and waiting trauma room bed, provide the physician with a full report, and are back in service 15 minutes after initially arriving at the hospital.

Fill-in-the-Patient Care Report

EMS Patient Care Report (PCR)					
Date:	Incident No.:	Nature of Call:		Location:	
Dispatched:	En Route:	At Scene:	Transport:	At Hospital:	In Service:
Patient Information					
Age: Sex: Weight (in kg [lb]):			Allergies: Medications: Past Medical History: Chief Complaint:		
Vital Signs					
Time:	BP:	Pulse:		Respirations:	SpO$_2$:
Time:	BP:	Pulse:		Respirations:	SpO$_2$:
Time:	BP:	Pulse:		Respirations:	SpO$_2$:
EMS Treatment (circle all that apply)					
Oxygen @ ___ L/min via (circle one): NC NRM BVM		Assisted Ventilation	Airway Adjunct		CPR
Defibrillation	Bleeding Control	Bandaging	Splinting		Other:
Narrative					

PREPARATORY

CHAPTER

7

Life Span Development

General Knowledge

Matching

Match each of the items in the left column to the appropriate definition in the right column.

_____ **1.** Preschoolers	**A.** Capillaries that filter blood within the kidneys
_____ **2.** Anxious-avoidant attachment	**B.** Cholesterol and calcium buildup inside the walls of the blood vessels that forms plaque
_____ **3.** Nephrons	**C.** Persons who are 19 to 40 years of age
_____ **4.** Toddlers	**D.** Areas where the infant's skull has not fused together
_____ **5.** Atherosclerosis	**E.** Persons who are 1 to 3 years of age
_____ **6.** School age	**F.** A bond between an infant and his or her parents in which the infant understands that the parents will be responsive to his or her needs
_____ **7.** Conventional reasoning	**G.** Persons who are 41 to 60 years of age
_____ **8.** Early adults	**H.** An infant reflex in which the infant opens his or her arms wide, spreads the fingers, and seems to grab at things
_____ **9.** Moro reflex	**I.** A type of reasoning in which a child bases decisions on his or her conscience
_____ **10.** Postconventional reasoning	**J.** A bond between an infant and his or her caregiver in which the infant is repeatedly rejected and develops an isolated lifestyle
_____ **11.** Rooting reflex	**K.** A type of reasoning in which a child looks for approval from peers and society
_____ **12.** Fontanelles	**L.** Persons who are 3 to 6 years of age
_____ **13.** Secure attachment	**M.** An infant reflex that occurs when something touches an infant's cheek, and the infant instinctively turns his or her head toward the touch
_____ **14.** Middle adults	**N.** Persons who are 6 to 12 years of age

Multiple Choice

Read each item carefully and then select the one best response.

_____ **1.** What is the decline in kidney filtration ability between the ages of 20 and 90 years?

    A. 10%

    B. 50%

    C. 45%

    D. 20%

_____ **2.** What is the typical age range for an adolescent?

    A. 6 to 12 years

    B. 3 to 6 years

    C. 12 to 18 years

    D. 10 to 19 years

_____ **3.** Children who make decisions based on their conscience are using what type of reasoning?

    A. Postconventional

    B. Psychosocial

    C. Conventional

    D. Preconventional

_____ **4.** Which of the following is a nervous system change commonly found in older adults?

    A. Increase in brain weight

    B. Increase in peripheral nerve functioning

    C. Less space for cerebral spinal fluid

    D. Deterioration of nerve endings

_____ **5.** Maturation of the reproductive system usually takes place during:

    A. early adulthood

    B. preschool

    C. middle adulthood

    D. adolescence

_____ **6.** What term is used to identify a person who is from birth to 1 month old?

    A. Infant

    B. Toddler

    C. Neonate

    D. Newborn

_____ **7.** What is the current estimated average life expectancy for humans?

    A. 120

    B. 78

    C. 67

    D. 56

_____ **8.** When encountering a patient with depressed fontanelles, you should suspect:

    A. respiratory distress

    B. dehydration

    C. atherosclerosis

    D. nephrosis

_____ **9.** What is "vital capacity"?

    A. The volume of blood moved by each contraction of the heart

    B. The maximum thickness of the meninges

    C. The volume of air moved during the deepest points of respiration

    D. The amount of air left in the lungs following exhalation

_____ **10.** Clingy behavior and the fear of unfamiliar people or places are normal among 10- to 18-month-old children and are commonly caused by _____ anxiety.

    A. bonding

    B. separation

    C. avoidant

    D. mistrust

_____ **11.** Diastolic blood pressure tends to _____ with age.

    A. decrease

    B. compensate

    C. increase

    D. decompensate

_____ **12.** Into what age range do toddlers and preschoolers fit?
  A. 1 to 6 years
  B. 2 to 8 years
  C. 2 to 7 years
  D. 0 to 5 years

_____ **13.** Empty nest syndrome is typically seen in which stage of life?
  A. middle adulthood
  B. adolescence
  C. late adulthood
  D. early adulthood

_____ **14.** At what age can an infant normally start tracking objects with his or her eyes and recognize familiar faces?
  A. 7 months
  B. 2 months
  C. 4 months
  D. 10 months

True/False

If you believe the statement to be more true than false, write the letter "T" in the space provided. If you believe the statement to be more false than true, write the letter "F."

_____ **1.** The majority of older adults live in assisted living facilities.

_____ **2.** The rooting reflex takes place when an infant's lips are stroked.

_____ **3.** Toddlers should have pulse rates between 90 and 150 beats/min.

_____ **4.** Men can produce sperm well into their 80s.

_____ **5.** The older the patient is, the thicker his or her lens will be.

_____ **6.** Typically, antisocial behavior will peak around age 13.

_____ **7.** Language is usually mastered by the 24th month.

_____ **8.** Breastfeeding helps to boost an infant's immune system.

_____ **9.** Teething in an infant typically begins around 6 months of age.

_____ **10.** Adolescents rarely struggle with their sense of identity or conflict among peers.

Fill-in-the-Blank

Read each item carefully and then complete the statement by filling in the missing words.

1. _____ adults are those who are age 19 to _____ years.

2. In toddlers, the pulse rate is _____ to _____ beats/min, and the respiratory rate is _____ to _____ breaths/min.

3. The leading cause of death in persons age 45 years to 64 years is _____.

4. Many older adults have remarkably good _____ and _____.

5. Rebellious behavior can be part of an adolescent trying to find his or her own _____.

6. A(n) _____ usually weighs 6 to _____ pounds at birth, and the head accounts for _____% of its body weight.

7. An infant's lungs are _____, and providing bag-mask device ventilations that are too forceful can result in trauma from pressure, or _____.

8. By _____ to 24 months, toddlers begin to understand cause and _____.

9. Changes in gastric and intestinal function may inhibit _____ intake and utilization in _____ adults.

10. Among older adults, _____ function in the 5 years preceding death is presumed to decline.

Critical Thinking

Multiple Choice

Read each critical-thinking item carefully and then select the one best response.

You are dispatched to a public park in the middle of a sprawling subdivision for an arm injury. You arrive to find a crying 8-year-old boy cradling his swollen and deformed left forearm. His friends tell you that he was holding on to the bars of the play structure and that his arm "snapped" when he jumped into the sand below.

_____ **1.** What would you expect this boy's normal pulse to be?
   A. Between 70 and 120 beats/min
   B. Higher than 150 beats/min
   C. Most likely below 70 beats/min
   D. Around 60 beats/min

_____ **2.** An adult bystander tells you that the boy kept trying to impress his friends with more and more dangerous stunts on the play structure prior to the injury. This is an indication of _____ reasoning.
   A. conventional
   B. preconventional
   C. unconventional
   D. postconventional

_____ **3.** You would expect to find a respiratory rate of between _____ and _____ breaths/min with this patient.
   A. 12, 20
   B. 15, 20
   C. 10, 15
   D. 20, 30

Short Answer

Complete this section with short written answers using the space provided.

1. Explain why breathing can become more labor intensive among older adults.

_____

_____

_____

2. Describe conventional reasoning.

_____

_____

_____

3. Explain the stage of development known as "trust versus mistrust."

_____

_____

_____

4. What is atherosclerosis, and how does it affect older adults?

_____

_____

_____

5. List the nine basic stages of life.

_____

_____

_____

Ambulance Calls

The following case scenarios provide an opportunity to explore the concerns associated with patient management and to enhance critical-thinking skills. Read each scenario and answer each question to the best of your ability.

1. You are dispatched to a residential care facility for a "fall from bed" and arrive to find a 96-year-old man refusing assistance, even though he has a large, darkening hematoma above his left ear. He keeps telling the care facility staff and you that he doesn't want any of you "yahoos" touching him.

What would you be most concerned about with this patient?

_____

_____

_____

2. You respond to a local residence for a toddler who burned her arm by knocking a lit candle off a shelf. You have responded to numerous abuse situations as an EMT and now find yourself suspicious of any child's injury. You would like to speak to this 16-month-old patient alone, but both parents stay nearby and seem very concerned about the child's well-being.

Would you try to speak to the child alone? Explain your reasoning.

_____

_____

_____

3. You and your partner are requested to a high school for a teenage boy who fell from the stage while rehearsing a play. You arrive to find him surrounded by concerned classmates. He is guarding the left side of his chest and breathing shallowly, but he refuses assistance and insists that he is doing fine.

How would you best manage this situation?

_____

_____

_____

Fill-in-the-Patient Care Report

Read the incident scenario and then complete the following patient care report (PCR).

The dispatch tones awaken you from a light sleep, and you instinctively pull a notepad from your pocket and write down the key components of the following dispatch:

0345

Geary Residential Home

16654 Geary Street

Respiratory distress

Note: All ALS units are tied up on calls.

Within 3 minutes, you and your partner, Leticia, are pulling the ambulance from the fire station and moving off through the silent, early-morning streets. At 0359, you arrive at the front entrance of the building and are escorted down several long, carpeted hallways to a small, dimly lit room.

"This is Mrs. Gershon," your escort tells you. "She started complaining about her breathing 20 minutes ago, and it's just getting worse."

Mrs. Gershon is a 93-year-old woman who has been living at Geary for nearly 17 years. She used to share the room with her husband, Ronald, until his death 3 years ago. She has had three myocardial infarctions in the past and takes medication to regulate blood pressure. Based on her wristband, you see that she is allergic to penicillin. She is sitting on the edge of her bed in the tripod position, breathing through pursed lips, and you can clearly see accessory muscle use in her neck.

"Hello, Mrs. Gershon. We are from the fire department, and we are here to help," you say to her. You speak loudly and clearly because her nurse told you that she has difficulty hearing. She looks up at you, inhales shallowly once, and then stops breathing.

"Mrs. Gershon, don't stop breathing now," you say while Leticia quickly hands you the bag-mask device, hissing with 15 L/min of oxygen. You begin ventilating the older woman, who is obviously exhausted after struggling to breathe for such a long period. You find no resistance to your assisted ventilations, and Mrs. Gershon just stares up at you as you continue squeezing the bag. Leticia and several nurses from the facility move the 44-kg (97-lb) patient onto the gurney and out to the ambulance as you continue ventilations. Before climbing into the driver's seat, Leticia takes a radial pulse of 110 irregular and places the pulse oximetry finger clip onto the patient. She then calls in your departure for the hospital at 0410 and provides a brief report to the receiving facility through dispatch. Within 7 minutes, you hear the truck's backup alarm, and the patient care compartment is flooded with the bright yellow light of the hospital's ambulance bay. The SpO_2 readout is showing 95%.

Several nurses and the emergency department physician come out to the ambulance and assist with getting Mrs. Gershon inside, where she is quickly sedated and intubated while you provide a verbal report to the charge nurse.

Eighteen minutes after arriving at the hospital, your ambulance is cleaned, stocked, and ready for the next call.

Fill-in-the-Patient Care Report

EMS Patient Care Report (PCR)			
Date:	Incident No.:	Nature of Call:	Location:
Dispatched:	En Route:	At Scene:	Transport:	At Hospital:	In Service:

Patient Information	
Age: Sex: Weight (in kg [lb]):	Allergies: Medications: Past Medical History: Chief Complaint:

Vital Signs				
Time:	BP:	Pulse:	Respirations:	SpO$_2$:
Time:	BP:	Pulse:	Respirations:	SpO$_2$:
Time:	BP:	Pulse:	Respirations:	SpO$_2$:

EMS Treatment (circle all that apply)				
Oxygen @ ____ L/min via (circle one): NC NRM BVM	Assisted Ventilation	Airway Adjunct	CPR
Defibrillation	Bleeding Control	Bandaging	Splinting	Other:

Narrative

CHAPTER

8 Lifting and Moving Patients

General Knowledge

Matching

Match each of the items in the left column to the appropriate definition in the right column.

_____ 1. Extremity lift
_____ 2. Flexible stretcher
_____ 3. Stair chair
_____ 4. Basket stretcher
_____ 5. Scoop stretcher
_____ 6. Backboard
_____ 7. Direct ground lift
_____ 8. Portable stretcher
_____ 9. Wheeled ambulance stretcher
_____ 10. Bariatrics

A. Separates into two halves and then inserted under the patient for carrying

B. A tubular-framed stretcher with rigid fabric stretched across it

C. Used for patients who are supine or sitting without an extremity or spinal injury; especially helpful in narrow spaces

D. A specifically designed stretcher that can be rolled along the ground and secured into the patient compartment

E. Used to carry patients across uneven terrain from remote locations; commonly used in technical and water rescues; Stokes litter

F. Used for patients who are found lying supine with no suspected spinal injury

G. A medical specialty focusing on the management of obesity

H. Used to carry patients up and down stairs

I. A spine board or longboard

J. Can be folded or rolled up; particularly useful in confined spaces

Multiple Choice

Read each item carefully and then select the one best response.

_____ 1. _____ safety depends on the use of proper lifting techniques and maintaining a proper hold when lifting or carrying a patient.
   A. Your
   B. Your team's
   C. The patient's
   D. All of the above

_____ 2. An urgent move would be required in which of the following circumstances:
   A. if a patient has a normal level of consciousness
   B. if the patient is complaining of neck pain
   C. in extreme weather conditions
   D. if a patient has normal vital signs

_____ 3. You may injure your back if you lift:
   A. with your back straight
   B. using a power lift technique
   C. with the shoulder girdle anterior to the pelvis
   D. keeping the weight close to you

_____   **4.** When lifting, you should:
    A. spread your legs past shoulder width
    B. lift a patient while reaching far in front of your torso
    C. keep the weight that you are lifting as close to your body as possible
    D. use your back muscles by bending at the waist

_____   **5.** When lifting a patient, proper technique involves which of the following?
    A. Leaning forward over the patient
    B. Avoiding bending at the waist
    C. Holding the weight away from your body
    D. Keeping the legs and knees locked straight

_____   **6.** In lifting with the palm down, the weight is supported by the _____ rather than the palm.
    A. fingers
    B. forearm
    C. lower back
    D. wrist

_____   **7.** When you must carry a patient up or down a flight of stairs or other significant incline, use a _____ if possible.
    A. backboard
    B. stair chair
    C. stretcher
    D. short backboard

_____   **8.** Most of a patient's weight will be distributed on which part of a backboard or stretcher?
    A. Head
    B. Foot
    C. Side
    D. Center

_____   **9.** A backboard is a device that provides support to patients who you suspect have all of the following EXCEPT:
    A. hip injuries
    B. pelvic injuries
    C. spinal injuries
    D. symptoms of heart attack

_____   **10.** Which of the following team leader actions is NOT required to safely lift and move a patient?
    A. Giving a command of execution
    B. Indicating where each team member is to be located
    C. Giving an abbreviated overview of the lifting and moving stages
    D. Completing all documentation prior to moving the patient

_____   **11.** Special _____ stretchers are usually required to move any patient who weighs more than 650 pounds (295 kg) to an ambulance.
    A. orthopedic
    B. pediatric
    C. geriatric
    D. bariatric

_____   **12.** Which of the following statements is FALSE regarding the use of a stair chair?
    A. Keep your back in a locked-in position.
    B. Lean back to help distribute the weight.
    C. Keep the patient's weight and your arms as close to your body as possible.
    D. Flex at the hips, not at the waist.

_____ **13.** When you use a body drag to move a patient:
   A. your back should always be locked in a slight curve
   B. twist so that the vertebrae can flex during the move
   C. consider hyperextending to gain more leverage
   D. drag the patient by the ankles

_____ **14.** When pulling a patient, you should do which of the following:
   A. extend your arms no more than about 15 inches to 20 inches (38 cm to 50 cm)
   B. stagger your feet so that the force of pull will be distributed toward your dominant hand
   C. move both yourself and the patient simultaneously
   D. pull the patient in rapid bursts of movement

_____ **15.** When log rolling a patient, you should do which of the following:
   A. avoid kneeling too closely to the patient's side
   B. hyperextend the back to reach completely across the patient
   C. refrain from using the belt loops or belt as a grab point
   D. use your shoulder muscles to help with the roll

_____ **16.** If the weight you are pushing is lower than your waist, you should push from:
   A. the waist
   B. a kneeling position
   C. the shoulder
   D. a squatting position

_____ **17.** If you are alone and must remove an unconscious patient from a car, you should first move the patient's:
   A. legs
   B. head
   C. torso
   D. pelvis

_____ **18.** Situations in which you should use an emergency move include all of the following EXCEPT:
   A. when fire, explosives, or hazardous materials are present
   B. when the patient feels like he or she might pass out
   C. when you are unable to gain access to others in a vehicle who need lifesaving care
   D. when you are unable to protect the patient from other hazards

_____ **19.** You can move a patient on his or her back along the floor or ground by using all of the following methods EXCEPT:
   A. pulling on the patient's clothing in the neck and shoulder area
   B. placing the patient on a blanket, coat, or other item that can be pulled
   C. pulling the patient by the legs if they are the most accessible part
   D. placing your arms under the patient's shoulders and through the armpits, and while grasping the patient's arms, dragging the patient backward

_____ **20.** The _____ is both the mechanical weight-bearing base of the spinal column and the fused central posterior section of the pelvic girdle.
   A. lumbar spine
   B. sacrum
   C. coccyx
   D. ileum

_____ **21.** Which of the following is NOT an indication for use of the rapid extrication technique?
   A. The patient is in severe pain.
   B. The patient's condition cannot be properly assessed before being removed from the vehicle.
   C. The patient blocks access to another seriously injured patient.
   D. The vehicle or the scene is unsafe.

_____ **22.** To avoid the strain of unnecessary lifting and carrying, you should use _____ or assist an able patient to the stretcher whenever possible.
  A. the direct ground lift
  B. the extremity lift
  C. the draw sheet method
  D. a scoop stretcher

_____ **23.** You should use a rigid _____, also called a Stokes litter, to carry a patient across uneven terrain from a remote location that is inaccessible by ambulance or other vehicle.
  A. basket stretcher
  B. scoop stretcher
  C. molded backboard
  D. flotation device

_____ **24.** Which of the following is true regarding the lifting and moving of geriatric patients?
  A. They generally have no fear or anxiety when being transported.
  B. Many will require additional padding or support to transport comfortably.
  C. They tend to have more flexibility than younger patients.
  D. They have less risk of skin tears or bruising than younger patients.

_____ **25.** Bariatrics is:
  A. the branch of medicine concerned with the elderly
  B. the branch of medicine concerned with the obese
  C. the branch of medicine concerned with infants
  D. the method used to assess blood pressure

Questions 26–29 are derived from the following scenario: You have been called to the scene of a high-speed motor vehicle collision involving two compact cars. The first vehicle was a rollover, ejecting the driver. The second vehicle contained both a driver and a front-seat passenger who cannot be reached because the door is up against a building. You note that the second vehicle is beginning to smoke, and flames can be seen from under the hood.

_____ **26.** What device will you use to put the rollover victim onto the wheeled ambulance stretcher?
  A. Extremity lift
  B. Scoop stretcher
  C. Short backboard
  D. Backboard

_____ **27.** For the passenger in the second vehicle, you may need to perform a(n) _____ on the driver in order to reach the patient.
  A. extremity lift
  B. emergency move
  C. short backboard
  D. You should do nothing different; treat each patient the same.

_____ **28.** Which of the following is an advantage of the diamond carry?
  A. It uses an even number of people (less likely to drop).
  B. It can be done with one person, freeing up others for patient care.
  C. The patient can be slid along the ground.
  D. It provides the best means of spinal immobilization.

_____ **29.** You'll likely use the _____ to transfer the patient from your stretcher to the hospital bed.
  A. diamond carry
  B. scoop stretcher
  C. portable stretcher
  D. draw sheet method

True/False

If you believe the statement to be more true than false, write the letter "T" in the space provided. If you believe the statement to be more false than true, write the letter "F."

_____ **1.** A portable stretcher is typically a lightweight folding device that does not have the undercarriage and wheels of a true ambulance stretcher.

_____ **2.** The term *power lift* refers to a posture that is safe and helpful for EMTs when they are lifting.

_____ **3.** If you find that lifting a patient is a strain, try to move the patient to the ambulance as quickly as possible to minimize the possibility of back injury.

_____ **4.** It is not important that you and your team use the correct lifting technique to lift a stretcher.

_____ **5.** One-person techniques for moving patients should be used only when immediate patient movement is necessary due to a life-threatening hazard and only one EMT is available.

_____ **6.** When carrying a patient down stairs or on an incline, make sure the stretcher is carried with the head end first.

_____ **7.** The rapid extrication technique is the preferred technique to use on all sitting patients with possible spinal injuries.

_____ **8.** It is unprofessional for you to discuss and plan a lift at the scene in front of the patient.

_____ **9.** Bariatrics is a medical specialty that deals with the care of the obese.

_____ **10.** An isolette is used to transport neonatal patients.

_____ **11.** The flexible stretcher is useful for moving patients through confined spaces.

_____ **12.** Pneumatic stretchers were developed to decrease the risk for EMS provider back injuries.

_____ **13.** Bariatric stretchers are the same as standard ambulance stretchers except for added lifting capacity.

Fill-in-the-Blank

Read each item carefully and then complete the statement by filling in the missing words.

1. To avoid injury to you, the patient, or your partners, you will have to learn how to lift and carry the patient properly, using proper _____ _____ and a power grip.

2. The key rule of lifting is to always keep the back in a straight, _____ position and to lift without twisting.

3. The safest and most powerful way to lift, lifting by extending the properly placed flexed legs, is called a(n) _____ _____.

4. The arm and hand have their greatest lifting strength when facing _____ up.

5. Be sure to pick up and carry the backboard with your back in the _____ position.

6. During a body drag where you and your partner are on each side of the patient, you will have to alter the usual pulling technique to prevent pulling _____ and producing adverse lateral leverage against your lower back.

7. When you are rolling the wheeled ambulance stretcher, your back should be _____, straight, and untwisted.

8. A patient on a backboard or stretcher can be lifted and carried by four providers in a(n) _____ carry.

9. Whenever a patient has been placed onto the stretcher, one EMT must hold the main frame to prevent

   _____.

10. The manual support and immobilization that you provide when using the rapid extrication technique produce

    a greater risk of _____ _____.

11. The _____ _____ _____ is used for patients with no suspected spinal injury who are found lying

    supine on the ground.

12. The _____ _____ may be especially helpful when the patient is in a very narrow space or when there

    is not enough room for the patient and a team of EMTs to stand side by side.

13. The mattress on a stretcher must be _____ _____ so that it does not absorb any type of potentially

    infectious material, including water, blood, or other body fluids.

14. It is essential that you _____ your equipment after use.

Critical Thinking

Short Answer

Complete this section with short written answers using the space provided.

1. List the nine different one-rescuer emergency moves.

   _____

   _____

   _____

2. List six situations where using a rapid extrication technique would be appropriate.

   _____

   _____

   _____

3. List three guidelines for loading the stretcher into the ambulance.

   _____

   _____

   _____

4. List five guidelines for carrying a patient on a stretcher.

   _____

   _____

   _____

5. Identify the key rule of lifting.

_____

_____

_____

Ambulance Calls

The following case scenarios provide an opportunity to explore the concerns associated with patient management and to enhance critical-thinking skills. Read each scenario and answer each question to the best of your ability.

1. You are dispatched to a construction site for a 26-year-old man who fell into a ravine. He is approximately 35 feet (11 m) down a rocky ledge. He is alert, with an unstable pelvis and weak radial pulses. You have all the help you need from the construction crew and the volunteer fire department.

How would you best manage this patient?

_____

_____

_____

2. You are dispatched to an "unknown medical problem" at a local residence. You are met at the door by the wife of the patient, who tells you that her husband is in the bathroom and is not acting right. You find the 350-pound (159-kg) patient lying in the bathroom, stuck between the toilet and the wall. He is not breathing and has no pulse.

How would you best manage this patient?

_____

_____

_____

3. You are dispatched to "difficulty breathing" at a nearby apartment complex. The patient's apartment is located on the top floor of a three-story building, is accessed through an exterior entryway, and no elevators are available. Your patient is morbidly obese and cannot walk.

How would you best manage this patient?

_____

_____

_____

Skills

Skill Drills
Skill Drill 8-1: Performing the Power Lift

Test your knowledge of this skill by filling in the correct words in the photo captions.

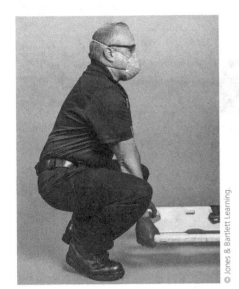

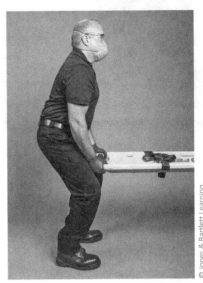

1. Lock your back in a(n) _____ curve. _____ and bend your legs. Grasp the backboard, palms up and just in front of you. _____ and _____ the weight between your arms.

2. Position your feet, _____ the object, and _____ your weight evenly. Lift by _____ your legs, keeping your back locked in.

Skill Drill 8-2: Performing the Diamond Carry

Test your knowledge of this skill by placing the following photos in the correct order. Number the first step with a "1," the second step with a "2," etc.

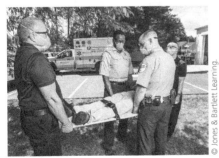

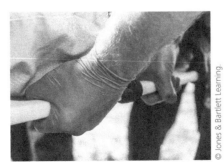

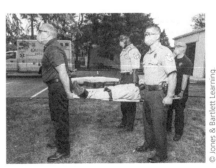

1. _____ The providers at each side turn the head-end hand palm down and release the other hand.

2. _____ The providers at each side turn toward the foot end. The provider at the foot end turns to face forward.

3. _____ Position yourselves facing the patient.

Skill Drill 8-3: Performing the One-Handed Carry

Test your knowledge of this skill by filling in the correct words in the photo captions.

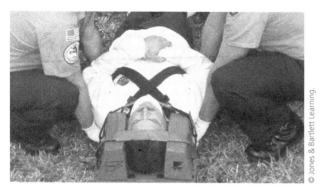

© Jones & Bartlett Learning.

1. _____ each other and use both _____.

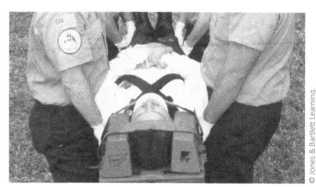

© Jones & Bartlett Learning.

2. Lift the backboard to _____ _____.

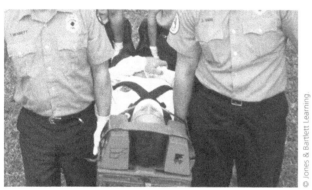

© Jones & Bartlett Learning.

3. _____ in the direction you will walk, and _____ to using one hand.

Skill Drill 8-7: Performing the Rapid Extrication Technique

Test your knowledge of this skill by placing the following photos in the correct order. Number the first step with a "1," the second step with a "2," etc.

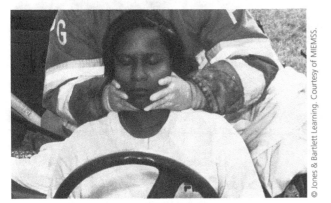

1. _____ The second provider supports the torso. The third provider frees the patient's legs from the pedals and moves the legs together, without moving the pelvis or spine.

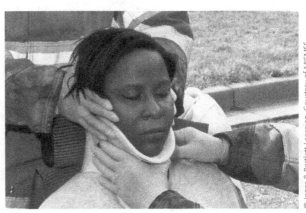

2. _____ The first provider provides in-line manual support of the head and cervical spine.

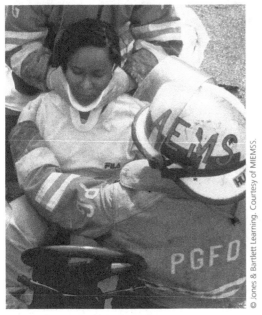

3. _____ The third provider exits the vehicle, moves to the backboard opposite the second provider, and they continue to slide the patient until the patient is fully on the board.

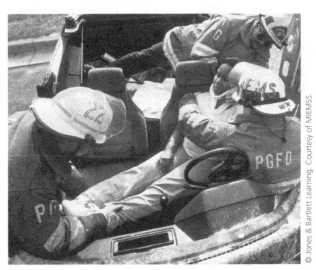

4. _____ The first (or fourth) provider places the backboard on the seat against the patient's buttocks. (Use of a backboard may depend on local protocols.)

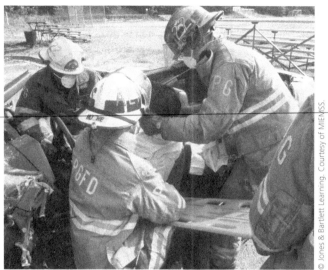

© Jones & Bartlett Learning. Courtesy of MIEMSS.

5. _____ The third provider moves to an effective position for sliding the patient. The second and the third providers slide the patient along the backboard in coordinated, 8- to 12-inch (20- to 30-cm) moves until the patient's hips rest on the backboard.

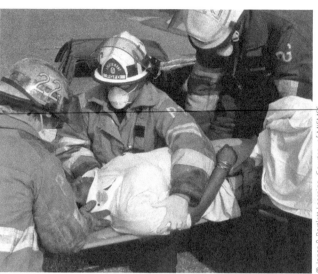

© Jones & Bartlett Learning. Courtesy of MIEMSS.

6. _____ The first (or fourth) provider continues to stabilize the head and neck while the second provider and the third provider carry the patient away from the vehicle and onto the prepared stretcher.

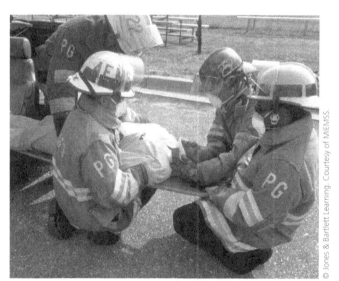

© Jones & Bartlett Learning. Courtesy of MIEMSS.

7. _____ The second provider and the third provider rotate the patient as a unit in several short, coordinated moves. The first provider (relieved by the fourth provider as needed) supports the patient's head and neck during rotation (and later steps).

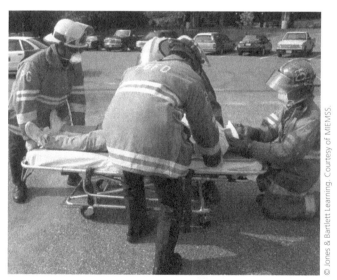

© Jones & Bartlett Learning. Courtesy of MIEMSS.

8. _____ The second provider gives commands, applies a cervical collar, and performs the primary assessment.

Skill Drill 8-9: Extremity Lift

Test your knowledge of this skill by filling in the correct words in the photo captions.

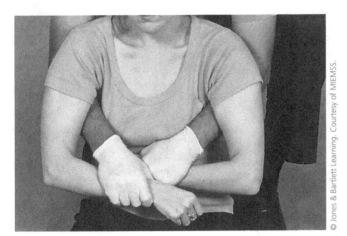

1. The patient's hands are _____ over the chest. Grasp the patient's wrists or _____ and pull the patient to a(n) _____ position.

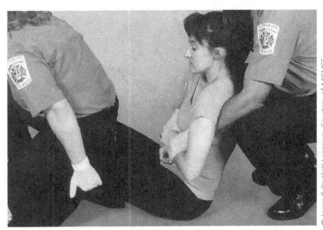

2. Your partner moves to a position between the patient's _____, facing in the _____ direction as the patient, and places his or her hands under the _____.

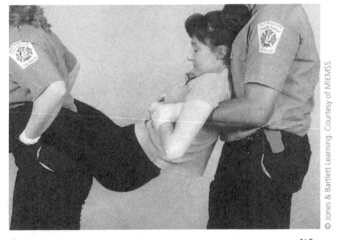

3. Rise to a(n) _____ position. On _____, lift and begin to move.

Skill Drill 8-10: Direct Carry

Test your knowledge of this skill by filling in the correct words in the photo captions.

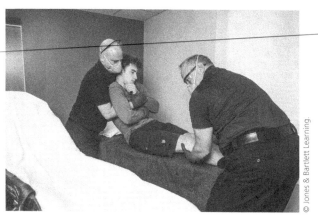

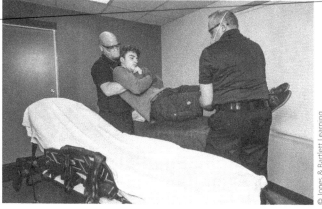

1. Position the stretcher _____ to the bed. Secure the _____ to prevent movement. Face the patient while standing between the _____ and the _____. Position your arms under the patient's _____ and _____. Your partner should position his or her hands under the patient's _____.

2. Lift the patient from the bed in a smooth, _____ fashion.

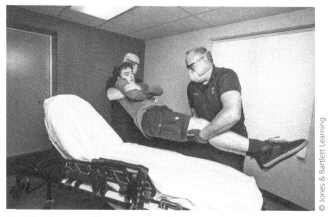

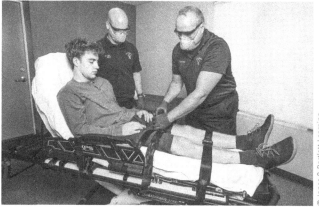

3. Slowly carry the patient to the _____.

4. _____ lower the patient onto the stretcher and secure with _____.

CHAPTER

9

The Team Approach to Health Care

General Knowledge

Matching

Match each of the items in the left column to the appropriate definition in the right column.

_____ **1.** Dependent groups

_____ **2.** Independent groups

_____ **3.** Situational awareness

_____ **4.** Team leader

_____ **5.** MIH model

_____ **6.** Group

A. Each individual is responsible for his or her own area

B. The knowledge and understanding of one's surroundings

C. A team member who provides role assignments, coordination, oversight, etc.

D. Each individual is told what to do

E. Consists of individual health care providers working independently to help the patient

F. Health care is provided in the community rather than at a physician's office or hospital

Multiple Choice

Read each item carefully and then select the one best response.

_____ **1.** A(n) _____ consists of a group of health care providers who are assigned specific roles and are working interdependently in a coordinated manner under a designated leader.

  A. group

  B. team

  C. dependent group

  D. independent group

_____ **2.** The "C" in the PACE mnemonic stands for:

  A. choose

  B. communication

  C. challenge

  D. clear

_____ **3.** A(n) _____ consists of individual health care providers working independently to help the patient.

  A. group

  B. team

  C. dependent group

  D. independent group

_____ **4.** When conflicts arise among health care teams, you should remember all of the following EXCEPT:

  A. that the patient comes first

  B. to separate the person from the issue

  C. to choose your battles

  D. it is acceptable to shout at other providers

_____ **5.** _____ entails emergency health care providers recognizing that by working together as a unified team from first patient contact to patient discharge, it is possible to improve individual and team performance, patient and provider safety, and ultimately, patient outcome.

    A. Mobile integrated health care

    B. Standard of care

    C. Continuum of care

    D. Community paramedicine

_____ **6.** In the _____ model, health care is provided within the community rather than at a physician's office or hospital.

    A. fire-based EMS

    B. continuum of care

    C. mobile integrated health care

    D. team health care

_____ **7.** Pit crew CPR consists of defining each intervention that needs to be addressed during cardiac arrest and training providers before the call to _____ any areas that are not being addressed as soon as they arrive on scene.

    A. rapidly identify

    B. prioritize

    C. take over

    D. rapidly identify, prioritize, and take over

_____ **8.** The best way for a team to be effective during an emergency call is to practice with one another and become familiar with each other's _____ and preferences.

    A. tools

    B. techniques

    C. capabilities

    D. tools, techniques, capabilities,

_____ **9.** It is your responsibility to understand what is allowed by the _____ where you work.

    A. scope of practice

    B. standard of care

    C. local protocols

    D. scope of practice, standard of care, and local protocols

_____ **10.** In _____, each individual is told what to do, and how often to do it, by his or her supervisor or group leader.

    A. groups

    B. teams

    C. dependent groups

    D. independent groups

_____ **11.** The team is NOT forced to move backward, resulting in a loss of valuable time and effort, if:

    A. incorrect information is handed off

    B. information is miscommunicated

    C. care is interrupted

    D. a proper transfer of patient care occurs

_____ **12.** The "P" in the PACE mnemonic stands for:

    A. practice

    B. probe

    C. prepare

    D. provide

_____ **13.** Assisting with an ALS skill does NOT include:
  A. patient preparation
  B. equipment set up
  C. continuing care
  D. performing skills for which you are not authorized

_____ **14.** All of the following are special teams EXCEPT:
  A. HazMat team
  B. MIH technicians
  C. Extracurricular EMS team
  D. EMS bike team

True/False

If you believe the statement to be more true than false, write the letter "T" in the space provided. If you believe the statement to be more false than true, write the letter "F."

_____ **1.** Team members who train and work together infrequently rarely need more explicit verbal direction to accomplish their tasks.

_____ **2.** Temporary teams are composed of crew members who regularly work together.

_____ **3.** EMS providers often have varying levels of certification or licensure.

_____ **4.** When using any advanced tool or technique, the focus is always on achieving a goal rather than on simply completing a procedure.

_____ **5.** If a conflict arises from the behavior of another team member and the conflict cannot be delayed or avoided, then focus on the individual rather than on the behavior itself.

_____ **6.** To successfully stabilize and treat the patient's condition, you must carefully coordinate your efforts with the advanced tools and techniques used by ALS providers.

_____ **7.** Excellent communication skills and teamwork are essential elements of emergency medicine.

Fill-in-the-Blank

Read each item carefully and then complete the statement by filling in the missing words.

1. The National Incident Management System defines a(n) _____ as "the organizational level that divides the incident according to functional levels of operation."

2. Team members who frequently _____ and _____ together are more likely to move smoothly from one step in the procedure to the next, performing as one seamless unit.

3. _____ _____ _____ is a way for team members to work together with the team leader to develop and maintain a shared understanding of the emergency situation.

4. While each provider may still be assigned to a particular area or task, everyone in a(n) _____ _____ works together, with shared responsibilities, accountability, and a common goal, as opposed to focusing on the goals of their own individual areas.

5. The _____ _____ is the team member who provides role assignments, coordination, oversight, centralized decision making, and support for the team to accomplish its goals and achieve desired results.

6. _____ _____ and mobile integrated health care teams may be the best example of the team concept of continuum of care.

Critical Thinking

Short Answer

Complete this section with short written answers using the space provided.

1. List the five techniques for handling team conflicts.

_____

_____

_____

2. List the five essential elements of a group that people must share, as defined by the Research Center for Group Dynamics.

_____

_____

_____

Ambulance Calls

The following case scenarios provide an opportunity to explore the concerns associated with patient management and to enhance critical-thinking skills. Read each scenario and answer each question to the best of your ability.

1. You are dispatched to assist with a patient who is experiencing chest pain and dizziness. You notice another EMT on the scene assisting with the application of the ECG. As the paramedic's attention is focused on starting an intravenous (IV) line, you see that the EMT has forgotten to attach one of the leads. The paramedic now begins assessing the patient's cardiac rhythm, but he appears confused by what he sees.

   How would you best manage this situation?

   _____

   _____

   _____

2. You are dispatched to a pulseless, apneic 45-year-old man. After assessing the patient, your paramedic partner decides to perform endotracheal intubation. This is the first field intubation that your partner has attempted. Your partner tells you that he "thinks" he passed through the cords. As you auscultate the chest, you do not hear breath sounds, but you do hear gurgling over the epigastrium.

   How would you best manage this situation?

   _____

   _____

   _____

3. You are in the patient compartment with your AEMT partner who is caring for a patient with congestive heart failure. Your partner has initiated IV therapy and is now giving a radio report to the receiving hospital. You notice that the IV tubing is still running wide open and that nearly the entire liter of fluid has been administered over a few minutes. The patient states his shortness of breath is worsening.

How would you best manage this situation?

_____

_____

_____

Patient Assessment

General Knowledge

Matching

Match each of the items in the left column to the appropriate definition in the right column.

_____	**1.** Triage	**A.** Sounds produced as air moves into and out of the lungs
_____	**2.** Cyanosis	**B.** The delicate membrane lining of the eyelid
_____	**3.** Subcutaneous emphysema	**C.** The indentation above the clavicles and in the spaces between the ribs during breathing
_____	**4.** Tachycardia	**D.** The white of the eyes
_____	**5.** Conjunctiva	**E.** The mental status of a patient
_____	**6.** Symptom	**F.** Mnemonic for gathering information about a patient's symptoms
_____	**7.** Accessory muscles of respiration	**G.** A yellow skin color due to liver disease or dysfunction
_____	**8.** Breath sounds	**H.** A crackling or grinding sound
_____	**9.** Chief complaint	**I.** To examine by touch
_____	**10.** Diaphoretic	**J.** Damage to tissues as the result of exposure to cold
_____	**11.** Jaundice	**K.** The way in which a patient responds to external stimuli
_____	**12.** Orientation	**L.** Neck, chest, and abdominal muscles used when difficulty breathing is present
_____	**13.** OPQRST	**M.** Air under the skin
_____	**14.** Palpate	**N.** The motion of a segment of chest wall that is opposite the normal movement during breathing
_____	**15.** Responsiveness	**O.** The most serious thing the patient is concerned about
_____	**16.** Retractions	**P.** The process of sorting patients based on severity of condition
_____	**17.** Sclera	**Q.** A blue-gray skin color associated with reduced oxygen levels
_____	**18.** Frostbite	**R.** Profuse sweating
_____	**19.** Crepitus	**S.** A subjective finding that the patient tells you about
_____	**20.** Paradoxical motion	**T.** A heart rate greater than 100 beats/min

Match the question with the corresponding assessment tool.

_____	**21.** What does the symptom feel like?	**A.** Signs and symptoms
_____	**22.** How long have you had the symptom?	**B.** Allergies
_____	**23.** Are you taking any medications?	**C.** Medications
_____	**24.** Did you eat this morning?	**D.** Past medical history

_____ **25.** Does anything make the symptoms better or worse?

E. Last oral intake

_____ **26.** On a scale of 1 to 10, how do you rate your symptom?

F. Events leading up to illness

_____ **27.** What were you doing before this happened?

G. Onset

_____ **28.** What type of reaction do you have when you take medication?

H. Provocation/palliation

_____ **29.** Does the pain move anywhere?

I. Quality

_____ **30.** When did the problem begin?

J. Region/radiation

_____ **31.** Does your chest hurt?

K. Severity

_____ **32.** Have you been recently ill?

L. Timing

Multiple Choice

Read each item carefully and then select the one best response.

_____ **1.** Which of the following is NOT considered part of the scene size-up?

A. Determining the mechanism of injury

B. Requesting additional assistance

C. Determining the level of responsiveness

D. Determining the need for personal protective equipment (PPE)/standard precautions

_____ **2.** You should consider all women of childbearing years who are complaining of lower abdominal pain to be:

A. pregnant until proven otherwise

B. experiencing cramps associated with menstruation

C. victims of sexual assault

D. suffering from a urinary tract infection

_____ **3.** With _____, the force of the injury occurs over a broad area, and the skin is usually not broken.

A. motor vehicle collisions

B. blunt trauma

C. penetrating trauma

D. gunshot wounds

_____ **4.** Which of the following conditions is NOT known to cause a slow capillary refill?

A. Vasoconstriction

B. Hypothermia

C. Age

D. Abdominal pain

_____ **5.** _____ is the measure of the amount of air that is moved into and out of the lungs in one breath.

A. Residual volume

B. Tidal volume

C. Vital capacity

D. Minute volume

_____ **6.** There are three elements to the physical exam. Which of the following is NOT one of those elements?

A. Puncture

B. Inspection

C. Palpation

D. Auscultation

_____ 7. When determining the initial general impression, you should note all of the following EXCEPT:
   A. the patient's age
   B. the level of distress
   C. the events leading up to the incident
   D. the patient's sex

_____ 8. Which of the following is included in the primary assessment?
   A. Blood pressure
   B. Palpating a pulse
   C. Oxygen saturation
   D. Pupil size

_____ 9. Which of the following conditions would be considered "high priority" when determining the priority of transport?
   A. Uncomplicated childbirth
   B. Mild abdominal pain
   C. Difficulty breathing
   D. Pink skin color

_____ 10. What does the "P" on the AVPU scale represent?
   A. Responsive to palpation
   B. Responsive to pain
   C. Responsive to provocation
   D. Responsive to palliation

_____ 11. A normal respiratory rate for an adult is typically:
   A. 5 to 10 breaths per minute
   B. 12 to 20 breaths per minute
   C. 15 to 30 breaths per minute
   D. 20 to 30 breaths per minute

_____ 12. For children younger than 1 year, you should palpate the _____ artery when assessing the pulse.
   A. carotid
   B. radial
   C. femoral
   D. brachial

_____ 13. When there are low levels of oxygen in the blood, the lips and mucous membranes appear blue or gray. What is the name of this condition?
   A. Cyanosis
   B. Pallor
   C. Jaundice
   D. Ashen

_____ 14. Your first consideration when assessing a pulse is to determine:
   A. how fast the rate is
   B. the quality
   C. if one is present
   D. if the rhythm is regular

_____ 15. To obtain the pulse rate in most patients, you should count the number of pulses felt in a _____ period and then multiply by two.
   A. 15-second
   B. 20-second
   C. 25-second
   D. 30-second

_____ **16.** In a patient with deeply pigmented skin, where should you look for changes in color?
  A. Ear canals
  B. External eyelids
  C. Groin
  D. Mucous membranes of the mouth

_____ **17.** With _____, the force of the injury occurs at a small point of contact between the skin and the object piercing the skin.
  A. motor vehicle collisions
  B. blunt trauma
  C. penetrating trauma
  D. falls

_____ **18.** Which of the following is NOT considered a method for controlling external bleeding?
  A. Direct pressure
  B. Tourniquet
  C. Cold water
  D. Elevation

_____ **19.** The _____ is/are the most serious thing that the patient is concerned about, the reason why they called 9-1-1.
  A. chief complaint
  B. pertinent negatives
  C. severity
  D. past medical history

_____ **20.** The four items used to assess the orientation of a patient's mental status include all of the following EXCEPT:
  A. person
  B. place
  C. history
  D. events

_____ **21.** An integral part of the rapid exam is evaluation using the mnemonic:
  A. AVPU
  B. DCAP-BTLS
  C. OPQRST
  D. SAMPLE

_____ **22.** In the absence of light, the pupils will:
  A. constrict
  B. stay fixed
  C. dilate
  D. become unequal

_____ **23.** When assessing the respiratory system, which of the following is NOT considered essential to the assessment?
  A. Respiratory rate
  B. Depth of breathing
  C. Quality/character of breathing
  D. Breath odor

_____ **24.** Which of the following statements regarding assessment of the airway is TRUE?
  A. The body will not be supplied the necessary oxygen if the airway is not managed.
  B. You should use the head tilt–chin lift maneuver to open the airway in trauma patients.
  C. The tongue is generally not a cause of airway obstruction.
  D. A conscious patient who cannot speak or cry is most likely hyperventilating.

_____ **25.** Which of the following is NOT considered a type of breath sound?
   A. Rhonchi
   B. Vibration
   C. Wheeze
   D. Stridor

_____ **26.** You are examining a 40-year-old female who you suspect might be a victim of abuse. Which of the following supports your suspicion?
   A. Mechanism of injury that matches the patient's history
   B. Unremarkable medical history with no previous injuries
   C. Multiple injuries in various stages of healing
   D. Consistent history reporting by the patient

_____ **27.** When caring for a patient who is unable to speak or understand English, you should:
   A. raise the volume of your voice
   B. give the hospital advance notice in your radio report
   C. feel free to make derogatory remarks
   D. encourage the patient to learn English

_____ **28.** _____ is an assessment tool used to evaluate the effectiveness of oxygenation.
   A. Capnography
   B. Capnometry
   C. Pulse oximetry
   D. Blood glucose

_____ **29.** The pressure felt along the wall of the artery when the ventricles of the heart contract is referred to as the:
   A. asystolic pressure
   B. diastolic pressure
   C. idiopathic pressure
   D. systolic pressure

_____ **30.** A blood pressure cuff that's too large for the patient:
   A. may result in a falsely low reading
   B. may result in a falsely high reading
   C. will not affect the reading
   D. should be used in patients with arm pain

_____ **31.** Which of the following is NOT typically found on an abdominal exam?
   A. Guarding
   B. Crepitation
   C. Tenderness
   D. Rigidity

_____ **32.** Crackling sounds produced by air bubbles under the skin are known as:
   A. subcutaneous ecchymosis
   B. subcutaneous emphysema
   C. subcutaneous erythema
   D. subcutaneous emboli

_____ **33.** Unstable patients should be reassessed every _____ minutes.
   A. 5
   B. 10
   C. 15
   D. 20

_____ **34.** In the _____ position, the patient sits leaning forward on outstretched arms with the head and chin thrust slightly forward.

    A. Fowler's

    B. tripod

    C. sniffing

    D. lithotomy

_____ **35.** In an unresponsive adult patient, the primary location to assess the pulse is the _____ artery.

    A. carotid

    B. femoral

    C. radial

    D. brachial

_____ **36.** Liver disease or dysfunction may cause _____, resulting in the patient's skin and sclera turning yellow.

    A. cyanosis

    B. jaundice

    C. diaphoresis

    D. lack of perfusion

_____ **37.** When obtaining a blood pressure by palpation in the arm, you should place your fingertips on the _____ artery.

    A. carotid

    B. brachial

    C. radial

    D. posterior tibial

_____ **38.** The _____ is performed at regular intervals during the assessment process, and its purpose is to identify and treat changes in a patient's condition.

    A. primary assessment

    B. reassessment

    C. secondary assessment

    D. scene size-up

_____ **39.** Which of the following is NOT considered a sign?

    A. Dizziness

    B. Marked deformities

    C. External bleeding

    D. Wounds

_____ **40.** When blood pressure drops, the body compensates to maintain perfusion to the vital organs by:

    A. decreasing the pulse rate

    B. dilating the arteries

    C. decreasing the respiratory rate

    D. decreasing the blood flow to the skin and extremities

_____ **41.** When assessing and treating a patient who is visually impaired, it is important that you do all of the following EXCEPT:

    A. speak loudly into the patient's ear because he or she can't see you

    B. announce yourself when entering the residence

    C. put items that were moved back into their previous position

    D. explain to the patient what is happening

_____ **42.** Which of the following statements is false regarding the assessment of patients with a language barrier?

    A. You should find an interpreter.

    B. You should determine whether the patient understands you.

    C. Your questioning should be lengthy and complex.

    D. You should be aware of the language diversity in your community.

True/False

If you believe the statement to be more true than false, write the letter "T" in the space provided. If you believe the statement to be more false than true, write the letter "F."

_____ **1.** Responsiveness is evaluated with the mnemonic DCAP-BTLS.

_____ **2.** Reassessment is not necessary for stable patients.

_____ **3.** An assessment of the patient's musculoskeletal system typically is done because of a chief complaint associated with some type of trauma.

_____ **4.** The apparent absence of a palpable pulse in an unresponsive patient is not a cause for concern.

_____ **5.** A patient with a poor general impression is considered a priority patient.

_____ **6.** When assessing the head, you should assess the patient's ears and nose for fluid.

_____ **7.** Paradoxical motion of the chest wall is commonly associated with upper respiratory infections.

_____ **8.** The abdomen is broken into six areas for assessment at the EMT level.

_____ **9.** In the reassessment process, you should reevaluate everything that has been done to this point in the patient assessment process.

_____ **10.** Law enforcement personnel may be needed at scenes to control traffic or intervene in domestic violence situations.

_____ **11.** Determining the mental status and the level of consciousness of a patient take a great deal of time while on scene.

_____ **12.** Depressed brain function can result from trauma or stroke.

_____ **13.** PEARRL is used to describe skin color.

_____ **14.** You should consider providing positive pressure ventilation in a conscious patient who has a respiratory rate of 14 breaths/min.

_____ **15.** When documenting vital signs, you should note whether the patient's respirations are regular or irregular.

_____ **16.** Patients with difficulty breathing, severe chest pain, and signs of poor perfusion should be transported immediately.

_____ **17.** Correct identification of high-priority patients is an essential aspect of the primary assessment and helps to improve patient outcome.

_____ **18.** You should not interrupt patients when speaking, and you should be empathetic to their situations.

_____ **19.** Being openly judgmental of patients who may have a chemical dependency is acceptable as long as you remain professional.

_____ **20.** Scenes involving domestic violence can be extremely dangerous for EMS personnel.

_____ **21.** You should consider all females of childbearing age who are reporting lower abdominal pain to be pregnant unless ruled out by history or other information.

_____ **22.** Once you have allowed a talkative patient a chance to express himself or herself, you should allow the patient to continue talking about whatever he or she wants.

_____ **23.** EMTs can expect anxious patients to exhibit signs of psychological shock.

_____ **24.** It is unusual for a patient, family member, or friend to vent hostility toward EMS.

_____ **25.** Information gathered from an intoxicated patient may be unreliable.

_____ **26.** Your presence may make a crying patient feel more secure.

_____ **27.** Depression is not a common reason for patients to call for EMS.

_____ **28.** When assessing a patient, you should inspect the pelvis for symmetry and any obvious signs of injury, bleeding, and deformity.

_____ **29.** Pulse and motor and sensory functions are typically assessed when examining a patient's extremities.

Fill-in-the-Blank

Read each item carefully and then complete the statement by filling in the missing words.

1. A(n) _____ is an objective condition that you can observe about the patient.

2. _____ _____ are protective measures for dealing with blood and bodily fluids.

3. When there are multiple patients, you should use the _____ _____ _____ to help organize the triage, logistics, and treatment of patients.

4. _____ _____ _____ should be requested for patients with severe injuries or complex medical problems.

5. Identifying and initiating treatment of immediate, potentially life-threatening conditions is the goal of the _____ _____.

6. You should think of the _____ _____ as a visual assessment, gathering information as you approach the patient.

7. _____ is the flow of blood through body tissues and vessels.

8. _____ tests the mental status of the patient by checking memory and thinking ability.

9. When light is shined into the eyes, the pupils should _____.

10. A brassy, crowing sound that is prominent on inspiration, suggesting a mildly occluded airway, is referred to as _____.

11. If there is a potential for trauma, use the _____ _____ _____ to open the airway.

12. During _____ the chest muscles relax, and air is released out of the lungs.

13. If a patient seems to develop difficulty breathing after your primary assessment, you should immediately reevaluate the _____.

14. If you hear fluid in the airway during your assessment, you should immediately _____ the airway to prevent aspiration.

15. A patient who coughs up thick yellow or green sputum most likely has a(n) _____ _____.

16. _____ _____ and seesaw breathing in a pediatric patient indicate inadequate breathing.

17. If you cannot palpate a pulse in an unresponsive patient, you should begin _____.

18. _____ is a heart rate greater than 100 beats/min.

19. The _____ is the delicate membrane lining the eyelids, and it covers the exposed surface of the eye.

20. Skin that is cool, clammy, and pale in your primary assessment typically indicates _____.

21. When the skin is bathed in sweat, it is described as _____.

22. A capillary refill time should be less than _____ second(s).

23. Direct pressure stops bleeding and helps the blood to _____, or clot, naturally.

24. A rapid scan to identify immediate threats should take no more than _____ second(s).

25. The _____ _____ refers to the time from injury to definitive care.

26. The goal of the primary assessment is to identify and treat _____ _____.

27. _____ _____ provides details about the patient's chief complaint and an account of the patient's signs and symptoms.

28. You should use _____ questions when taking a history of a patient.

29. _____ is a mnemonic used to gather past medical or trauma history.

30. _____ _____ are negative findings used to help identify a patient's problem.

31. _____ _____ should be assessed in all known diabetic patients and all patients who are unresponsive for an unknown reason.

32. _____ describes the process of touching or feeling the patient for abnormalities.

33. _____ is a noninvasive method that can quickly and efficiently provide information on a patient's ventilatory status, circulation, and metabolism.

34. _____ _____ is the residual pressure that remains in the arteries during the relaxation phase of the heart.

35. A(n) _____ assessment should be performed anytime you are confronted with a patient who has a change in mental status, a possible head injury, or syncope.

Critical Thinking

Short Answer
Complete this section with short written answers using the space provided.

1. What is the single goal of primary assessment?

_____

_____

_____

2. What is the general impression based on?

_____

_____

_____

3. What do the letters ABC stand for in the assessment process?

_____

_____

_____

4. What four kinds of questions are asked when assessing orientation, and what purpose do these questions serve?

_____

_____

_____

5. What three questions should you ask yourself when assessing a patient's breathing?

_____

_____

_____

6. List the elements of DCAP-BTLS.

_____

_____

_____

7. What three questions should you ask yourself to determine if additional resources are needed at a scene?

_____

_____

_____

8. Define the acronym PEARRL.

_____

_____

_____

9. Explain the difference between a sign and a symptom.

_____

_____

_____

10. You are caring for a 24-year-old male with a pertinent sexual history. What questions should he be asked as part of your history taking?

_____

_____

_____

Ambulance Calls

The following case scenarios provide an opportunity to explore the concerns associated with patient management and to enhance critical-thinking skills. Read each scenario and answer each question to the best of your ability.

1. You are dispatched to a motor vehicle collision where you find a 32-year-old man with extensive trauma to the face and gurgling in his airway. He is responsive only to pain. You also note that the windshield is spider-webbed and that there is deformity to the steering wheel. He is not wearing a seat belt.

How would you best manage this patient? What clues tell you the transport status?

_____

_____

_____

2. You are dispatched to a local residence for "difficulty breathing." You find a man standing in his kitchen, leaning against a counter in a tripod position, and holding a metered-dose inhaler. As you question him, you see that he is working very hard to breathe, hear wheezing, and note that he can answer you with only one- or two-word responses.

What is the transport status of this patient?

_____

_____

_____

3. You are dispatched to "man fallen" at a private home. You arrive to find an older man who appears to have fallen down a flight of wooden stairs onto a cement basement floor. He is responsive to painful stimuli, has bruising, and has a small laceration above his left eye.

How would you best manage this patient?

_____

_____

_____

Skills

Skill Drills

Skill Drill 10-1: Performing a Rapid Exam to Identify Life Threats

Test your knowledge of this skill by placing the following photos in the correct order. Number the first step with a "1," the second step with a "2," etc.

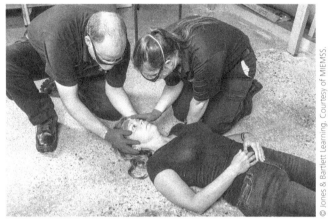

1. _____ Assess the chest. Listen to breath sounds on both sides of the chest.

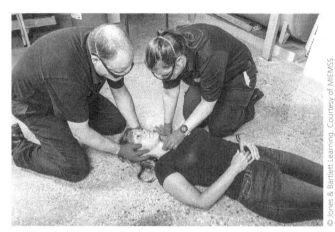

2. _____ Assess the back. If spinal immobilization is indicated, do so with minimal movement to the patient's spine by log rolling the patient in one motion.

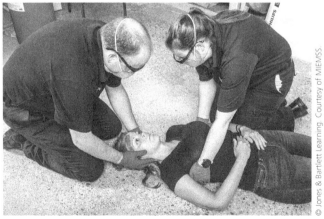

3. _____ Assess the head. Have your partner maintain in-line stabilization if indicated.

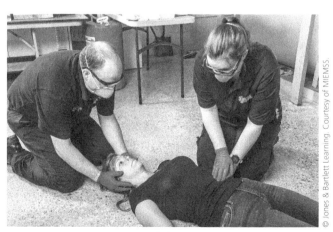

4. _____ Assess the abdomen.

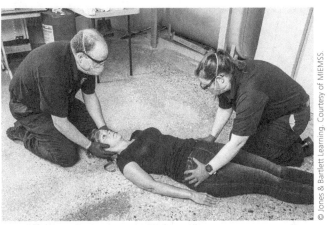

5. _____ Assess all four extremities. Assess pulse and motor and sensory function.

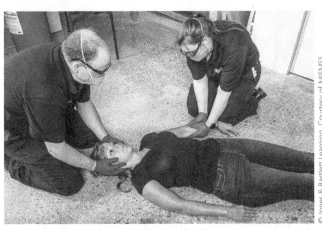

6. _____ Assess the neck.

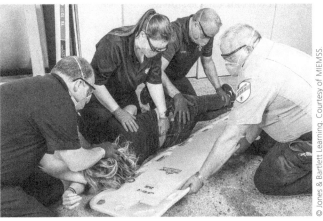

7. _____ Assess the pelvis. If there is no pain, gently compress the pelvis downward and inward to look for tenderness and instability.

Skill Drill 10-3: Obtaining Blood Pressure by Auscultation

Test your knowledge of this skill by placing the following photos in the correct order. Number the first step with a "1," the second step with a "2," etc.

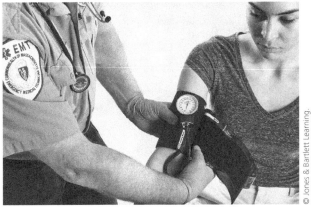

1. _____ Support the exposed arm at the level of the heart. Palpate the brachial.

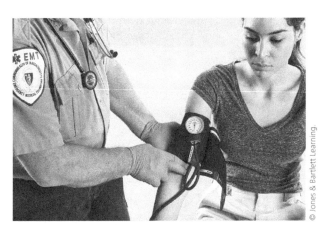

2. _____ Open the valve, and quickly release remaining air.

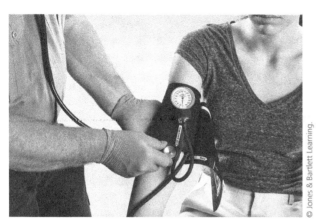

© Jones & Bartlett Learning.

3. _____ Follow standard precautions. Check for a dialysis fistula, central line, previous mastectomy, and injury to the arm. If any are present, use the brachial artery on the other arm. Apply the cuff snugly. The lower border of the cuff should be about 1 inch (2.5 cm) above the antecubital space.

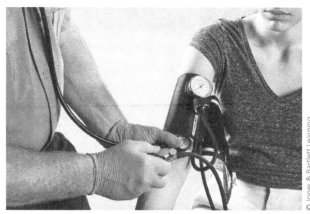

© Jones & Bartlett Learning.

4. _____ Close the valve, and pump to 30 mm Hg above the point at which you stop hearing pulse sounds. Note the systolic and diastolic pressures as you let air escape slowly.

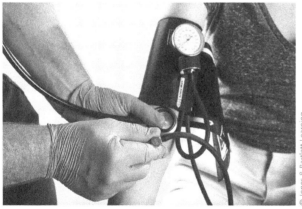

© Jones & Bartlett Learning.

5. _____ Place the stethoscope over the brachial artery, and grasp the ball-pump and turn-valve.

Airway Management

General Knowledge

Matching

Match each of the items in the left column to the appropriate definition in the right column.

_____ 1. Inhalation
_____ 2. Exhalation

_____ 3. Alveoli
_____ 4. Mediastinum

_____ 5. Hypoxic drive
_____ 6. Tidal volume
_____ 7. Diaphragm

_____ 8. Intercostal muscle
_____ 9. Ventilation
_____ 10. Larynx
_____ 11. Hypoxia
_____ 12. Cheyne-Stokes

A. Moves downward with contraction
B. An irregular breathing pattern with increased rate and depth followed by apnea
C. An active part of breathing
D. A complex structure made of cartilage, marking where the upper airway ends and the lower airway begins
E. The amount of air moved during one breath
F. Raises ribs when it contracts
G. The space between the lungs that contains the heart, great vessels, trachea, main bronchi, esophagus, and many nerves
H. The functional site of oxygen and carbon dioxide exchange
I. A passive process not requiring muscular effort
J. Insufficient oxygen for cells and tissues
K. A secondary system for control of breathing
L. The exchange of air between lungs and the environment

Multiple Choice

Read each item carefully and then select the one best response.

_____ 1. What percentage of the air that we breathe is made up of oxygen?
   A. 78%
   B. 12%
   C. 16%
   D. 21%

_____ 2. What concentration of inspired oxygen is provided by a nasal cannula when the flowmeter is set at 1 to 6 L/min?
   A. 10% to 18%
   B. 24% to 44%
   C. 52% to 84%
   D. 89% to 98%

_____ 3. Which of the following statements regarding respiratory rate is TRUE?
   A. The respiratory rate is about equal to the person's heart rate.
   B. The normal rate is 12 to 20 breaths/min.
   C. The rate is faster when the person is sleeping.
   D. The rate is the same in infants and children.

_____   **4.** Which of the following is a sign of inadequate breathing in an adult?
- **A.** Respiratory rate of 18 breaths/min
- **B.** Diminished breath sounds
- **C.** Equal chest expansion
- **D.** Warm, pink skin

_____   **5.** The brainstem normally triggers breathing by increasing respirations when:
- **A.** carbon dioxide levels increase
- **B.** oxygen levels increase
- **C.** carbon dioxide levels decrease
- **D.** nitrogen levels decrease

_____   **6.** Which of the following is a contraindication for placement of an oropharyngeal airway?
- **A.** Intact gag reflex
- **B.** Severe head injury
- **C.** Unconsciousness
- **D.** Fractured nasal bone

_____   **7.** The proper technique for sizing an oropharyngeal airway before insertion is to measure the device from:
- **A.** the tip of the nose to the earlobe
- **B.** the bridge of the nose to the tip of the chin
- **C.** the earlobe or angle of the jaw to the corner of the mouth
- **D.** the center of the jaw to the earlobe

_____   **8.** What is a common problem when a single EMT uses a bag-mask device?
- **A.** Overinflation of the lungs
- **B.** Delivering an inappropriate rate of ventilations
- **C.** Environmental conditions
- **D.** Maintaining an airtight mask seal

_____   **9.** When ventilating a patient with a bag-mask device, you should:
- **A.** look for inflation of the cheeks
- **B.** squeeze the bag hard and fast
- **C.** look for rise and fall of the chest
- **D.** only perform this with an advanced airway

_____   **10.** When the airway is not clear, suctioning the oral cavity before positive pressure ventilation is initiated is important because it:
- **A.** stimulates the patient to breathe
- **B.** prevents gagging
- **C.** helps reduce the risk of aspiration
- **D.** prevents tachycardia

_____   **11.** Which of the following is the most common method of assisting ventilations in the field?
- **A.** Mouth-to-mask with one-way valve
- **B.** Continuous positive airway pressure (CPAP)
- **C.** Flow-restricted, oxygen-powered ventilation device
- **D.** Bag-mask device with oxygen reservoir and supplemental oxygen

_____   **12.** When a person goes _____ minutes without oxygen, brain damage is very likely.
- **A.** 0 to 4
- **B.** 4 to 6
- **C.** 6 to 10
- **D.** more than 10

_____ 13. What is the most common airway obstruction in the unconscious patient?
  A. Food
  B. Tonsils
  C. Blood
  D. Tongue

_____ 14. What are agonal gasps?
  A. Occasional gasping breaths but adequate to maintain life
  B. Occasional gasping breaths but unable to maintain life
  C. Painful respirations due to broken ribs
  D. Another name for ataxic respirations

_____ 15. Which of the following could result in an inaccurate pulse oximetry reading?
  A. Warm extremities
  B. Carbon monoxide poisoning
  C. Vasodilation
  D. Hyperthermia

True/False

If you believe the statement to be more true than false, write the letter "T" in the space provided. If you believe the statement to be more false than true, write the letter "F."

_____ **1.** Nasopharyngeal airways physically keep the tongue from blocking the upper airway and facilitate suctioning of the oropharynx.

_____ **2.** Nasal cannulas can deliver a maximum of 44% oxygen at 6 L/min.

_____ **3.** Oropharyngeal airways should be measured from the tip of the nose to the earlobe.

_____ **4.** Compressed gas cylinders pose no unusual risk.

_____ **5.** The pin-indexing system is used to allow any gas regulator to be connected to an oxygen cylinder.

Fill-in-the-Blank

Read each item carefully and then complete the statement by filling in the missing words.

1. The upper airway consists of all anatomic airway structures above the level of the _____ _____.

2. In exhalation, air pressure in the lungs is _____ than the pressure outside.

3. The air we breathe contains _____ % oxygen and _____ % nitrogen.

4. The primary mechanism for triggering breathing is the level of _____ _____ in the blood.

5. During inhalation, the _____ and _____ _____ contract, causing the thorax to enlarge.

6. Continuous _____ airway _____ has proven to be immensely beneficial to patients experiencing respiratory distress from acute pulmonary edema or obstructive pulmonary disease.

7. Insufficient oxygen in the cells and tissues is called _____.

8. _____ _____ is the act of air moving in and out the lungs during chest compressions.

Labeling

Label the following diagrams with the correct terms.

1. Upper and Lower Airways

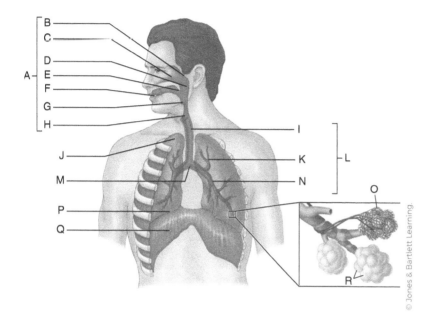

A. _____

B. _____

C. _____

D. _____

E. _____

F. _____

G. _____

H. _____

I. _____

J. _____

K. _____

L. _____

M. _____

N. _____

O. _____

P. _____

Q. _____

R. _____

2. Oral Cavity

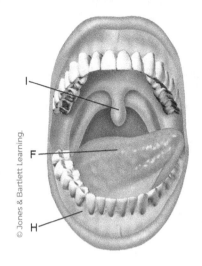

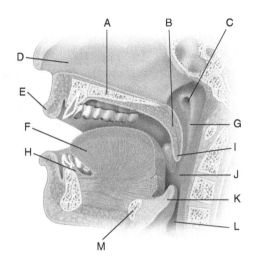

A. _____

B. _____

C. _____

D. _____

E. _____

F. _____

G. _____

H. _____

I. _____

J. _____

K. _____

L. _____

M. _____

3. Thoracic Cavity

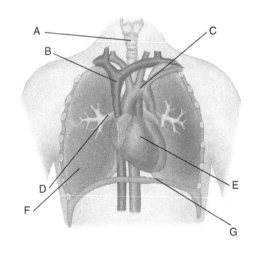

A. _____

B. _____

C. _____

D. _____

E. _____

F. _____

G. _____

© Jones & Bartlett Learning.

Critical Thinking

Multiple Choice

Read each critical-thinking item carefully and then select the one best response.

Questions 1–5 are derived from the following scenario: You respond to a construction site and find a worker lying supine in the dirt. He was struck by a heavy construction vehicle and flew more than 15 feet (4.6 m) before landing in his current position. There is discoloration and distention of his abdomen about the right upper quadrant (RUQ). He is unconscious, and his respirations are 10 breaths/min and shallow, with noisy gurgling sounds.

_____ 1. What airway technique will you use to open his airway?
   A. Head tilt–neck lift maneuver
   B. Jaw-thrust
   C. Head tilt–chin lift maneuver
   D. Cross-finger technique

_____ 2. After opening the airway, your next priority is to:
   A. provide oxygen at 6 L/min via a nonrebreathing mask
   B. provide oxygen at 15 L/min via a nasal cannula
   C. assist respirations
   D. suction the airway

_____ 3. What method will you use to keep his airway open?
   A. Nasal cannula
   B. Jaw thrust maneuver
   C. Oropharyngeal airway
   D. Head tilt–chin lift maneuver

_____ 4. While assisting with respirations, you note gastric distention. In order to prevent or alleviate the distention, you should do all of the following EXCEPT:
   A. ensure that the patient's airway is appropriately positioned
   B. ventilate the patient at the appropriate rate
   C. ventilate the patient at the appropriate volume
   D. ventilate the patient at a faster rate

_____ 5. The patient is now apneic. What is the correct ventilation rate for assisting this adult patient?
   A. One breath every 6 seconds
   B. One breath every 3 to 5 seconds
   C. One breath every 10 to 12 seconds
   D. There is no need to assist with ventilations for this patient.

Short Answer

Complete this section with short written answers using the space provided.

   1. List five contraindications for CPAP.

   _____

   _____

   _____

2. What are the normal respiratory rates for adults, children, and infants?

_____

_____

_____

3. How can you avoid gastric distention while performing artificial ventilation?

_____

_____

_____

4. List six signs of inadequate breathing.

_____

_____

_____

5. What are accessory muscles? Name three.

_____

_____

_____

6. When should extreme caution be used while inserting a nasal airway?

_____

_____

_____

7. List the four steps in nasal airway insertion.

_____

_____

_____

8. What is the best suction tip for suctioning infants and children? Why

_____

_____

_____

Ambulance Calls

The following case scenarios provide an opportunity to explore the concerns associated with patient management and to enhance critical-thinking skills. Read each scenario and answer each question to the best of your ability.

1. You are dispatched to a motor vehicle collision with multiple patients early one morning near the end of your shift. Your patient was the unrestrained driver of one of the vehicles. She is 38 years old and struck her face against the steering wheel and windshield. There is a large laceration on her nose, and several teeth are missing. Although unconscious, she has vomited a large amount of food and blood, which is pooling in her mouth. You note gurgling noises as she attempts to breathe.

   How would you best manage this patient?

   _____

   _____

   _____

2. You are dispatched to a local restaurant for an unconscious woman. As you arrive, you are greeted by a frantic restaurant manager. She tells you that one of her staff members went into the restroom to complete the hourly cleaning routine and found a woman lying on the floor, motionless and apparently not breathing. You and your partner enter the cramped ladies' bathroom to find an older woman who is apneic and cyanotic but who has a carotid pulse. You attempt to ventilate the patient using a bag-mask device but are unsuccessful.

   How should you manage this patient?

   _____

   _____

   _____

3. You are outside doing some yard work when you hear one of your neighbors call for help. As you cross the street, you see a husband standing over his wife, who is lying on the ground. He tells you that she complained of feeling lightheaded, and then she suddenly passed out. He further tells you that he was able to help her to the ground without injury. When you assess her, you hear snoring sounds as she breathes.

   How do you manage this patient?

   _____

   _____

   _____

Fill-in-the-Patient Care Report

Read the incident scenario and then complete the following patient care report (PCR).

It is 1530, and you have just been dispatched to Market Street High School for a possible drug overdose. As your partner steers the ambulance into the nearly empty school parking lot at 1543, you see a woman waving her arms from near one of the low, gray buildings. You and your partner pull the equipment-laden gurney from the back of the truck and hurry across the grass.

"The janitor found her in the stall," the woman's voice trembles as you arrive at the restroom entrance where she is standing. "She's kind of breathing, but I can't wake her up . . . she's had some troubles in the past with drugs."

You find the 14-year-old girl lying on her left side on the tile floor in the middle of three stalls, unresponsive to pain and with slow, snoring respirations.

"You see that?" your partner says, unzipping the airway bag and pointing toward the girl's bluish lips and fingernails.

"I'm going to drag her out of here so we have room while you get the bag-mask device set up," you say, carefully pulling the 110-pound (50-kg) girl from the stall and resting her on her back. You immediately open her airway with the head tilt–chin lift maneuver, which stops the snoring sound, but you still note that her breathing is very shallow. Just then, your partner finishes assembling the oxygen tank and bag-mask device and inserts an oropharyngeal airway. Within 2 minutes of the time that you got out of the ambulance, your partner is assisting the patient's respirations, getting adequate chest rise, and you are getting a quick set of vital signs.

You note that her blood pressure is 124/86 mm Hg, pulse is 112 beats/min and regular, respirations (with assistance) are 12 breaths/min, and her oxygen saturation is 93%.

Just as you are finishing vitals, the local fire crew arrives and helps place the patient onto the gurney and into the back of the ambulance. One of the firefighters even jumps into the back to continue assisting the girl's ventilations so that your partner can complete the assessment and obtain a second set of vitals en route to the receiving hospital.

You notify dispatch at 1556 that you are pulling away from the scene and heading to the hospital 12 minutes south of the school. The patient's second set of vitals, obtained 4 minutes after going en route, were as follows: blood pressure 122/86 mm Hg, pulse 110 beats/min, respirations 12 breaths/min (still being assisted), and a pulse oximetry reading of 96%.

On arrival at the hospital, you transfer the patient to the emergency department staff and clean and restock your equipment. Fifty-five minutes after receiving the initial dispatch, you go back in service.

Fill-in-the-Patient Care Report

EMS Patient Care Report (PCR)					
Date:	Incident No.:		Nature of Call:		Location:
DIspatched:	En Route:	At Scene:	Transport:	At Hospital:	In Service:

Patient Information	
Age: Sex: Weight (in kg [lb]):	Allergies: Medications: Past Medical History: Chief Complaint:

Vital Signs				
Time:	BP:	Pulse:	Respirations:	SpO$_2$:
Time:	BP:	Pulse:	Respirations:	SpO$_2$:
Time:	BP:	Pulse:	Respirations:	SpO$_2$:

EMS Treatment (circle all that apply)				
Oxygen @ ___ L/min via (circle one): NC NRM BVM		Assisted Ventilation	Airway Adjunct	CPR
Defibrillation	Bleeding Control	Bandaging	Splinting	Other:

Narrative

Skills

Skill Drills

Test your knowledge of these skills by filling in the correct words in the photo captions.

Skill Drill 11-2: Positioning the Unconscious Patient

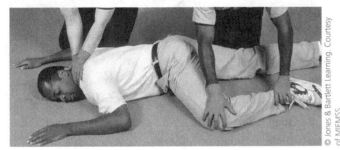

1. Support the _____ while your partner straightens the patient's legs.

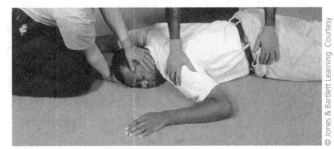

2. Have your partner place his or her _____ on the patient's far _____ and hip.

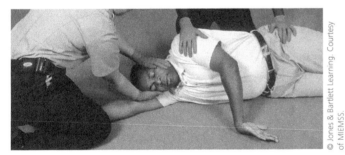

3. _____ the patient as a unit with the EMT at the patient's _____ calling the count to begin the move.

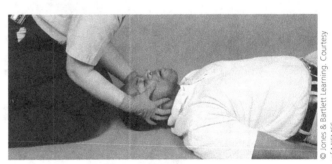

4. _____ and _____ the patient's airway and _____ status.

Skill Drill 11-4: Inserting an Oral Airway

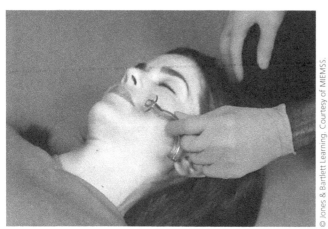

1. Size the _____ by measuring from the patient's _____ to the corner of the _____.

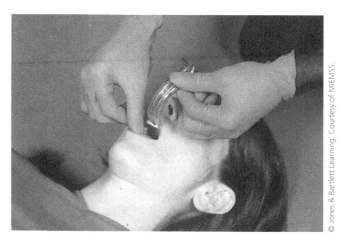

2. Open the patient's _____ with the _____ -finger technique. Hold the _____ upside down with your other hand. Insert the airway with the tip facing the _____ of the mouth.

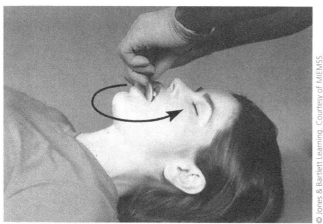

3. _____ the airway _____. Insert the airway until the _____ rests on the patient's lips and teeth. In this position, the airway will hold the _____ forward.

Skill Drill 11-7: Placing an Oxygen Cylinder Into Service

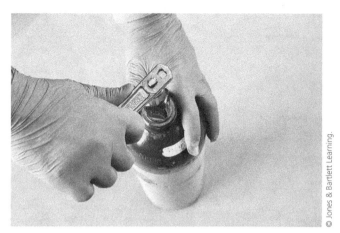

1. Using an oxygen _____, turn the valve _____ to slowly "crack" the cylinder.

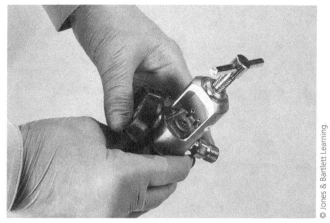

2. Attach the regulator/flowmeter to the _____ stem using the two pin- _____ holes, and make sure that the _____ is in place over the larger hole.

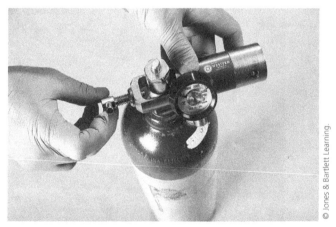

3. Align the _____ so that the pins fit snugly into the correct holes on the _____ stem, and hand tighten the _____.

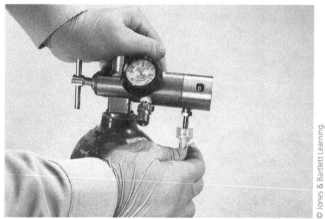

4. Attach the _____ connective tubing to the _____.

Skill Drill 11-8: Performing One-Rescuer Bag-Mask Ventilation (page 465)

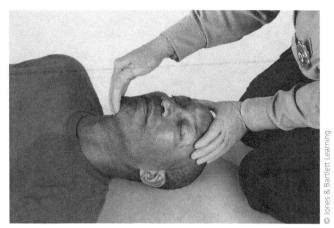

1. Assemble the necessary equipment and position yourself _____ the patient's _____. Open the airway using the appropriate maneuver.

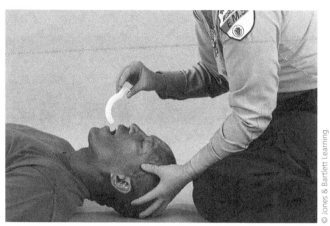

2. _____ as necessary to clear away any _____. Insert an appropriate basic airway _____.

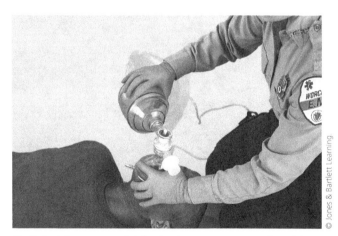

3. Select the appropriately sized _____ and position it properly on the patient's face. Use the _____ technique to make a seal. Avoid the fleshy soft tissue of the neck.

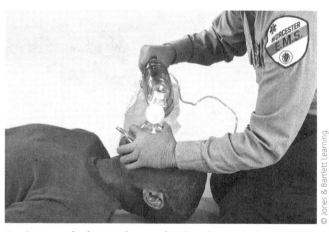

4. Squeeze the bag with your free hand. Watch for adequate _____ _____. Squeeze at the appropriate rate based on the patient's age.

CHAPTER

12

Principles of Pharmacology

General Knowledge

Matching

Match each of the items in the left column to the appropriate definition in the right column.

_____ **1.** Absorption

_____ **2.** Contraindication

_____ **3.** Adverse effect

_____ **4.** Dose

_____ **5.** Indication

_____ **6.** Action

_____ **7.** Pharmacology

_____ **8.** Capsules

_____ **9.** Topical medications

A. Lotions, creams, ointments

B. Intended therapeutic effect that a drug is supposed to have

C. The science of drugs and their ingredients, uses, and actions

D. The amount of medication given

E. Gelatin shells filled with powdered or liquid medication

F. Any action of a drug other than the desired one

G. Reasons or conditions for which a medication is given

H. The process by which medications travel through body tissues until they reach the bloodstream

I. A situation in which a drug should not be given

Multiple Choice

Read each item carefully and then select the one best response.

_____ **1.** Which of the following is taken into consideration when determining the dose of a medicine?

A. Sex

B. Occupation

C. Ability to swallow

D. Age

_____ **2.** Nitroglycerin relieves the squeezing or crushing pain associated with angina by:

A. dilating the arteries to increase the oxygen supply to the heart muscle

B. causing the heart to contract harder and increase cardiac output

C. causing the heart to beat faster to supply more oxygen to the heart

D. causing the heart to beat faster and more efficiently

_____ **3.** The brand name that a manufacturer gives to a medication is called the_____ name.

A. trade

B. generic

C. chemical

D. prescription

_____ **4.** The fastest way to deliver a chemical substance is by the _____ route.

A. intravenous

B. oral

C. sublingual

D. intramuscular

_____   **5.** Which of the following is considered a relative contraindication to administration of aspirin?

  A. Hypersensitivity to aspirin

  B. History of asthma

  C. Preexisting liver damage

  D. History of nausea

_____   **6.** The most common technique for naloxone administration is via the:

  A. oral route

  B. intramuscular route

  C. intranasal route

  D. intravenous route

_____   **7.** Outside a hospital, a(n) _____ is the preferred method of giving oxygen to patients who are experiencing significant respiratory distress.

  A. nasal cannula

  B. nonrebreathing mask

  C. bag-mask device

  D. endotracheal tube

_____   **8.** Which of the following is NOT a characteristic of epinephrine?

  A. Dilating passages in the lungs

  B. Secreted naturally by the pituitary gland

  C. Increasing the heart rate and blood pressure

  D. Dilating blood vessels

_____   **9.** What medication is commonly administered in a metered-dose inhaler (MDI)?

  A. Nitroglycerine

  B. Albuterol

  C. Activated charcoal

  D. Naloxone

_____   **10.** Nitroglycerin relieves pain because its purpose is to increase blood flow by relieving the spasms or causing the arteries to:

  A. dilate

  B. constrict

  C. thicken

  D. contract

_____   **11.** Which of the following routes of administration involves medication being absorbed in the fat tissue between the skin and muscle?

  A. Intravenous

  B. Intramuscular

  C. Subcutaneous

  D. Intranasal

Questions 12–16 are derived from the following scenario: You are called to a home of a 34-year-old male who is unresponsive. When you arrive, you find the patient supine and unconscious on the living room floor, with snoring respirations.

_____   **12.** Which of the following medications might be useful in this situation?

  A. Nitroglycerin

  B. Albuterol

  C. Naloxone

  D. Aspirin

_____ **13.** Which medication commonly comes in gel form?

  A. Naloxone

  B. Epinephrine

  C. Glucose

  D. Activated charcoal

_____ **14.** The government publication listing all drugs in the United States is called the:

  A. _United States Pharmacopoeia_

  B. _Department of Transportation Reference Guide_

  C. _US Pharmacology_

  D. _Nursing Drug Reference_

_____ **15.** Oral glucose is _____ for this patient.

  A. indicated

  B. contraindicated

  C. not normally given

  D. prescribed

_____ **16.** Which of the following statements about oxygen is FALSE?

  A. It is the most commonly administered medication in the prehospital setting.

  B. It should be administered to all patients.

  C. It is not safe to use around open flames.

  D. The nonrebreathing mask is the preferred route of administration for shock.

True/False

If you believe the statement to be more true than false, write the letter "T" in the space provided. If you believe the statement to be more false than true, write the letter "F."

_____ **1.** Oxygen is a catalyst for combustion.

_____ **2.** Oral glucose may be administered to an unconscious patient in order to save his or her life.

_____ **3.** Epinephrine is a hormone produced by the pancreas.

_____ **4.** Nitroglycerin can decrease blood pressure.

_____ **5.** Sublingual medications are rapidly absorbed into the digestive tract.

_____ **6.** Parenteral medications enter the body through the digestive tract.

_____ **7.** Enteral medications enter the body through the skin.

_____ **8.** Nitroglycerin should be administered only when the patient's systolic blood pressure is above 100 mm Hg.

Fill-in-the-Blank

Read each item carefully and then complete the statement by filling in the missing words.

1. _____ is a simple sugar that is readily absorbed by the bloodstream.

2. _____ is the main hormone that controls the body's fight-or-flight response.

3. Nitroglycerin is usually taken _____.

4. _____ _____ are the effects that are undesirable but pose little risk to the patient.

5. When given by mouth, _____ may be absorbed from the stomach fairly quickly because the medication is already dissolved.

6. A(n) _____ is a chemical substance that is used to treat or prevent disease or relieve pain.

Critical Thinking

Multiple Choice

Read each critical-thinking item carefully and then select the one best response.

_____ **1.** You and your partner are dispatched to a home on the east side of town for a possible heart attack. On arrival, you are met by a distressed wife who says her husband began having chest pain while mowing the lawn. After obtaining the patient's vital signs, you begin to take a SAMPLE history. When you ask about medications, the patient begins listing off all of the medications he has been prescribed by his doctor. Nitroglycerin may be contraindicated if the patient was currently taking which of the following medications?

    A. Albuterol

    B. Aspirin

    C. Oxygen

    D. Sildenafil

_____ **2.** Your patient is a 73-year-old man who complains of severe chest pressure with trouble breathing while having dinner at a local diner. He has a small vial of nitroglycerin in his pocket but says that he has not taken any in several days and needs you to help him to get the vial open. After administering oxygen, what is the first thing that you should do?

    A. Obtain the patient's blood pressure and ensure that his systolic pressure is not below 100 mm Hg.

    B. Begin assisting the patient's ventilations.

    C. Place him in the recovery position.

    D. Check his blood glucose level.

_____ **3.** You are called to the beach for a 15-year-old boy who is having trouble breathing. He tells you between gasps that he was stung by something and that his body feels "swollen." Just then, his mother runs up to you and puts an EpiPen into your hand. "Here," she says breathlessly. "This is his EpiPen. He needs this!" Would you administer epinephrine to this patient?

    A. Yes. Push the EpiPen firmly against the patient's thigh for several seconds.

    B. No. The EpiPen will make his condition worse.

    C. Yes. Use the sublingual route.

    D. No. His signs and symptoms contraindicate an epinephrine injection.

_____ **4.** "I think she's drunk!" a bystander yells as you and your partner arrive on the scene of an unknown medical problem. You observe an approximately 45-year-old woman stumbling between several cars in the parking lot of a grocery store. As you catch up to the woman, you ask her if she is diabetic. She nods clumsily and leans against one of the cars. You test her blood glucose and obtain a reading of 49 mg/dL. What should you do?

    A. Administer glucose gel orally.

    B. Contact medical control for further instructions.

    C. Restrain her onto the gurney and insert a nasopharyngeal airway.

    D. Wait for an ALS response so that glucose can be administered intravenously.

_____ **5.** You are dispatched to the county fair for a 54-year-old woman complaining of chest pain. You arrive to find her pressing on the center of her chest and note that she has pale, clammy skin. You ask if she has any cardiac history, and she tells you, "No, I just have arthritis, and my doctor says that I am prediabetic." Her vital signs are: pulse 112 beats/minute, respiratory rate 18 breaths/minute, blood pressure 94/62 mm Hg, and oxygen saturation 99% on room air. Would you give this patient aspirin?

    A. No. Nitroglycerin would be more appropriate.

    B. Yes. Her signs and symptoms indicate a cardiac problem, and aspirin could help.

    C. No. Aspirin is contraindicated for arthritis.

    D. Yes. Its analgesic properties may help with the discomfort.

Short Answer

Complete this section with short written answers using the space provided.

1. List seven routes of medication administration.

   _____

   _____

   _____

2. What are the "nine rights" of medication administration?

   _____

   _____

   _____

3. List three characteristics of epinephrine.

   _____

   _____

4. What are the steps for administering intranasal naloxone?

   _____

   _____

   _____

5. List four effects of nitroglycerin.

   _____

   _____

   _____

6. Explain why metered-dose inhalers are often used with a spacer.

   _____

   _____

   _____

Ambulance Calls

The following case scenarios provide an opportunity to explore the concerns associated with patient management and to enhance critical-thinking skills. Read each scenario and answer each question to the best of your ability.

1. You are dispatched to "difficulty breathing" at one of your town's many parks. As you near the park entrance, you see a crowd of people who frantically wave for you. You arrive to find a city employee who was apparently mowing the park grounds when he accidentally mowed over a yellow jacket nest. He was wearing coveralls, but he was repeatedly stung around his neck and face. He appears to be somewhat confused; you can hear stridor with each inspiration, and his blood pressure is 80/40 mm Hg. Your local protocols allow EMTs to carry EpiPens.

   How do you best manage this patient?

   _____

   _____

   _____

2. You are dispatched to an "unknown medical problem" at the Crosstown Mall. You were called after police were summoned to subdue a combative male shopper. Police officers were able to calm him down but felt that something was "not right" about him. You arrive to find a calm but confused man who is sweaty and pale. He has no complaints but keeps repeating, "I have to get home now." You notice a medical ID bracelet indicating that this patient is an insulin-dependent diabetic.

   How do you best manage this patient?

   _____

   _____

   _____

3. You are dispatched to the residence of a 68-year-old man who is complaining of "crushing" chest pain radiating down his left arm and trouble breathing for the past hour. He is pale, cool, diaphoretic, and is very nauseated. He tells you he had a heart attack several years ago and takes nitroglycerin as needed. He took two tablets prior to your arrival and reports no relief.

   How would you best manage this patient?

   _____

   _____

   _____

Fill-in-the-Patient Care Report

Read the incident scenario and then complete the following patient care report (PCR).

"Hey, you! Medic!" It's 1300, and you are just finishing lunch at one of the picnic tables in Northern Park when you hear someone yelling from across the small duck pond. "This lady needs help!"

You whistle at your partner, who is sitting in the ambulance reading a biology textbook, and then begin the short walk to where a small crowd is gathering near an ivy-covered gazebo.

"I think she's having trouble breathing," a man says, moving aside so you can see a 38-year-old woman sitting in the tripod position on a wooden park bench. Her eyes are bulging, her lips and fingernails are beginning to turn blue, and you can immediately see accessory muscles moving in her neck as she struggles to breathe. You kneel in front of the bench, making eye contact with the panicked woman, and say, "I'm an EMT, and I'm going to help you, okay?" She nods her head frantically.

"Does anyone know her?" you shout, looking at the confused faces around you. A teenaged girl appears and says, "I don't know her, but she dropped this when she first started to freak out." The girl then hands you a blue plastic metered-dose inhaler labeled for asthma.

Approximately 4 minutes since first being alerted to the problem, you quickly shake the metered-dose inhaler and hand it to the woman, who claws for it and pumps it once into her mouth and inhales weakly. Right then, your partner arrives with the gurney and the equipment bags from the ambulance, and you instruct him to initiate oxygen therapy immediately with a nonrebreathing mask.

As you are helping the 45-kg (100-lb) woman onto the gurney, you notice that her lips and fingernails are returning to normal and that although she is still struggling to breathe, she is moving more air with each respiratory cycle. The high-concentration oxygen, set at 15 L/min, seems to be helping. Four minutes after the patient first used her inhaler, you and your partner load her into the ambulance for the 10-minute drive to the closest emergency department.

You obtain the patient's vital signs as soon as the ambulance rolls away from the scene, noting a blood pressure of 142/98 mm Hg, a heart rate of 110 beats/min, 28 labored respirations per minute, and a pulse oximetry reading of 88%. You are able to complete two more sets of vitals at 5-minute intervals prior to pulling into the hospital ambulance bay (138/90 mm Hg, 102 beats/min, 24 breaths/min labored, 92%; and 132/88 mm Hg, 96 beats/min, 20 breaths/min with good tidal volume, 96%), and between one more puff from the inhaler and the high-flow oxygen, the patient has improved tremendously.

You and your partner transfer the patient to an emergency department bed, provide the charge nurse with a full report, and are ready to go back into service 40 minutes from first being alerted to the emergency.

Fill-in-the-Patient Care Report

EMS Patient Care Report (PCR)			
Date:	Incident No.:	Nature of Call:	Location:
Dispatched:	En Route:	At Scene:	Transport:	At Hospital:	In Service:

Patient Information	
Age: Sex: Weight (in kg [lb]):	Allergies: Medications: Past Medical History: Chief Complaint:

Vital Signs				
Time:	BP:	Pulse:	Respirations:	SpO$_2$:
Time:	BP:	Pulse:	Respirations:	SpO$_2$:
Time:	BP:	Pulse:	Respirations:	SpO$_2$:

EMS Treatment (circle all that apply)				
Oxygen @ ___ L/min via (circle one): NC NRM BVM	Assisted Ventilation	Airway Adjunct	CPR
Defibrillation	Bleeding Control	Bandaging	Splinting	Other:

Narrative

Shock

General Knowledge

Matching

Match each of the items in the left column to the appropriate definition in the right column.

_____ **1.** Shock

_____ **2.** Perfusion

_____ **3.** Sphincters

_____ **4.** Autonomic nervous system

_____ **5.** Blood pressure

_____ **6.** Anaphylactic shock

_____ **7.** Septic shock

_____ **8.** Syncope

_____ **9.** Compensated shock

A. Widespread vascular dilation after exposure to an allergen

B. Inadequate cellular perfusion

C. Regulates involuntary body functions

D. Early stage of shock where blood pressure can still be maintained

E. The pressure of blood within the vessels at a given moment in time

F. Widespread vascular dilation in response to severe infection

G. Adequate circulation of blood to the tissues

H. Regulate blood flow in capillaries

I. Fainting or loss of consciousness

Multiple Choice

Read each item carefully and then select the one best response.

_____ **1.** What is the basic definition of shock?

    A. A state of inadequate cellular perfusion

    B. The loss of blood from the body

    C. An inadequate supply of oxygen in the lungs

    D. A state of low blood pressure

_____ **2.** Blood flow through the capillary beds is regulated by:

    A. systolic pressure

    B. the capillary sphincters

    C. perfusion

    D. diastolic pressure

_____ **3.** The autonomic nervous system regulates functions such as:

    A. running

    B. digestion

    C. eye movement

    D. walking

_____ **4.** Regulation of blood flow is determined by:

    A. oxygen intake

    B. systolic pressure

    C. cellular need

    D. diastolic pressure

_____ **5.** Patients in cardiogenic shock should NOT receive:

    A. oxygen

    B. positive pressure ventilation

    C. ALS care

    D. nitroglycerine

_____ **6.** Which of the following is a cause of obstructive shock?

    A. Hemorrhage

    B. Infection

    C. Myocardial infarction

    D. Tension pneumothorax

_____ **7.** Which of the following is NOT a basic cause of shock?

    A. Poor pump function

    B. Blood or fluid loss

    C. Blood vessel dilation

    D. Release of norepinephrine

_____ **8.** Which of the following molecules is the primary carrier of oxygen in the bloodstream?

    A. Albumin

    B. Iron

    C. Hemoglobin

    D. Thyroglobulin

_____ **9.** _____ develops when the heart muscle can no longer generate enough pressure to circulate the blood to all organs.

    A. Pump failure

    B. Cardiogenic shock

    C. A myocardial infarction

    D. Congestive heart failure

_____ **10.** Neurogenic shock usually results from damage to the spinal cord at the:

    A. cervical level

    B. thoracic level

    C. lumbar level

    D. sacral level

_____ **11.** Which of the following statements about septic shock is FALSE?

    A. There is an insufficient volume of fluid in the container.

    B. The fluid that has leaked out often collects in the respiratory system.

    C. There is a larger-than-normal vascular bed to contain the smaller-than-normal volume of intravascular fluid.

    D. There is damage to the spinal cord, resulting in vasodilation.

_____ **12.** Neurogenic shock causes hypoperfusion due to:

    A. widespread dilation of the vascular system

    B. massive vasoconstriction

    C. low circulating blood volume

    D. obstruction of blood flow from the heart

_____ **13.** Hypovolemic shock is a result of:

    A. widespread vasodilation

    B. low circulating blood volume

    C. massive vasoconstriction

    D. pump failure

_____ **14.** _____ is often the last vital sign to change in decompensated shock.

    A. Blood pressure

    B. Heart rate

    C. Respiratory rate

    D. Oxygen saturation

_____ **15.** Which of the following statements about anaphylactic shock is TRUE?

    A. There is no blood loss in anaphylactic shock.

    B. It is caused by a lack of red blood cells.

    C. It is associated with bronchodilation.

    D. It can result from myocardial pump failure.

_____ **16.** In which of the following scenarios would you LEAST suspect shock?

    A. a mild allergic reaction

    B. multiple severe fractures

    C. a severe infection

    D. abdominal or chest injury

_____ **17.** When treating a suspected unstable shock patient, vital signs should be recorded approximately every _____ minutes.

    A. 2

    B. 5

    C. 10

    D. 15

_____ **18.** Which of the following is NOT a sign of cardiogenic shock?

    A. Cyanosis

    B. Strong, bounding pulse

    C. Nausea

    D. Anxiety

_____ **19.** _____ is a sudden reaction of the nervous system that produces temporary vascular dilation and fainting.

    A. Neurogenic shock

    B. Psychogenic shock

    C. Vascular shock

    D. Cardiogenic shock

True/False

If you believe the statement to be more true than false, write the letter "T" in the space provided. If you believe the statement to be more false than true, write the letter "F."

_____ **1.** Life-threatening allergic reactions can occur even when a patient has previously tolerated a substance without having an allergic reaction.

_____ **2.** Bleeding is a common cause of cardiogenic shock.

_____ **3.** Shock occurs when oxygen and nutrients cannot get to the body's cells.

_____ **4.** A person in shock, left untreated, will survive.

_____ **5.** Compensated shock will present with falling blood pressure.

_____ **6.** An injection of epinephrine is the most effective treatment for anaphylactic shock.

_____ **7.** Septic shock occurs as a result of a severe infection.

_____ **8.** Metabolism is the cardiovascular system's circulation of blood and oxygen to all cells in different tissues and organs of the body.

_____ **9.** Shock occurs only with massive blood loss from the body.

_____ **10.** Decompensated shock is a late phase of shock and indicates progression of shock is irreversible.

Fill-in-the-Blank

Read each item carefully and then complete the statement by filling in the missing words.

1. _____ refers to inadequate cellular perfusion.

2. Pressure in the arteries during cardiac _____ is known as systolic pressure.

3. The body responds to shock by directing blood flow away from organs that are more _____ of low flow.

4. Pulse pressure represents the force generated with each _____ of the heart.

5. Blood contains red blood cells, white blood cells, _____, and a liquid called _____.

6. Inadequate circulation that does not meet the body's needs is known as _____.

7. _____ are circular muscle walls in capillaries, causing the walls to _____ and_____.

8. _____ pressure occurs during cardiac relaxation, while _____ pressure occurs during cardiac contractions.

9. As a result of the aging process, older patients generally have more serious _____ than younger patients.

10. The autonomic nervous system controls the _____ actions of the body.

Critical Thinking

Multiple Choice

Read each critical-thinking item carefully and then select the one best response.

_____ 1. You are called to the residence of a 67-year-old man who is complaining of chest pain. He is alert and oriented. During your assessment, the patient tells you he has had two previous heart attacks. He is taking medication for fluid retention. As you listen to his lungs, you notice that he has fluid in his lungs. This is known as pulmonary:
   A. edema
   B. overload
   C. cessation
   D. failure

_____ 2. You are called to a construction site where a 27-year-old worker has fallen from the second floor. He landed on his back and is drifting in and out of consciousness. A quick assessment reveals no bleeding or blood loss. His blood pressure is 90/60 mm Hg with a pulse rate of 110 beats/min. His airway is open, and his breathing is within normal limits. You realize the patient is in shock. Based on this information, the patient's shock is most likely due to an injury to the:
   A. thoracic vertebrae
   B. skull
   C. spinal cord
   D. peripheral nerves

_____ **3.** You respond to the local nursing home for an 85-year-old woman who has altered mental status. During your assessment, you notice that the patient has a fever. She is hypotensive, and her pulse is tachycardic. The nursing staff tells you that she has been sick for several days and that they called because her mental status continued to decline. You suspect the patient is in septic shock. This type of shock is due to:

    A. pump failure

    B. massive vasoconstriction

    C. Release of bacterial toxins

    D. increased volume

_____ **4.** You are called to a motor vehicle collision. Your patient is a 19-year-old woman who was not wearing her seat belt. She is conscious but confused. Her airway is open, and respirations are within normal limits. Her pulse is slightly tachycardic. Her blood pressure is within normal limits. She is complaining of being thirsty and appears very anxious. What is the last measurable factor to change that would indicate shock?

    A. Mental status

    B. Blood pressure

    C. Pulse rate

    D. Respirations

_____ **5.** You respond to a 17-year-old football player who was hit by numerous opponents. While walking off the field, he became unconscious. You take cervical spine control and start your assessment. You know that in the treatment of shock, you must do all of the following EXCEPT:

    A. secure and maintain an airway

    B. provide respiratory support

    C. assist ventilations

    D. use hot water bottles or heating pads to keep the patient warm

Short Answer

Complete this section with short written answers using the space provided.

1. List the causes, signs and symptoms, and treatment of anaphylactic shock.

_____

_____

_____

2. List the causes, signs and symptoms, and treatment of cardiogenic shock.

_____

_____

_____

3. List the causes, signs and symptoms, and treatment of hypovolemic shock.

_____

_____

_____

4. List the causes, signs and symptoms, and treatment of neurogenic shock.

_____

_____

_____

5. List the causes, signs and symptoms, and treatment of psychogenic shock.

_____

_____

_____

6. List the causes, signs and symptoms, and treatment of septic shock.

_____

_____

_____

7. List the three basic physiologic causes of shock.

_____

_____

_____

8. List the signs and symptoms of decompensated shock.

_____

_____

_____

Ambulance Calls

The following case scenarios provide an opportunity to explore the concerns associated with patient management and to enhance critical-thinking skills. Read each scenario and answer each question to the best of your ability.

1. You are dispatched to the victim of a fall at the local community college theater. One of the students involved in rigging the theater backgrounds fell from the platform above the stage. He landed directly on his back and is now complaining of numbness and tingling in his lower body.

How would you best manage this patient?

_____

_____

_____

2. You are dispatched to a local long-term care facility for an older man with a fever. You arrive to find an 80-year-old man who is responsive to painful stimuli and has the following vital signs: blood pressure of 80/40 mm Hg, weak radial pulse of 140 beats/min and irregular, respirations of 60 breaths/min and shallow, and pulse oximetry of 80% on 4 L/min nasal cannula. His temperature is 101.8°F (38.8°C).

How would you best manage this patient?

_____

_____

_____

3. You are dispatched to a residence where a 16-year-old girl was stung by a bee. Her mother tells you she is severely allergic to bees. She is voice responsive, covered in hives, and wheezing audibly. She has a very weak radial pulse and is blue around the lips.

How would you best manage this patient?

_____

_____

_____

Fill-in-the-Patient Care Report

Read the incident scenario and then complete the following patient care report (PCR).

You look at the glowing face of your watch in the darkness of the ambulance cab and realize that you have 4 hours until the end of your shift at 0200. At that moment, the dispatcher's voice bursts from the radio with a call for a motorcyclist down in the eastbound lanes of Highway 62 at exit 19, a 5-minute drive from your current location. Your partner copies the dispatch as you activate the lights and siren and pull out of the parking lot, en route to the scene.

As you pull past the highway patrol's vehicle barricade, you see pieces of metal and plastic scattered down the freeway and a man lying motionless across both closed lanes. You and your partner approach to find the man responsive and coherent but complaining of "feeling odd" and not being able to move his legs. Along with the help of a responding fire crew, you and your partner are able to quickly remove the patient's helmet, apply a cervical collar, and immobilize the approximately 143-pound (65-kg) 18-year-old man to a long backboard after initiating oxygen therapy.

"Eight-minute scene time!" your partner whistles, shutting you into the back of the ambulance with the immobilized patient. As your partner pulls away from the accident scene en route to the local trauma center, minutes away, you obtain a set of vital signs (blood pressure 98/62 mm Hg; pulse 110 beats/min and weak; respirations 18 breaths/min, shallow but adequate; a pulse oximetry reading of 94% on high-flow oxygen via a nonrebreathing mask; and pale, cool, moist skin). You cut away the patient's clothing to look for concealed injuries and find that both of his legs are pale, cooler than his torso, and not diaphoretic.

"I'm really feeling weird," the man says, panic evident in his eyes. "Am I dying?"

"We're doing everything we can to make sure that doesn't happen," you say, before asking your partner to upgrade to lights and siren while you cover the patient with blankets. Exactly 5 minutes after leaving the scene, you unload the patient and push him through the automatic doors of the university hospital, where he is quickly enveloped by the trauma team.

Approximately 15 minutes later, you and your partner pull out of the ambulance bay and advise dispatch that you are back and available for another call.

Fill-in-the-Patient Care Report

EMS Patient Care Report (PCR)					
Date:	Incident No.:		Nature of Call:		Location:
Dispatched:	En Route:	At Scene:	Transport:	At Hospital:	In Service:
Patient Information					
Age: Sex: Weight (in kg [lb]):			Allergies: Medications: Past Medical History: Chief Complaint:		
Vital Signs					
Time:	BP:		Pulse:	Respirations:	SpO$_2$:
Time:	BP:		Pulse:	Respirations:	SpO$_2$:
Time:	BP:		Pulse:	Respirations:	SpO$_2$:
EMS Treatment (circle all that apply)					
Oxygen @ ____ L/min via (circle one): NC NRM BVM		Assisted Ventilation	Airway Adjunct		CPR
Defibrillation	Bleeding Control	Bandaging	Splinting		Other:
Narrative					

Assessment Review

Answer the following questions pertaining to the assessment of the types of emergencies discussed in this chapter.

_____ 1. In the scene size-up for a patient(s) who you think may be susceptible to shock, your initial step is to:
  A. ensure scene safety
  B. splint all potential fractures first
  C. ask the patient if he or she has an EpiPen
  D. immediately obtain a patient history

_____ 2. During the primary assessment of a patient in shock, you should:
  A. treat any immediate life threats
  B. obtain a SAMPLE history
  C. get a complete set of vital signs
  D. inform medical control of the situation

_____ 3. You have completed your primary assessment of an embarrassed patient who fainted after seeing a coworker injure himself. Your next step should be:
  A. a rapid secondary assessment
  B. to obtain a medical history
  C. a detailed physical examination
  D. a reassessment

_____ 4. Interventions for the treatment of shock should include:
  A. giving the patient something to drink
  B. maintaining normal body temperature
  C. withholding high-flow oxygen
  D. delaying transport to splint fractures

_____ 5. You are transporting an unstable patient who you feel is going into shock. How often do you recheck his vital signs?
  A. Every 3 minutes
  B. Every 10 minutes
  C. Every 5 minutes
  D. Every 15 minutes

CHAPTER

14 BLS Resuscitation

General Knowledge

Matching

Match each of the items in the left column to the appropriate definition in the right column.

_____	**1.** Mechanical piston device	**A.** The steps used to reestablish artificial ventilation and circulation in a patient who is not breathing and has no pulse
_____	**2.** Abdominal-thrust maneuver	**B.** Opening the airway without causing manipulation to the cervical spine
_____	**3.** Basic life support (BLS)	**C.** Noninvasive emergency lifesaving care used to treat airway obstructions, respiratory arrest, and cardiac arrest
_____	**4.** Advanced life support (ALS)	**D.** Procedures such as cardiac monitoring, intravenous (IV) medications, and advanced airway adjuncts
_____	**5.** Cardiopulmonary resuscitation (CPR)	**E.** The method of dislodging food or other material from the throat of a conscious choking victim
_____	**6.** Gastric distention	**F.** The stomach becoming filled with air
_____	**7.** Impedance threshold device	**G.** Depresses the sternum via a plunger mounted on a backboard
_____	**8.** Head tilt–chin lift maneuver	**H.** Used to maintain an open airway in an adequately breathing patient with a decreased level of consciousness
_____	**9.** Jaw-thrust maneuver	**I.** Opening the airway in a patient who has not sustained trauma to the cervical spine
_____	**10.** Recovery position	**J.** A valve device that helps to draw more blood back to the heart during chest compressions

Multiple Choice

Read each item carefully and then select the one best response.

_____ **1.** After _____ without oxygen, brain damage is very likely.
  A. 1 minute
  B. 3 minutes
  C. 4 minutes
  D. 6 minutes

_____ **2.** All of the following are considered advanced lifesaving procedures EXCEPT:
  A. cardiac monitoring
  B. bag-mask ventilation
  C. administration of IV fluids and medications
  D. use of advanced airway adjuncts

_____ **3.** In a conscious infant who is choking, you would first give five back slaps, followed by:
  A. attempting to breathe
  B. five chest thrusts
  C. checking the pulse
  D. five abdominal thrusts

_____ **4.** In addition to checking level of consciousness, it is also important to protect the _____ from further injury while assessing the patient and performing CPR.

    A. neck

    B. ribs

    C. internal organs

    D. facial structures

_____ **5.** In most cases, cardiac arrest in infants and children results from:

    A. toxic ingestion

    B. anaphylaxis

    C. congenital heart disease

    D. respiratory arrest

_____ **6.** Common causes of respiratory arrest in infants and children include:

    A. foreign body obstruction

    B. vomiting

    C. poor feeding

    D. chronic obstructive pulmonary disease (COPD)

_____ **7.** Resuscitation would NOT be initiated if which of the following obvious signs of death were present:

    A. bleeding

    B. dependent edema

    C. decapitation

    D. pale skin

_____ **8.** Once you begin CPR in the field, you must continue until:

    A. the fire department arrives

    B. the funeral home arrives

    C. a person of equal or higher training relieves you

    D. law enforcement arrives and assumes responsibility

_____ **9.** If you encounter a pregnant patient in cardiac arrest, your priorities are to provide high-quality CPR and:

    A. relieve pressure off the aorta and vena cava

    B. rapid transport for emergency caesarian section

    C. intermittent abdominal thrusts

    D. increase pressure on the aorta and vena cava

_____ **10.** To perform a _____, place your fingers behind the angles of the patient's lower jaw and then move the jaw forward.

    A. head tilt–chin lift maneuver

    B. jaw-thrust maneuver

    C. tongue–jaw lift maneuver

    D. head–jaw tilt maneuver

_____ **11.** Providing fast, aggressive ventilations could result in:

    A. excessive bleeding

    B. rupture of the bronchial tree

    C. gastric distention

    D. damage to the oral pharynx

_____ **12.** A(n) _____ is an opening that connects the trachea directly to the skin.

    A. ileostomy

    B. stoma

    C. laryngectomy

    D. colostomy

_____ 13. _____ position helps to maintain a clear airway in a patient with a decreased level of consciousness who has not had traumatic injuries and is breathing on his or her own.

   A. The recovery
   B. The lithotomy
   C. Trendelenburg's
   D. Fowler's

_____ 14. In the adult, cardiac arrest is determined by the absence of the pulse at the _____ artery.

   A. femoral
   B. radial
   C. ulnar
   D. carotid

_____ 15. In the adult, the proper hand placement for chest compressions is accomplished by placing the heel of one hand:

   A. on the lower half of the sternum
   B. near the clavicles
   C. over the xiphoid process
   D. between the nipples

_____ 16. Which of the following is NOT a common complication from performing chest compressions?

   A. Fractured ribs
   B. Lacerated liver
   C. Fractured sternum
   D. Lacerated pancreas

_____ 17. When checking for a pulse in an infant, you should palpate the _____ artery.

   A. radial
   B. brachial
   C. carotid
   D. femoral

_____ 18. The rate of compressions for an infant is _____ compressions per minute.

   A. 70 to 80
   B. 80 to 100
   C. 100 to 120
   D. 120 to 150

_____ 19. The ratio of compression to ventilation for infants and children is _____ when performing two-rescuer CPR.

   A. 1:5
   B. 5:1
   C. 15:2
   D. 2:15

_____ 20. Sudden airway obstruction is usually easy to recognize in someone who is eating or has just finished eating because they suddenly:

   A. are able to speak clearly
   B. turn pink
   C. make exaggerated efforts to breathe
   D. start screaming

_____ 21. You should suspect an airway obstruction in the unresponsive patient if:

   A. the patient is breathing
   B. you do not produce visible chest rise with ventilations
   C. there is no pulse
   D. you have adequate chest rise with each ventilation

_____ **22.** You should use _____ for women in advanced stages of pregnancy who are conscious and suffering from a foreign body airway obstruction.

    A. the blind finger sweep

    B. back slaps

    C. the abdominal-thrust maneuver

    D. chest thrusts

_____ **23.** For a patient with a mild airway obstruction, you should:

    A. begin chest compressions

    B. attempt a finger sweep to remove the foreign body

    C. not interfere with the patient's attempt to expel the foreign body

    D. immediately perform abdominal thrusts

True/False

If you believe the statement to be more true than false, write the letter "T" in the space provided. If you believe the statement to be more false than true, write the letter "F."

_____ **1.** During the primary assessment, you need to quickly evaluate the patient's airway, breathing, circulation, and level of consciousness.

_____ **2.** All unconscious patients need all elements of BLS.

_____ **3.** A person who is unresponsive may or may not need CPR.

_____ **4.** The recovery position should be used to maintain an open airway in a patient with a head or spinal injury.

_____ **5.** You should use a bag-mask device when providing artificial ventilations in the prehospital environment.

_____ **6.** You should not start CPR if the patient has obvious signs of irreversible death.

_____ **7.** When performing CPR, you must allow the chest to fully recoil between each compression.

_____ **8.** The ratio of compressions to ventilations for one-person CPR on an adult is 2:1.

_____ **9.** Short, jabbing compressions are more effective than rhythmic compressions.

_____ **10.** A mask with a one-way valve or other barrier device can be used to provide rescue breathing to a child or infant with a stoma if a bag-mask device is unavailable.

_____ **11.** Families typically expect EMS providers to stop resuscitation and leave their loved one on scene.

_____ **12.** When an AED with adult pads is used on an infant, it may be necessary to use anterior-posterior pad placement based on the manufacturer's recommendations.

_____ **13.** In the adult, the sternum should be depressed 2 to 2.4 inches (5 to 6 cm) during chest compressions.

_____ **14.** In adults, the compression-to-breath ratio is always 30:2 in two-rescuer CPR.

_____ **15.** A Physician Orders for Life-Sustaining Treatment (POLST) must be signed by an authorized medical provider to be valid.

Fill-in-the-Blank

Read each item carefully and then complete the statement by filling in the missing words.

1. Permanent brain damage is possible if the brain is without oxygen for _____ to _____ minutes.

2. If the patient's chest is _____, then the electrical current may move across the _____ rather than between the pads to the patient's heart.

3. Because of the urgent need to start CPR in a pulseless, nonbreathing patient, you must complete a primary assessment as soon as possible and begin CPR with _____ _____.

4. If you encounter a patient who has a hard lump beneath the skin in the chest near the heart, you should assume the patient has a(n) _____.

5. _____ _____, such as living wills, may express the patient's wishes, but these documents are not binding for all health care providers.

6. For CPR to be effective, the patient must be lying supine on a(n) _____, _____ surface.

7. Without an open _____, rescue breathing will not be effective.

8. The _____ _____ _____ should be applied to an adult cardiac arrest patient as soon as it is available.

9. Assess for a pulse in an adult patient by palpating the _____ artery.

10. A(n) _____ _____ _____ is a device that depresses the sternum via a compressed gas-powered or electric-powered plunger mounted on a backboard.

Critical Thinking

Short Answer

Complete this section with short written answers using the space provided.

1. List the four obvious signs of death, in addition to absence of pulse and breathing, that are used as a general rule against starting CPR.

_____

_____

_____

2. List the six components of the American Heart Association's chain of survival.

_____

_____

_____

3. List five respiratory problems leading to cardiac arrest in children.

_____

_____

_____

4. Describe how to perform the head tilt–chin lift maneuver.

_____

_____

_____

5. Describe how to perform the jaw-thrust maneuver.

_____

_____

_____

6. Describe the process of chest compressions during one-rescuer adult CPR.

_____

_____

_____

7. List and describe the method for "switching positions" during two-rescuer adult CPR.

_____

_____

_____

8. Describe the process of abdominal thrusts for a standing patient with a foreign body airway obstruction.

_____

_____

_____

9. Describe the process for chest thrusts on a standing and a supine patient.

_____

_____

_____

10. Describe the process for removing a foreign body airway obstruction in a responsive infant.

_____

_____

_____

Ambulance Calls

The following case scenarios provide an opportunity to explore the concerns associated with patient management and to enhance critical-thinking skills. Read each scenario and answer each question to the best of your ability.

1. You are dispatched to a "person down." The dispatcher informs you that the caller said the patient is not breathing. On arrival, you find a 78-year-old woman in bed, apneic, and pulseless. In the process of moving the patient to place a CPR board underneath her, you note the discoloration of her back and hips known as extreme dependent lividity.

   How would you best manage this patient?

   _____

   _____

   _____

2. You are off-duty when you hear a dispatch for "chest pain" at a private residence near you. You arrive to find the patient's family members attempting to apply an AED they bought over the Internet. The patient currently has a pulse and is breathing.

   How would you best manage this situation?

   _____

   _____

   _____

3. You are dispatched to an "unconscious man" at a private residence. You arrive to find the man lying in the grass in the backyard. There is a ladder and equipment on the rooftop. It appears he was working on the roof of his two-story home. No one witnessed the event. The man is breathing and has a pulse.

   How would you best manage this patient?

   _____

   _____

   _____

Skills

Skill Drills

Skill Drill 14-1: Performing Chest Compressions

Test your knowledge of this skill by filling in the correct words in the photo captions.

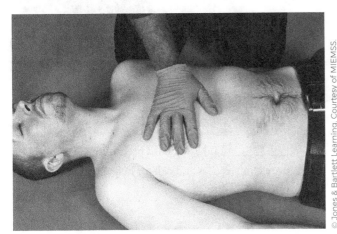

1. Take standard precautions. Place the _____ of one hand on the _____ of the chest.

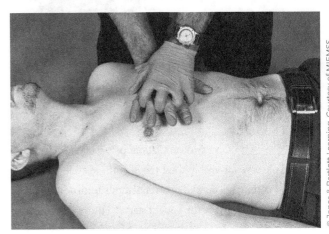

2. Place the _____ of your other _____ over the first hand.

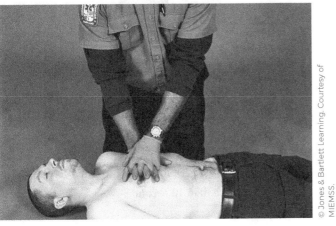

3. With your arms straight, lock your _____, and position your shoulders directly over your _____. Depress the sternum at a rate of _____ to _____ compressions per minute, and to a depth of _____ to _____ using a direct downward movement. Allow the chest to return to its normal position; do not lean on the chest between compressions. _____ and relaxation should be of equal duration.

Skill Drill 14-2: Performing One-Rescuer Adult CPR

Test your knowledge of this skill by placing the following photos in the correct order. Number the first step with a "1," the second step with a "2," etc.

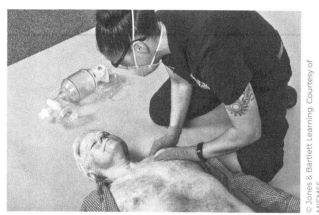

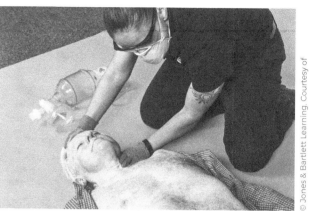

1. _____ Give two ventilations of 1 second each and observe for visible chest rise. Continue cycles of 30 chest compressions and two ventilations until additional personnel arrive or the patient starts to move.

2. _____ Take standard precautions. Establish unresponsiveness and call for help. Use your cell phone if needed.

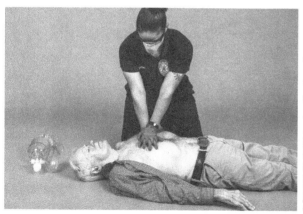

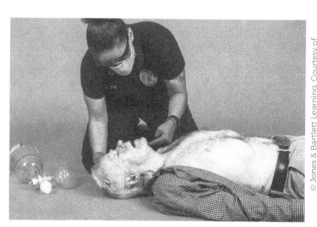

3. _____ Open the airway according to your suspicion of spinal injury.

4. _____ Check for breathing and a carotid pulse for no more than 10 seconds.

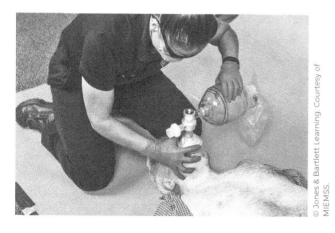

5. _____ If breathing and pulse are absent, begin CPR until an AED is available. Give 30 chest compressions at a rate of 100 to 120 per minute.

Skill Drill 14-3: Performing Two-Rescuer Adult CPR

Test your knowledge of this skill by filling in the correct words in the photo captions.

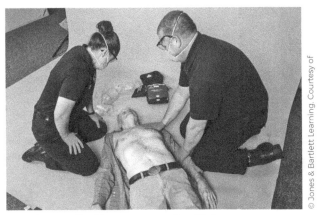

1. Take standard _____. Establish _____ and take positions.

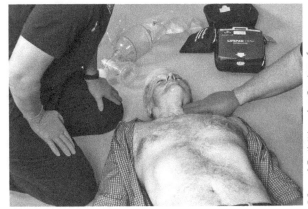

2. Check for breathing and a(n) _____ pulse.

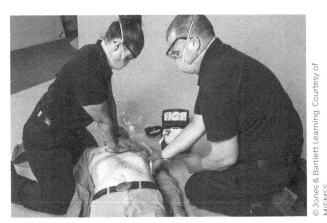

3. Begin CPR, starting with _____ _____. Give 30 chest compressions at a rate of _____ to _____ per minute. If the AED is available, then apply it and follow the voice prompts.

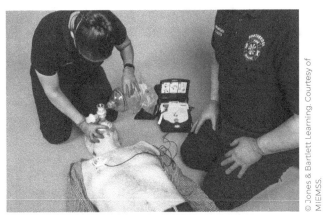

4. _____ the airway according to your suspicion of spinal injury.

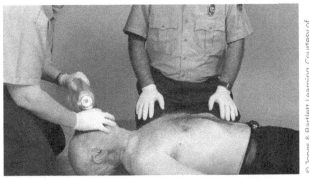

5. Give _____ _____ of 1 second each and observe for _____ _____ _____. Continue cycles of 30 chest compressions and two ventilations (switch roles every five cycles [2 minutes]) until ALS providers take over or the patient starts to move. Reanalyze the patient's cardiac rhythm with the AED every 2 minutes and deliver a shock if indicated.

Medical Overview

General Knowledge

Matching

Match each of the items in the left column to the related term in the right column.

_____	**1.** Asthma	**A.** Respiratory
_____	**2.** Hemophilia	**B.** Cardiovascular
_____	**3.** Congestive heart failure	**C.** Neurologic
_____	**4.** Substance abuse	**D.** Gastrointestinal
_____	**5.** Chronic bronchitis	**E.** Urologic
_____	**6.** Diabetes mellitus	**F.** Endocrine
_____	**7.** Pelvic inflammatory disease	**G.** Hematologic
_____	**8.** Syncope	**H.** Immunologic
_____	**9.** Depression	**I.** Toxicologic
_____	**10.** Kidney stones	**J.** Psychiatric
_____	**11.** Emphysema	**K.** Gynecologic
_____	**12.** Appendicitis	
_____	**13.** Anaphylactic reaction	
_____	**14.** Heart attack	
_____	**15.** Sickle cell disease	
_____	**16.** Pancreatitis	
_____	**17.** Vaginal bleeding	
_____	**18.** Diverticulitis	
_____	**19.** Plant poisoning	
_____	**20.** Seizure	

Multiple Choice

Read each item carefully and then select the one best response.

_____ **1.** The most important aspect of the scene size-up is:

  A. determining the number of patients

  B. calling for additional resources

  C. ensuring scene safety

  D. determining the nature of the illness

_____ **2.** The _____ is your awareness of and concern for potentially serious underlying and unseen injuries or illnesses.

  A. nature of illness

  B. index of suspicion

  C. general impression

  D. clinical impression

_____ 3. If your patient is alone and unresponsive, in order to obtain some form of medical history, you should:
   A. ask people in the neighborhood
   B. go through the patient's wallet
   C. survey the scene for medication containers or medical devices
   D. search through the patient's bedroom drawers for hidden illegal drugs

_____ 4. "Has this ever happened before?" helps to determine the:
   A. chief complaint
   B. history of present illness
   C. medications
   D. provocation of pain

_____ 5. You should assess pulse, motor, and sensation in all of the extremities and check for pupillary reactions if you suspect a(n) _____ problem.
   A. cardiovascular
   B. endocrine
   C. neurologic
   D. psychological

_____ 6. When palpating the chest and abdomen, you are attempting to identify areas of:
   A. bruising
   B. tenderness
   C. crepitus
   D. nausea

_____ 7. Patients with altered mental status should be considered _____ when determining transport options.
   A. nonemergency
   B. low priority
   C. moderate priority
   D. high priority

_____ 8. A patient suffering from a heart attack should be transported to:
   A. a local clinic, 5 minutes away
   B. a community hospital with no catheterization lab, 10 minutes away
   C. a university hospital with a catheterization lab, 15 minutes away
   D. a trauma center, 20 minutes away

_____ 9. Which statement regarding HIV is FALSE?
   A. It is not easily transmitted in your work environment.
   B. It is not considered a hazard when deposited on mucous membranes.
   C. You should always wear gloves when treating a patient with HIV.
   D. Many patients with HIV do not show symptoms.

_____ 10. If you have been exposed to an HIV-positive patient's blood, you should:
   A. not worry about it because transmission rates are low
   B. immediately notify your infectious disease officer
   C. wait until your next doctor visit to seek evaluation
   D. wash the area thoroughly and get an updated tetanus shot

_____ 11. The incubation period for the Ebola virus is approximately:
   A. 1 to 3 days after exposure
   B. 2 to 6 days after exposure
   C. 6 to 12 days after exposure
   D. 2 to 4 weeks after exposure

_____ **12.** The incubation period for hepatitis B is typically:
  A. 1 to 2 weeks
  B. 5 to 10 weeks
  C. 4 to 12 weeks
  D. 1 to 10 weeks

_____ **13.** Vaccinations are NOT available for which form of hepatitis?
  A. Hepatitis A
  B. Hepatitis B
  C. Hepatitis C
  D. All forms of hepatitis

_____ **14.** Which of the following statements about tuberculosis is FALSE?
  A. It is found in open, uncrowded living spaces.
  B. It can be found in crowded environments with poor ventilation.
  C. It is spread through the air via droplets.
  D. The primary infection is typically not serious.

_____ **15.** _____ is a bacterium that causes infections and is resistant to many antibiotics.
  A. Meningitis
  B. Tuberculosis
  C. Hepatitis C
  D. MRSA

_____ **16.** A(n) _____ is an outbreak that occurs on a global scale.
  A. epidemic
  B. pandemic
  C. endemic
  D. transdemic

True/False

If you believe the statement to be more true than false, write the letter "T" in the space provided. If you believe the statement to be more false than true, write the letter "F."

_____ **1.** You are obligated as a medical professional to refrain from labeling patients and displaying personal biases.

_____ **2.** In an unconscious adult patient, you should assess for a pulse in the carotid artery.

_____ **3.** An epidemic occurs when new cases of a disease in the human population exceed the number of expected cases.

_____ **4.** History taking may be the only way to determine what the problem is or what may be causing the problem.

_____ **5.** Conscious medical patients will always need a full-body scan.

_____ **6.** The use of lights and siren during transport should be limited to situations where a life-threatening injury is present and it would meaningfully accelerate transport time.

_____ **7.** Exposure to the virus that causes AIDS is a risk that EMTs face on a regular basis.

_____ **8.** EMTs can receive a vaccination against HIV to protect them from exposure.

_____ **9.** Middle East respiratory syndrome coronavirus (MERS-CoV) is a virus most commonly found in bats and camels living in the Middle East.

_____ **10.** Hepatitis A can only be transmitted from a patient who has an acute infection.

_____ **11.** HIV is far more contagious than hepatitis B.

_____ **12.** If you are exposed to a patient with pulmonary tuberculosis, you should be tested with a tuberculin skin test to see if you have been infected.

_____ **13.** MRSA is believed to be transmitted from patient to patient via the unwashed hands of health care providers.

_____ **14.** Whooping cough is an airborne disease caused by a virus.

_____ **15.** Meningococcal meningitis is highly contagious.

_____ **16.** All strains of influenza are transmitted through oral or fecal contamination.

_____ **17.** When examining the neck, you should assess for jugular vein distention and tracheal deviation.

_____ **18.** You should avoid asking family members for information regarding patient allergies and medication.

_____ **19.** Cardiac arrest patients are usually transported to the closest hospital with emergency facilities.

_____ **20.** Differentiating a high-priority transport from a low-priority transport is often a skill developed with experience.

_____ **21.** Herpes simplex is primarily an animal respiratory disease that has mutated to infect humans.

Fill-in-the-Blank

Read each item carefully and then complete the statement by filling in the missing words.

1. _____ _____ may be the result of sickle cell disease or various blood clotting disorders, such as hemophilia.

2. _____ _____ occurs when you become focused on one aspect of the patient's condition and exclude all others.

3. As you approach a patient, you should determine the level of consciousness by using the _____ scale.

4. You should assess vital signs every _____ minutes in an unstable patient and every _____ minutes in a stable patient.

5. Permission to administer certain medication is usually obtained from _____ _____.

6. A(n) _____ should be used on a patient who is apneic and pulseless.

7. _____ patients include those with altered mental status, airway and breathing difficulties, or any sign of circulatory compromise.

8. Modes of transportation ultimately come in two categories: _____ or _____.

9. A(n) _____ _____ is a medical condition caused by the growth and spread of small harmful organisms within the body.

10. _____ refers to inflammation of the liver.

11. _____ _____ is transmitted orally through oral or fecal contamination.

12. You should note any _____ _____ along the veins that indicate potential IV drug use when examining the extremities.

13. _____ is the strength or ability of a pathogen to produce disease.

14. _____ is a chronic mycobacterial disease that usually strikes the lungs.

15. Patients with a fever, headache, stiff neck, and altered mental status may be suffering from _____.

Fill-in-the-Table

Read each section of the chart and complete the missing areas.

Causes of Infectious Disease		
Type of Organism	**Description**	**Example**
Bacteria		*Salmonella*
	Smaller than bacteria; multiply only inside a host and die when exposed to the environment	
Fungi		
Protozoa (parasites)		Amoebas
	Invertebrates with long, flexible, rounded, or flattened bodies	

Critical Thinking

Short Answer

Complete this section with short written answers using the space provided.

1. List four examples of how you can contract HIV while taking care of patients in EMS.

_____

_____

_____

2. What are the five major components of patient assessment for medical emergencies?

_____

_____

_____

3. List three conditions that are deemed serious and require rapid transport.

_____

_____

_____

4. List at least three important questions to ask a patient who potentially recently traveled.

_____

_____

_____

Ambulance Calls

The following case scenarios provide an opportunity to explore the concerns associated with patient management and to enhance critical-thinking skills. Read each scenario and answer each question to the best of your ability.

1. You respond to a local apartment building in the downtown area for a 42-year-old man with respiratory distress. On arrival, you notice the patient sitting in a chair and has pale, diaphoretic skin. The patient tells you that he has been sick for several days and is too sick to drive himself to the hospital. When taking a history, the patient tells you that he has had night sweats and has been coughing up blood. His only complaint is fever and slight shortness of breath. He has no other significant history.

How would you best manage this patient?

_____

_____

_____

2. While driving back from a call, your unit is dispatched to a local recreation area for a 58-year-old woman with chest pain. On arrival, you notice a woman lying on the ground with several bystanders assisting her. The patient is alert and oriented and complains of chest pain.

What history-taking questions can you ask to help with your assessment of this patient?

_____

_____

_____

CHAPTER

16

Respiratory Emergencies

General Knowledge

Matching

Match each of the items in the left column to the appropriate definition in the right column.

_____	**1.** Respiration	**A.**	Ongoing irritation of the trachea and bronchi
_____	**2.** Pulmonary edema	**B.**	An acute spasm of the bronchioles, associated with excessive mucus production and swelling of the mucous lining
_____	**3.** Epiglottitis	**C.**	Accumulation of air in the pleural space
_____	**4.** Emphysema	**D.**	Fluid buildup within the alveoli and lung tissue
_____	**5.** Pleural effusion	**E.**	An infection of the lung tissue leading to impaired gas exchange
_____	**6.** Tuberculosis	**F.**	A substance that leads to an allergic reaction
_____	**7.** Dyspnea	**G.**	Difficulty breathing
_____	**8.** Pneumonia	**H.**	An infection that can produce severe inflammation of the upper airway
_____	**9.** Hypoxia	**I.**	A blood clot or other substance in the circulatory system that travels to a blood vessel where it causes a blockage
_____	**10.** Chronic bronchitis	**J.**	A disease of the lungs in which the alveoli lose elasticity due to chronic stretching
_____	**11.** Hyperventilation	**K.**	Overbreathing to the point that the level of carbon dioxide in the blood falls below normal
_____	**12.** Allergen	**L.**	Fluid outside the lung
_____	**13.** Embolus	**M.**	A condition in which the body's cells and tissues do not have enough oxygen
_____	**14.** Asthma	**N.**	The exchange of oxygen and carbon dioxide
_____	**15.** Pneumothorax	**O.**	A disease that can lay dormant in the lungs for decades, then reactivate

Multiple Choice

Read each item carefully and then select the one best response.

_____ **1.** A blood clot lodged in the pulmonary artery is referred to as a:

    A. myocardial infarction

    B. stroke

    C. pulmonary embolism

    D. pulmonary effusion

_____ **2.** The oxygen–carbon dioxide exchange takes place in the:

    A. trachea

    B. bronchial tree

    C. alveoli

    D. blood

_____ 3. The letter "S" in the pneumonic PASTE refers to:
   A. symptoms
   B. sputum
   C. severity
   D. sickness

_____ 4. If carbon dioxide levels drop too low, the person automatically breathes:
   A. normally
   B. rapidly and deeply.
   C. slower and less deeply.
   D. fast and shallow.

_____ 5. If the level of carbon dioxide in the arterial blood rises above normal, the patient breathes:
   A. normally
   B. rapidly and deeply
   C. slower and less deeply
   D. fast and shallow

_____ 6. Inflammation and swelling of the pharynx, larynx, and trachea resulting in a "seal bark" is typically caused by:
   A. emphysema
   B. chronic bronchitis
   C. croup
   D. epiglottitis

_____ 7. The rate of breathing is typically increased when:
   A. oxygen levels increase
   B. oxygen levels decrease
   C. carbon dioxide levels increase
   D. carbon dioxide levels decrease

_____ 8. _____ is a sign of hypoxia of the brain.
   A. Altered mental status
   B. Decreased pulse rate
   C. Decreased respiratory rate
   D. Delayed capillary refill time

_____ 9. An obstruction to the exchange of gases between the alveoli and the capillaries may result from:
   A. epiglottitis
   B. pneumonia
   C. a cold
   D. croup

_____ 10. Pulmonary edema can develop quickly after a major:
   A. heart attack
   B. episode of syncope
   C. brain injury
   D. trauma

_____ 11. Pulmonary edema may be produced by:
   A. cigarette smoking
   B. seasonal allergies
   C. inhaling toxic chemical fumes
   D. carbon monoxide poisoning

_____ **12.** _____ is a loss of the elastic material around the air spaces as a result of chronic stretching of the alveoli.

   A. Emphysema

   B. Bronchitis

   C. Pneumonia

   D. Diphtheria

_____ **13.** _____ is a genetic disorder that affects the lungs and digestive system.

   A. Chronic obstructive pulmonary disease

   B. Cystic fibrosis

   C. Pertussis

   D. Bronchiolitis

_____ **14.** Which of the following signs and symptoms will help distinguish chronic obstructive pulmonary disease (COPD) from congestive heart failure?

   A. Dyspnea

   B. Dependent edema

   C. Wheezing

   D. Skin color changes

_____ **15.** A pneumothorax is a partial or complete accumulation of air in the:

   A. pleural space

   B. alveoli

   C. abdomen

   D. subcutaneous tissue

_____ **16.** Asthma produces a characteristic _____ as patients attempt to exhale through partially obstructed air passages.

   A. rhonchi

   B. stridor

   C. wheezing

   D. rattle

_____ **17.** An allergic response to certain foods or some other allergen may produce an acute:

   A. bronchodilation

   B. asthma attack

   C. vasoconstriction

   D. insulin release

_____ **18.** In most cases, what is the treatment of choice for anaphylaxis?

   A. Epinephrine

   B. High-flow oxygen

   C. Antihistamines

   D. Albuterol

_____ **19.** A collection of fluid outside the lungs on one or both sides of the chest is called a:

   A. pulmonary edema

   B. subcutaneous emphysema

   C. pleural effusion

   D. tension pneumothorax

_____ **20.** Always consider _____ in patients who were eating just before becoming short of breath.

   A. upper airway obstruction

   B. spontaneous pneumothorax

   C. lower airway obstruction

   D. bronchoconstriction

_____   **21.** _____ is defined as overbreathing to the point that the level of arterial carbon dioxide falls below normal.

    A. Reactive airway syndrome

    B. Hyperventilation

    C. Tachypnea

    D. Pleural effusion

_____   **22.** Which of the following is NOT an indication of inadequate breathing?

    A. Accessory muscle use

    B. Cyanosis

    C. A regular pattern of inspiration and expiration

    D. Unequal chest expansion

Questions 23–27 are derived from the following scenario: You respond to the home of a 78-year-old man having difficulty breathing. He is sitting at the kitchen table in a classic tripod position, wearing a nasal cannula. He is cyanotic, smoking, and has his shirt unbuttoned. His respirations are 30 breaths/min and shallow, his pulse rate is 110 beats/min, and his blood pressure is 136/88 mm Hg.

_____   **23.** Your first thought as an EMT should be to:

    A. apply a nonrebreathing mask at 15 L/min.

    B. call for backup.

    C. assess the airway status.

    D. determine scene safety.

_____   **24.** His brainstem senses the elevated level of _____ in the arterial blood, causing the rapid respirations.

    A. carbon dioxide

    B. oxygen

    C. insulin

    D. tobacco

_____   **25.** Proper management of this patient might include:

    A. application of a CPAP device

    B. chest compressions

    C. suctioning

    D. epinephrine

_____   **26.** Which of the following is NOT a sign or symptom of his inadequate breathing?

    A. He was cyanotic.

    B. His blood pressure was 136/88.

    C. He was in a tripod position.

    D. His pulse rate was over 100 beats/min (tachycardia).

_____   **27.** What should you do during the reassessment of this patient?

    A. Assess vital signs every 2 minutes.

    B. Repeat the primary assessment.

    C. Reassess what time your shift ends.

    D. Repeat the initial history.

_____   **28.** Which of the following is a question you would NOT typically ask during the history taking of a patient with dyspnea?

    A. What has the patient already done for the breathing problem?

    B. Does the patient use a prescribed inhaler?

    C. Does the patient have any allergies?

    D. What time did the patient wake up this morning?

_____ **29.** Generic names for popular inhaled medications include:
  A. Ventolin
  B. Flovent
  C. Albuterol
  D. Atrovent

_____ **30.** Contraindications to helping a patient self-administer a metered-dose inhaler include all of the following EXCEPT:
  A. failure to obtain permission from medical control
  B. noticing that the patient is in the tripod position
  C. noticing that the patient has already taken the maximum dose of the medication
  D. noticing that the medication has expired

_____ **31.** Contraindications for CPAP include:
  A. being alert and able to follow commands
  B. a pulse oximetry reading of less than 90%
  C. a respiratory rate greater than 26 breaths/min
  D. hypotension

_____ **32.** A prolonged asthma attack that is unrelieved by epinephrine may progress into a condition known as:
  A. pleural effusion
  B. status epilepticus
  C. status asthmaticus
  D. reactive airway disease

_____ **33.** Which of the following statements is FALSE regarding influenza?
  A. It may worsen chronic medical conditions.
  B. It is primarily a human respiratory disease that has mutated to infect animals.
  C. It is transmitted by direct contact with nasal secretions and aerosolized droplets.
  D. It has the potential to become a pandemic.

_____ **34.** Pulse oximeters measure the percentage of hemoglobin saturated with:
  A. carbon dioxide
  B. carbon monoxide
  C. oxygen
  D. iron

_____ **35.** An acute spasm of the smaller airways associated with excessive mucus production and swelling is characteristic of:
  A. asthma
  B. chronic bronchitis
  C. emphysema
  D. severe acute respiratory syndrome (SARS)

True/False

If you believe the statement to be more true than false, write the letter "T" in the space provided. If you believe the statement to be more false than true, write the letter "F."

_____ **1.** Chronic bronchitis is characterized by spasm and narrowing of the bronchioles due to exposure to allergens.

_____ **2.** With pneumothorax, the lung collapses because the negative pressure in the pleural space is lost.

_____ **3.** Anaphylactic reactions occur only in patients with a previous history of asthma or allergies.

_____ **4.** Decreased breath sounds in asthma occur because fluid in the pleural space has moved the lung away from the chest wall.

_____ **5.** Patients with carbon monoxide poisoning initially complain of headache, fatigue, and nausea.

_____ **6.** Pulmonary edema is commonly associated with congestive heart failure.

_____ **7.** The distinction between hyperventilation and hyperventilation syndrome is straightforward and should guide the EMT's treatment choices.

_____ **8.** COPD most often results from cigarette smoking.

_____ **9.** COPD is characterized by long expiration phases.

_____ **10.** In cystic fibrosis, mucus becomes thick, sticky, and hard to move.

_____ **11.** When assessing a patient, the general impression will help you decide whether the patient's condition is stable or unstable.

_____ **12.** The pulse oximeter can be a valuable tool in evaluating oxygenation.

_____ **13.** Oxygen is typically withheld from COPD patients regardless of their breathing status.

_____ **14.** Side effects of inhalers used for acute shortness of breath include increased pulse rate, nervousness, and muscle tremors.

_____ **15.** Patients who are hyperventilating should be treated by having them breathe into a paper bag.

_____ **16.** Epiglottitis is seen in both the pediatric and adult populations.

_____ **17.** A respiratory syncytial virus (RSV) infection can cause respiratory illnesses such as bronchiolitis and pneumonia.

_____ **18.** When assisting a patient with a small-volume nebulizer, the oxygen flowmeter should be set to 10 L/min.

_____ **19.** Snoring sounds are indicative of a partial upper airway obstruction.

_____ **20.** Signs and symptoms of pulmonary emboli include dyspnea, hemoptysis, and tachycardia.

Fill-in-the-Blank

Read each item carefully and then complete the statement by filling in the missing words.

1. The level of _____ _____ sensed by the brainstem stimulates respiration.

2. The level of _____ in the blood is a secondary stimulus for respiration.

3. _____ passes from the blood through capillaries to tissue cells.

4. Carbon dioxide and oxygen are exchanged in the _____.

5. If you suspect a patient has tuberculosis, you should wear gloves, eye protection, and a(n) _____

_____.

6. Children with chronic pulmonary medical conditions may use a home ventilator that is connected by a(n)

_____ tube.

7. _____ _____ is an odorless, highly poisonous gas that results from incomplete oxidation of carbon in

combustion.

8. High-pitched sounds heard on inspiration as air tries to pass through an obstruction in the upper airway are

commonly referred to as _____.

9. _____ or _____ are the sounds of air trying to pass through fluid in the alveoli.

10. When asking questions about the present illness during the history and secondary assessment, use the mnemonics _____ and _____ to guide you in your general questioning.

11. _____ _____, or allergic rhinitis, causes coldlike symptoms, including a runny nose, sneezing, congestion, and sinus pressure.

12. Medication from a(n) _____ or small-volume _____ is delivered through the respiratory tract to the lung.

13. _____ is an airborne bacterial infection that is highly contagious and results in coughing attacks lasting longer than a minute.

14. _____ are lower-pitched sounds caused by secretions or mucus in the larger airways.

15. A patient with a barrel chest and a "puffing" style of breathing most likely has _____.

Labeling

Label the following diagrams with the correct terms.

1. Obstruction, Scarring, and Dilation of the Alveolar Sac

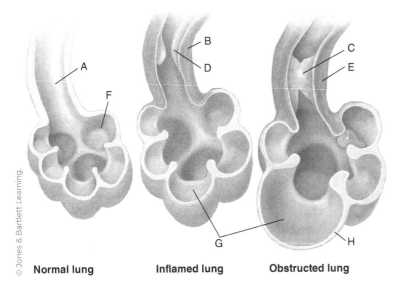

Normal lung   Inflamed lung   Obstructed lung

A. _____

B. _____

C. _____

D. _____

E. _____

F. _____

G. _____

H. _____

Critical Thinking

Short Answer

Complete this section with short written answers using the space provided.

1. List five characteristics of normal breathing.

_____

_____

_____

2. List six conditions where wheezing can be found.

_____

_____

_____

3. Under what conditions should you not assist a patient with a metered-dose inhaler?

_____

_____

_____

4. Describe chronic bronchitis.

_____

_____

_____

5. List complications associated with a tracheostomy tube.

_____

_____

_____

6. Explain carbon dioxide retention.

_____

_____

_____

7. When ventilating a patient, how would you determine whether your ventilations are adequate?

_____

_____

_____

Ambulance Calls

The following case scenarios provide an opportunity to explore the concerns associated with patient management and to enhance critical-thinking skills. Read each scenario and answer each question to the best of your ability.

1. You are called to the home of a young boy who is reportedly experiencing difficulty swallowing. You arrive to find concerned parents who tell you that their son seems to be "sick." He can't swallow, has a high fever, and refuses to lie down. As you enter the child's bedroom, you find him standing with arms outstretched onto the footboard of the bed, drooling, and with a very frightened look on his face.

How do you best manage this patient?

_____

_____

_____

2. You are dispatched to a 36-year-old woman complaining of shortness of breath. You arrive to find a slightly overweight woman who tells you that she "can't catch her breath." She is a smoker whose only medication is birth control pills.

How would you best manage this patient?

_____

_____

_____

3. You are called to the home of a 73-year-old man complaining of severe dyspnea. The patient has a history of COPD and is on home oxygen at 2 L/min via a nasal cannula. His family tells you that he has a long history of breathing problems and emphysema. He is cyanotic around his lips, and his respirations are 36 breaths/min and shallow.

How would you best manage this patient?

_____

_____

_____

4. You respond to a skilled nursing facility to find an 82-year-old man complaining of shortness of breath. The nursing staff tells you that the patient has a cardiac history. The patient is using accessory muscles and can speak in two- to three-word sentences. You notice pink froth produced when the patient coughs and hear crackles when listening to the lungs.

How would you best manage this patient?

_____

_____

_____

Skills

Skill Drills

Test your knowledge of this skill by filling in the correct words in the photo captions.

Skill Drill 16-1: Assisting a Patient With a Metered-Dose Inhaler

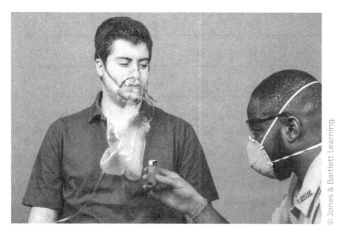

1. Check to make sure you have the correct medication for the correct patient. Check the expiration date. Ensure inhaler is at room temperature or _____.

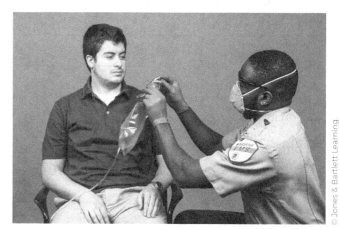

2. Remove oxygen mask. Hand inhaler to patient. Instruct about breathing and _____ _____.

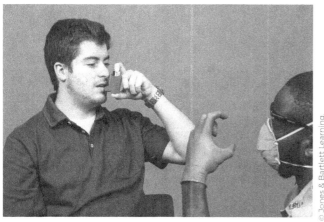

3. Instruct patient to press inhaler and inhale one puff. Instruct about _____ _____.

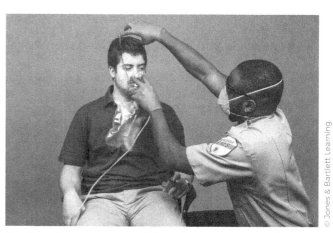

4. Reapply _____. After a few _____, have patient repeat _____ if order or protocol allows.

Skill Drill 16-2: Assisting a Patient With a Small-Volume Nebulizer

Test your knowledge of this skill by placing the following photos in the correct order. Number the first step with a "1," the second step with a "2," etc.

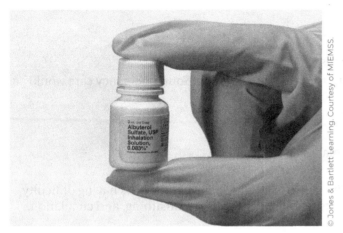

1. _____ Instruct the patient on how to breathe.

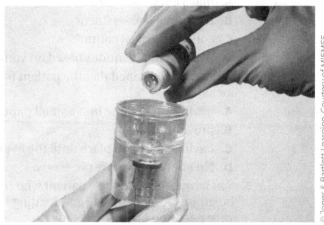

2. _____ Pour the medication into the container on the nebulizer. In some cases, sterile saline may be added (about 3 mL) to achieve the optimum volume of fluid for the nebulized application.

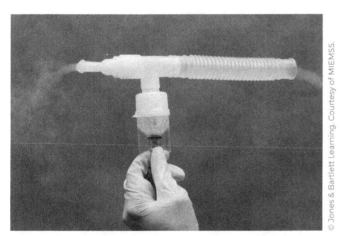

3. _____ Check to make sure you have the correct medication for the correct patient. Check the expiration date. Confirm you have the correct patient and correct dose.

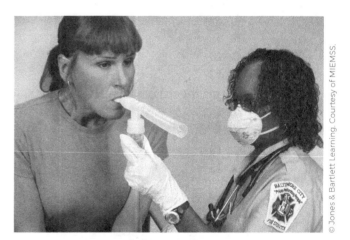

4. _____ Attach the medication container to the nebulizer, mouthpiece, and tubing. Attach oxygen tubing to the oxygen tank. Set the flowmeter at 6 L/min.

Assessment Review

Answer the following questions pertaining to the assessment of the types of emergencies discussed in this chapter.

_____ 1. You have been assessing a 17-year-old girl in respiratory distress, and you have just completed the secondary assessment. Your next step is to:
   A. make a transport decision
   B. perform a reassessment
   C. contact medical control
   D. perform interventions based on your findings

_____ 2. You have determined that the patient in Question 1 is hyperventilating. Your emergency care would include:
   A. having her breathe into a small paper sack
   B. providing oxygen
   C. having her run in place until the hyperventilation subsides
   D. No interventions are necessary.

_____ 3. You have been called to a patient who resides in a long-term care facility and who is having difficulty breathing. After assessing and treating life threats to the patient's airway, breathing, and circulation, your next step in this case is to:
   A. make a transport decision
   B. obtain a SAMPLE history
   C. obtain an OPQRST history
   D. obtain baseline vital signs

_____ 4. During the reassessment, vital signs should be taken every _____ minutes for the unstable patient.
   A. 3
   B. 5
   C. 10
   D. 15

_____ 5. During the reassessment, vital signs should be taken every _____ minutes for the stable patient.
   A. 3
   B. 5
   C. 10
   D. 15

Emergency Care Summary

Complete the statements pertaining to emergency care for the types of emergencies discussed in this chapter by filling in the missing word(s).

NOTE: While the following steps are widely accepted, be sure to consult and follow your local protocol.

General Management of Respiratory Emergencies
Managing life threats to the patient's _____ and ensuring the delivery of high-flow oxygen are the primary concerns with any respiratory emergency. Patients breathing at a rate of less than _____ breaths/min or greater than _____ breaths/min should receive _____-_____ _____. Continually assess the patient's mental status, and provide emotional support as needed. Transport in a position of comfort. For all respiratory emergencies, make sure you have taken the appropriate standard precautions, including the use of a(n) _____ _____ in a patient with suspected tuberculosis.

Upper or Lower Airway Infection
Dyspnea from an upper airway infection may be from _____ or _____. Patients should receive _____ oxygen if available. Patients who are sitting forward, seem lethargic, or are drooling may have _____. Do not force the patient to lie down or attempt to suction or insert a(n) _____ airway because this may cause a spasm and a complete airway obstruction. Transport should be rapid.
Lower airway infections may be from the common cold, bronchitis, or _____. Patients need supplemental oxygen, monitoring of vital signs, and transport to the hospital.

Asthma, Hay Fever, and Anaphylaxis
Not all wheezing is the result of asthma! Obtain a thorough _____ from the patient or family. If the patient is wheezing and has asthma, assist with the patient's prescribed _____ or administer a small-volume nebulizer containing _____. Provide supplemental oxygen and provide ventilatory support as needed. Patients whose asthma progresses to _____ _____ require immediate transportation. Be prepared to assist their ventilations because they may become too exhausted to breathe.
Hay fever usually requires only support and transport, but if the condition has worsened from generalized cold symptoms, the patient may require supplemental oxygen and _____ support.
Anaphylaxis is a true emergency that requires rapid intervention and _____. Airway, oxygen, and ventilatory support are paramount. Determine if the patient has a prescribed _____. Transport promptly. Reassess the patient's condition en route to the hospital.

Pneumothorax
A pneumothorax may occur spontaneously or may be the result of a(n) _____ _____. Place the patient in a position of comfort, and support the _____. Provide prompt transport, monitor the patient carefully, and be prepared to assist ventilations and provide _____ _____ if necessary.

Obstruction of the Airway
Managing an airway obstruction is a priority. Use age-appropriate _____ life support foreign body airway obstruction _____ to clear the airway. Administer supplemental oxygen, and transport the patient to the closest hospital. Some patients do not want to go to a hospital after the obstruction is cleared. Encourage them to be transported for evaluation of possible _____ to the airway.

Hyperventilation
Gather a thorough _____, and attempt to determine the _____ _____ because the hyperventilation may be the result of a serious problem. Do not have the patient breathe into a(n) _____ _____; this maneuver could make things worse. Instead, _____ the patient, administer supplemental oxygen, and provide prompt transport to the hospital.

CHAPTER

17 Cardiovascular Emergencies

General Knowledge

Matching

Match each of the items in the left column to the appropriate definition in the right column.

_____ 1. Atria

_____ 2. Coronary arteries

_____ 3. Atrioventricular node

_____ 4. Myocardium

_____ 5. Sinus node

_____ 6. Venae cavae

_____ 7. Ventricles

_____ 8. Aorta

_____ 9. Atherosclerosis

_____ 10. Dysrhythmia

_____ 11. Ischemia

_____ 12. Infarction

_____ 13. Tachycardia

_____ 14. Asystole

_____ 15. Bradycardia

_____ 16. Thromboembolism

A. An absence of heart electrical activity

B. Calcium and cholesterol buildup inside blood vessels

C. Blood vessels that supply blood to the myocardium

D. An abnormal heart rhythm

E. An unusually slow heart rhythm, less than 60 beats/min

F. Decreased blood flow and poor oxygenation

G. Heart muscle

H. Lower chambers of the heart

I. The death of tissue

J. A rapid heart rhythm, greater than 100 beats/min

K. Carry oxygen-poor blood back to the heart

L. Upper chambers of the heart

M. The body's main artery

N. Electrical impulses begin here

O. Electrical impulses slow here to allow blood to move from the atria to the ventricles

P. A blood clot floating through blood vessels until it reaches a narrow area and blocks blood flow

Match each of the medical conditions in the left column to the appropriate description in the right column.

_____ 17. Acute myocardial infarction

_____ 18. Cardiac arrest

_____ 19. Angina pectoris

_____ 20. Cardiogenic shock

_____ 21. Congestive heart failure

_____ 22. Hypertensive emergency

_____ 23. Dissecting aneurysm

A. A condition where the heart cannot effectively pump blood, leading to fluid backing up into the lungs and edema

B. The sudden tearing and separation of the inner layers of the aorta, with the potential for great blood loss

C. The heart lacks power to effectively pump blood to the body, resulting in low blood pressure

D. Systolic blood pressure greater than 180 mm Hg

E. A lack of cardiac pumping activity

F. Exertional chest pain, relieved by nitroglycerin

G. The complete blockage of a coronary artery

Multiple Choice

Read each item carefully and then select the one best response.

_____ 1. _____ allows a cardiac muscle cell to contract spontaneously without a stimulus from a nerve source.
- **A.** Repetition
- **B.** Reactivity
- **C.** Automaticity
- **D.** Autonomy

_____ 2. The aorta receives its blood supply from the:
- **A.** right atrium
- **B.** left atrium
- **C.** right ventricle
- **D.** left ventricle

_____ 3. Blood enters the right atrium from the body through the:
- **A.** vena cava
- **B.** aorta
- **C.** pulmonary artery
- **D.** pulmonary vein

_____ 4. The only vein(s) in the body that carry oxygenated blood is/are the:
- **A.** external jugular veins
- **B.** pulmonary veins
- **C.** subclavian veins
- **D.** inferior vena cava

_____ 5. Normal electrical impulses originate in the sinus node, in the upper part of the right:
- **A.** atrium
- **B.** ventricle
- **C.** superior vena cava
- **D.** aortic arch

_____ 6. Dilation of the coronary arteries _____ blood flow.
- **A.** shuts off
- **B.** increases
- **C.** decreases
- **D.** regulates

_____ 7. The _____ are tiny blood vessels that are approximately one cell thick.
- **A.** arterioles
- **B.** venules
- **C.** capillaries
- **D.** ventricles

_____ 8. _____ carry oxygen to the body's tissues and then remove carbon dioxide.
- **A.** Red blood cells
- **B.** White blood cells
- **C.** Platelets
- **D.** Veins

_____ 9. _____ is the maximum pressure exerted by the left ventricle as it contracts.
- **A.** Cardiac output
- **B.** Diastolic blood pressure
- **C.** Systolic blood pressure
- **D.** Stroke volume

_____ **10.** Atherosclerosis can lead to a complete _____ of a coronary artery.
  A. occlusion
  B. disintegration
  C. dilation
  D. contraction

_____ **11.** The lumen of an artery may be partially or completely blocked by the blood-clotting system due to a _____ that exposes the inside of the atherosclerotic wall.
  A. tear
  B. crack
  C. clot
  D. rupture

_____ **12.** Tissues downstream from a blood clot will suffer from lack of oxygen. If blood flow is resumed in a short time, the _____ tissues will recover.
  A. sclerotic
  B. hypoxic
  C. necrotic
  D. rheumatic

_____ **13.** Risk factors for myocardial infarction include all of the following EXCEPT:
  A. male gender
  B. high blood pressure
  C. stress
  D. increased activity level

_____ **14.** When, for a brief period of time, heart tissues do not get enough oxygen, the pain is called:
  A. necrosis
  B. angina
  C. ischemia
  D. atherosclerosis

_____ **15.** Angina pain may be felt in the:
  A. epigastrium
  B. legs
  C. lower back
  D. lower abdomen

_____ **16.** The underlying cause of a dissecting aortic aneurysm is:
  A. controlled hypertension
  B. uncontrolled hypertension
  C. transient hypertension
  D. benign hypertension

_____ **17.** Because the oxygen supply to the heart is diminished with angina, the _____ can become compromised, putting the person at risk for significant cardiac rhythm problems.
  A. respiratory system
  B. clotting cascade
  C. electrical system
  D. vasculature

_____ **18.** About _____ minutes after blood flow is cut off, some heart muscle cells begin to die.
  A. 10
  B. 20
  C. 30
  D. 40

_____ **19.** An acute myocardial infarction is more likely to occur in the larger, thick-walled left ventricle, which needs more _____ than the right ventricle.
- **A.** oxygen and glucose
- **B.** force to pump
- **C.** blood and oxygen
- **D.** electrical activity

_____ **20.** Which of the following statements regarding congestive heart failure (CHF) is FALSE?
- **A.** Stridor is a common lung sound heard on exam.
- **B.** It can be caused by diseased heart valves.
- **C.** It can be treated with nitroglycerin.
- **D.** Ankle edema is a common finding.

_____ **21.** Cardiogenic shock often occurs soon after a(n):
- **A.** hypertensive emergency
- **B.** acute myocardial infarction
- **C.** aortic aneurysm
- **D.** unstable angina attack

_____ **22.** Sudden death is usually the result of _____, in which the heart fails to generate an effective blood flow.
- **A.** acute myocardial infarction (AMI)
- **B.** atherosclerosis
- **C.** premature ventricular contractions (PVCs)
- **D.** cardiac arrest

_____ **23.** Disorganized, ineffective quivering of the ventricles is known as:
- **A.** ventricular fibrillation
- **B.** asystole
- **C.** ventricular standstill
- **D.** ventricular tachycardia

_____ **24.** Which of the following is NOT a cause of CHF?
- **A.** Chronic hypotension
- **B.** Heart valve damage
- **C.** Myocardial infarction
- **D.** Long-standing high blood pressure

_____ **25.** Signs and symptoms of shock include all of the following EXCEPT:
- **A.** elevated heart rate
- **B.** pale, clammy skin
- **C.** air hunger
- **D.** elevated blood pressure

_____ **26.** Which of the following changes in heart function occurs in patients with CHF?
- **A.** A decrease in heart rate
- **B.** Enlargement of the left ventricle
- **C.** Enlargement of the right ventricle
- **D.** A decrease in blood pressure

_____ **27.** Physical findings of AMI include skin that is _____ because of poor cardiac output and the loss of perfusion.
- **A.** pink
- **B.** white
- **C.** gray
- **D.** red

_____ **28.** All patient assessments begin by determining whether the patient:

    A. is breathing

    B. can talk

    C. is responsive

    D. has a pulse

_____ **29.** To assess chest pain, use the mnemonic:

    A. AVPU

    B. OPQRST

    C. SAMPLE

    D. CHART

_____ **30.** When using the mnemonic OPQRST, the "P" stands for:

    A. paresthesia

    B. pain

    C. provocation

    D. predisposing factors

_____ **31.** In addition to angina and myocardial infarction, nitroglycerin can be used to treat:

    A. CHF

    B. cardiogenic shock

    C. aortic aneurysm

    D. hypertensive emergency

_____ **32.** When administering nitroglycerin to a patient, you should make sure the patient has not taken any medications for _____ in the last 24 hours.

    A. angina

    B. erectile dysfunction

    C. migraine headaches

    D. gallbladder dysfunction

_____ **33.** In general, a maximum of _____ dose(s) of nitroglycerin is/are given for any one episode of chest pain.

    A. one

    B. two

    C. three

    D. four

_____ **34.** _____ are inserted when the electrical control system of the heart is so damaged that it cannot function properly.

    A. Stents

    B. Pacemakers

    C. Balloon angioplasties

    D. Defibrillations

_____ **35.** When the battery wears out in a pacemaker, the patient may experience:

    A. syncope

    B. chest pain

    C. nausea

    D. tachycardia

_____ **36.** The computer inside the AED is specifically programmed to recognize rhythms that require defibrillation to correct, most commonly:

    A. asystole

    B. ventricular tachycardia

    C. ventricular fibrillation

    D. supraventricular tachycardia

_____ **37.** The AED should be applied only to unresponsive patients with no:

    A. significant medical problems

    B. cardiac history

    C. pulse

    D. brain activity

_____ **38.** _____ usually refers to a state of cardiac arrest despite an organized electrical complex.

    A. Asystole

    B. Pulseless electrical activity

    C. Ventricular fibrillation

    D. Ventricular tachycardia

_____ **39.** The links in the chain of survival include all of the following EXCEPT:

    A. immediate high-quality CPR

    B. ALS and postarrest care

    C. administration of nitroglycerin

    D. rapid defibrillation

_____ **40.** Defibrillation works best if it takes place within _____ minutes of the onset of cardiac arrest.

    A. 2

    B. 4

    C. 6

    D. 10

Questions 41–45 are derived from the following scenario: At 0500, you respond to the home of a 76-year-old man complaining of chest pain. On arrival, the patient states that he had been sleeping in the recliner all night due to indigestion. He also tells you he has taken two nitroglycerin tablets. He continues to have pain and reports trouble breathing.

_____ **41.** Your first priority is to:

    A. apply an AED

    B. provide high-flow oxygen

    C. evaluate the need to administer a third nitroglycerin tablet

    D. size-up the scene

_____ **42.** His vital signs are as follows: respirations, 16 breaths/min; pulse, 98 beats/min; blood pressure, 92/76 mm Hg. He is still complaining of chest pain. What actions should you take to intervene?

    A. Provide high-flow oxygen.

    B. Administer a third nitroglycerin tablet.

    C. Apply an AED.

    D. Begin chest compressions.

_____ **43.** Your patient suddenly becomes unresponsive. Assessment reveals no breathing and no pulse. Your partner begins chest compressions while you apply the AED. When operating an AED, what is the first step in the defibrillation sequence?

    A. Plug the pads connector to the AED.

    B. Apply the AED pads to the patient's chest.

    C. Remove clothing from the patient's chest.

    D. Turn on the AED.

_____ **44.** After applying an AED to this patient, the AED states, "No shock advised." What is your next step of action?

    A. Load and transport the patient.

    B. Push to reanalyze.

    C. Perform CPR for 2 minutes, starting with chest compressions, then have the AED reanalyze.

    D. Consider termination.

_____ **45.** Your patient is now conscious, and you are en route to the hospital. You are six blocks away when the patient stops breathing again and no longer has a pulse. You should:
- **A.** continue to the hospital
- **B.** continue to the hospital and analyze the rhythm
- **C.** stop the vehicle and analyze the rhythm
- **D.** only perform chest compressions

True/False

If you believe the statement to be more true than false, write the letter "T" in the space provided. If you believe the statement to be more false than true, write the letter "F."

_____ **1.** The right side of the heart pumps oxygen-rich blood to the body.

_____ **2.** In the normal heart, the need for increased blood flow to the myocardium is easily met by an increase in heart rate.

_____ **3.** Atherosclerosis results in narrowing of the lumen of coronary arteries.

_____ **4.** Infarction is a temporary interruption of the blood supply to the tissues.

_____ **5.** Angina can result from a spasm of the artery.

_____ **6.** The pain of angina and the pain of AMI are easily distinguishable.

_____ **7.** Nitroglycerin works in most patients within 5 minutes to relieve the pain of AMI.

_____ **8.** If an AED malfunctions during use, you must report that problem to the manufacturer and the US Food and Drug Administration (FDA).

_____ **9.** Angina occurs when the heart's need for oxygen exceeds its supply.

_____ **10.** White blood cells are the most numerous cells in the blood and help the blood to clot.

_____ **11.** Cardiac arrest in children is less common than in adults and is usually caused by a breathing problem.

_____ **12.** An AED with special pediatric pads may be used on pediatric medical patients between the ages of 1 month and 8 years who have been assessed to be unresponsive, not breathing, and pulseless.

_____ **13.** Dissecting aortic aneurysms are rarely considered life threatening.

_____ **14.** Heart disease is the number-one killer of women in the United States.

_____ **15.** If a patient complaining of chest pain has a history of a previous AMI, you should ask if this pain feels similar to the previous AMI.

Fill-in-the-Blank

Read each item carefully and then complete the statement by filling in the missing words.

1. The heart is divided down the middle by a wall called the _____.

2. The _____ is the body's main artery.

3. The _____ ventricle pumps blood in through the pulmonary circulation.

4. Electrical impulses spread from the _____ node to the ventricles.

5. Blood supply to the heart is increased by _____ of the coronary arteries.

6. _____ _____ cells remove carbon dioxide from the body's tissues.

7. _____ blood pressure reflects the pressure on the walls of the arteries when the ventricle is at rest.

8. The heart has _____ chambers.

9. The _____ side of the heart is more muscular because it must pump blood into the aorta and all the other arteries of the body.

10. _____ is the most effective way to assist a person with CHF to breathe effectively and to prevent an invasive airway management technique.

11. The collection of fluid in the part of the body that is closest to the ground is called _____ _____.

12. A hypertensive emergency usually occurs only with a systolic pressure greater than _____.

13. In CHF, blood tends to back up in the _____ _____, increasing the pressure in the capillaries of the lungs.

14. A late finding in cardiogenic shock would be a systolic blood pressure of less than _____.

15. Damage to the _____ area of the heart often presents with bradycardia.

Labeling

Label the following diagrams with the correct terms.

1. Right and Left Sides of the Heart
Where arrows appear, also indicate the origin and destination of the blood.

A. _____

B. _____

C. _____

D. _____

E. _____

F. _____

G. _____

H. _____

I. _____

J. _____

K. _____

L. _____

© Jones & Bartlett Learning.

2. Electrical Conduction System

A. _____

B. _____

C. _____

D. _____

E. _____

F. _____

G. _____

H. _____

I. _____

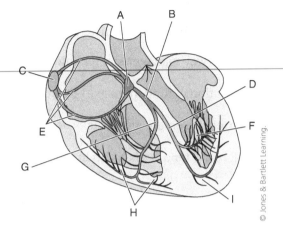

3. Pulse Points

State the name of the artery that is being assessed at each of the following pulse points:

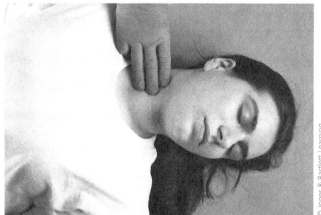

A

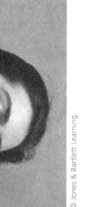

B

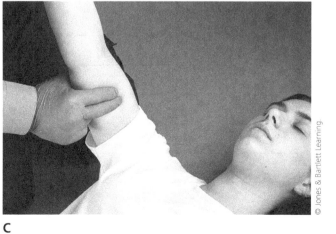

C

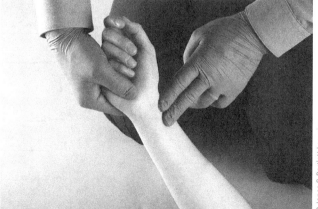

D

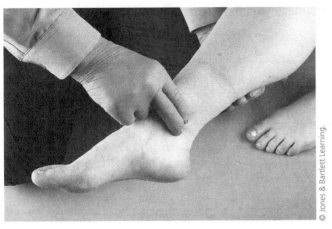

E

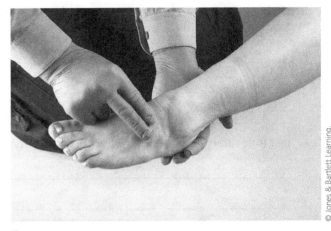

F

A. _____

B. _____

C. _____

D. _____

E. _____

F. _____

Critical Thinking

Short Answer

Complete this section with short written answers using the space provided.

1. Explain the differentiating features between an AMI and a dissecting aortic aneurysm.

_____

_____

_____

2. What are the three most common errors of AED use?

_____

_____

_____

3. If ALS is not responding to the scene, what are the three points at which transport should be initiated for a cardiac arrest patient?

_____

_____

_____

4. List four safety considerations for operating an AED.

_____

_____

_____

5. Explain the difference between stable angina and unstable angina.

_____

_____

_____

6. List three ways in which AMI pain differs from angina pain.

_____

_____

_____

7. List three serious consequences of AMI.

_____

_____

_____

8. Name at least five signs and symptoms associated with AMI.

_____

_____

_____

9. List six steps in the treatment of a patient with CHF.

_____

_____

_____

Ambulance Calls

The following case scenarios provide an opportunity to explore the concerns associated with patient management and to enhance critical-thinking skills. Read each scenario and answer each question to the best of your ability.

1. You are dispatched to the residence of a 58-year-old man complaining of chest pain. He states that it feels like "somebody is standing on my chest." He sat down when it started and took a nitroglycerin tablet. He is still a little nauseated and sweaty but feels better. He is very anxious.

   How would you best manage this patient?

   _____

   _____

   _____

2. You are dispatched to the home of a 45-year-old man experiencing chest pain. He told his wife that he was fine, but she decided to call 9-1-1. When you arrive, you find your patient sitting in the living room, looking anxious. He is sweaty and pale and admits the pain is worse than just a few moments ago. He tells you that he is a very athletic person, so the pain must just be stress related and will go away after he relaxes for a while. He tells you he does not want to be taken to the hospital.

   How would you best manage this patient?

   _____

   _____

   _____

3. You are dispatched to the home of a 60-year-old woman complaining of sudden weakness. She tells you that she usually has enough energy to perform daily tasks around the house, but today she's suddenly very tired, has some pain in her jaw, and has some nausea. She denies any history of recent illness, including cough, cold, or fever. She is otherwise healthy and does not take any medications.

   How would you best manage this patient?

   _____

   _____

   _____

Fill-in-the-Patient Care Report

Read the incident scenario and then complete the following patient care report (PCR).

Your shift ends at 1900, and you have 10 minutes to go. As you sit there daydreaming about your plans for the evening, the tones go off. "Unit 6291, respond to 1574 S. Main Street for a 58-year-old man with chest pain; time 1901."

You immediately acknowledge the call and note the incident number of 011543. You arrive on the scene 8 minutes later and notice a woman standing on the front porch. Your partner grabs the gear as you approach the woman. She tells you that her husband has had chest pain for about 30 minutes and has taken two nitroglycerin tablets but is not feeling any better.

As you enter the residence, you see a man sitting up on the living room couch. The man looks like he is having difficulty breathing. You introduce yourself to the patient and ask what is wrong. "I have horrible pressure in my chest," the patient replies. "Please help me." Because you are less than 5 minutes from the hospital, you elect not to request ALS.

"I was just sitting here on the couch when I began to feel incredible constant pressure in my chest. Then I began to get short of breath. I initially thought it was my angina, but this feels different and my nitro doesn't seem to be helping."

Your partner applies 15 L/min of oxygen via a nonrebreathing mask, and you note that you have been on scene for 2 minutes. You note that the patient has an intact airway, and although he is a little short of breath, he seems to be breathing adequately.

As you continue with your assessment, you note clear lung sounds and good pulses in all of his extremities.

"Does your pressure go anywhere?" you ask.

"No," replies the patient.

"On a scale from 1 to 10, can you rate that pressure for me?" The patient responds with a 5 out of 10.

Your partner hands you a piece of paper indicating the vital signs: pulse, 88 beats/min; respirations, 22 breaths/min; blood pressure, 136/88 mm Hg; SpO_2, 99%; time, 1914.

The patient tells you he has a history of hypertension, angina, and diabetes. He takes Lisinopril, nitroglycerin, metformin, and metoprolol. When you ask him about allergies, he says, "I can't have aspirin—my throat closes up."

Your local protocol allows you to assist with the administration of nitroglycerin. You check the patient's nitro and verify that it is indeed prescribed to him and that it is not expired. Because his systolic blood pressure is above 100 mm Hg, you elect to give the patient a nitro tablet. You explain to the patient that he is to place the tablet under his tongue and that he is not to chew or swallow it. You note the time as 1916.

You finish your secondary assessment and package the patient onto your litter.

The patient is loaded into your ambulance and transported to the local hospital. Just as you start en route to the hospital, you notice that it has been 5 minutes since you administered the nitro. You reassess his vital signs: pulse, 84 beats/min; respirations, 18 breaths/min; blood pressure, 122/74 mm Hg; SpO_2, 98%. The patient now rates his pain as a 4 out of 10.

In 5 minutes, you arrive at the local hospital with a stable patient and transfer care to the emergency department (ED) staff.

After giving your report to the ED staff and restocking/cleaning the unit, your partner looks at you and says, "Hey, you're only 35 minutes late." After his comment, you mark your unit available and return to the station.

Fill-in-the-Patient Care Report

EMS Patient Care Report (PCR)			
Date:	Incident No.:	Nature of Call:	Location:
Dispatched:	En Route:	At Scene:	Transport:	At Hospital:	In Service:

Patient Information	
Age: Sex: Weight (in kg [lb]):	Allergies: Medications: Past Medical History: Chief Complaint:

Vital Signs				
Time:	BP:	Pulse:	Respirations:	SpO$_2$:
Time:	BP:	Pulse:	Respirations:	SpO$_2$:
Time:	BP:	Pulse:	Respirations:	SpO$_2$:

EMS Treatment (circle all that apply)				
Oxygen @ ____ L/min via (circle one): NC NRM BVM	Assisted Ventilation	Airway Adjunct	CPR
Defibrillation	Bleeding Control	Bandaging	Splinting	Other:

Narrative

Skills

Skill Drills

Skill Drill 17-1: Administration of Nitroglycerin

Test your knowledge of this skill by filling in the correct words in the photo captions.

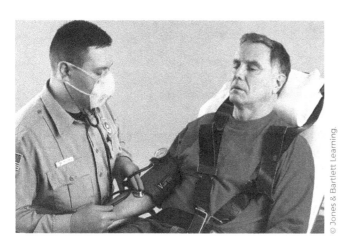

1. Obtain an order from _____ _____. Take the patient's blood pressure. Administer _____ only if the _____ blood pressure is greater than 100 mm Hg.

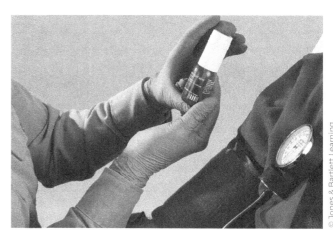

2. Check the medication and expiration date. Ask the patient about the last dose he or she took and its _____. Make sure that the patient understands the route of _____. Prepare to have the patient lie down to prevent _____.

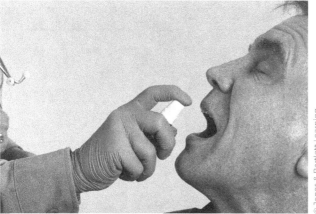

3. Ask the patient to lift his or her _____. Place the tablet or spray the dose under the _____ (while wearing gloves), or have the patient do so. Have the patient keep his or her mouth _____ with the tablet or spray under the tongue until it is dissolved and absorbed. Caution the patient against _____ or swallowing the tablet.

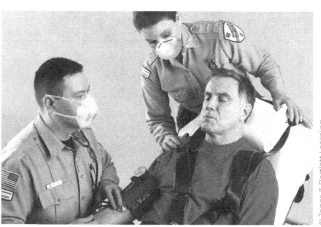

4. Recheck the blood pressure within _____ minutes. Record each medication and the time of administration. Reevaluate the _____ _____ and blood pressure, and repeat treatment, if necessary.

Skill Drill 17-3: Using an AED

Test your knowledge of this skill by placing the following photos in the correct order. Number the first step with a "1," the second step with a "2," etc.

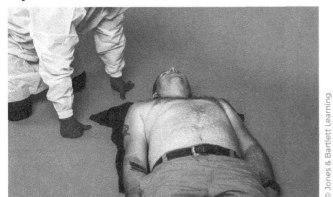

1. _____ Push the Analyze button, if there is one, and wait for the AED to determine whether a shockable rhythm is present. Stop CPR when the AED instructs you to.

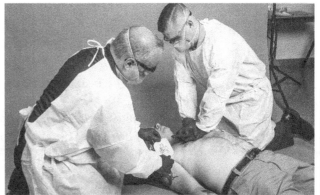

2. _____ If a shock is advised, state aloud, "Clear the patient," and ensure that no one is touching the patient. Reconfirm that no one is touching the patient and push the Shock button. Continue CPR for five cycles (2 minutes) after the shock is delivered.

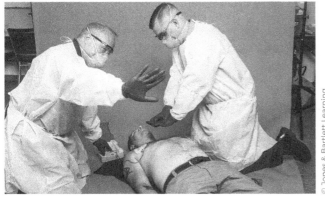

3. _____ Turn on the AED. Apply the AED pads to the chest and attach the pads to the AED.

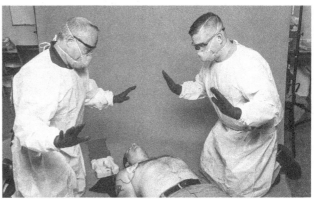

4. _____ Take standard precautions. Determine scene safety. Question bystanders. Determine responsiveness. Assess compression effectiveness if CPR is already in progress. If the patient is unresponsive and CPR has not been started yet, begin providing chest compressions and rescue breaths at a rate of 30 compressions to two breaths and a rate of 100 to 120 compressions per minute, continuing until an AED arrives and is ready for use.

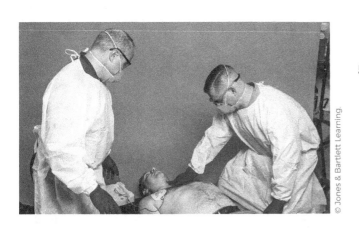

5. _____ After five cycles (2 minutes) of CPR, pause CPR and allow the AED to analyze the rhythm. If shock is advised, clear the patient, push the Shock button, and immediately resume CPR compressions. If no shock is advised, immediately resume CPR compressions and be sure to switch rescuers. Repeat the cycle of five cycles (2 minutes) of CPR, one shock (if indicated), and 2 minutes of CPR. Transport, and contact medical control as needed.

© Jones & Bartlett Learning.

Assessment Review

Answer the following questions pertaining to the assessment of the types of emergencies discussed in this chapter.

_____   **1.** What type of additional resource is typically required for someone with chest pain?

    A. Lift assistance

    B. Advanced life support

    C. Police

    D. Rescue team

_____   **2.** When taking a SAMPLE history of a conscious person with chest pain, what specific question should the EMT ask of the patient?

    A. Has he or she had a heart attack before?

    B. How long does he or she want to stay in the hospital?

    C. Did the patient's physician inform him or her of risk factors associated with heart disease?

    D. Does he or she exercise on a regular basis?

_____   **3.** Which step should NOT be taken to complete a history and physical exam on an unconscious patient with a suspected cardiac problem?

    A. Perform a full-body scan.

    B. Obtain vital signs.

    C. Obtain history from family or bystanders.

    D. Look through the patient's wallet for medical information.

_____   **4.** A patient taking medications such as Lasix or digoxin is likely to have which of the following underlying medical conditions?

    A. Hypertension

    B. Hyperglycemia

    C. CHF

    D. Cerebral vascular accident

_____   **5.** When assessing a cardiac arrest patient, you notice what appears to be a pacemaker implanted in the upper left chest. Care for this patient should include:

    A. attempting to deactivate the device by placing a magnet over it

    B. making sure the AED patches are not directly over the pacemaker device

    C. waiting for ALS to arrive before applying the AED

    D. not using the AED in this situation

MEDICAL

Neurologic Emergencies

General Knowledge

Matching

Match each of the items in the left column to the appropriate definition in the right column.

_____ **1.** Aneurysm	**A.** A period following a seizure that typically includes labored respirations and altered mental status
_____ **2.** Aphasia	**B.** Low blood glucose levels
_____ **3.** Aura	**C.** A surge of electrical activity in the brain, classified as generalized, partial, or status epilepticus
_____ **4.** Brainstem	**D.** Experiencing a warning sense prior to an event
_____ **5.** Cerebellum	**E.** Part of the brain located above the cerebellum; divided into right and left hemispheres
_____ **6.** Cerebrum	**F.** Loss of bowel or bladder control
_____ **7.** Hemiparesis	**G.** Stroke symptoms that go away in less than 24 hours
_____ **8.** Hypoglycemia	**H.** Weakness of one side of the body
_____ **9.** Incontinence	**I.** A seizure lasting longer than 30 minutes or multiple repetitive seizure episodes without regaining consciousness
_____ **10.** Ischemia	**J.** An interruption of blood flow to the brain that results in a loss of brain function
_____ **11.** Postictal state	**K.** Controls muscle and body coordination
_____ **12.** Seizure	**L.** A lack of oxygen that causes cells to not function properly
_____ **13.** Status epilepticus	**M.** A swelling or enlargement of part of an artery resulting from weakness of the arterial wall
_____ **14.** Stroke	**N.** An inability to produce or understand speech
_____ **15.** Transient ischemic attack	**O.** Controls basic functions of the body, such as breathing and blood pressure

Multiple Choice

Read each item carefully and then select the one best response.

_____ **1.** A _____ is typically characterized by unconsciousness and a generalized severe twitching of all of the body's muscles that lasts several minutes or longer.

    A. stroke

    B. postictal state

    C. simple partial seizure

    D. generalized seizure

_____ **2.** The _____ controls the most basic functions of the body, such as breathing, blood pressure, swallowing, and pupil constriction.
   A. brainstem
   B. cerebellum
   C. cerebrum
   D. spinal cord

_____ **3.** At each vertebra in the neck and back, _____ nerves, called spinal nerves, branch out from the spinal cord and carry signals to and from the body.
   A. two
   B. three
   C. four
   D. five

_____ **4.** All of the following are associated with altered mental status EXCEPT:
   A. coma
   B. seizure
   C. incontinence
   D. intoxication

_____ **5.** When blood flow to a particular part of the brain is cut off by a blockage inside a blood vessel, the result is:
   A. a hemorrhagic stroke
   B. atherosclerosis
   C. an ischemic stroke
   D. a cerebral embolism

_____ **6.** The patients who are at the highest risk of hemorrhagic stroke are those who have:
   A. untreated hypertension
   B. hypotension
   C. diabetes
   D. atherosclerosis

_____ **7.** Patients with a ruptured aneurysm typically complain of a sudden severe:
   A. bout of dizziness
   B. headache
   C. altered mental status
   D. thirst

_____ **8.** The plaque that builds up in atherosclerosis obstructs blood flow and interferes with the vessel's ability to:
   A. constrict
   B. dilate
   C. diffuse
   D. exchange gases

_____ **9.** A transient ischemic attack (TIA), or mini-stroke, is the name given to a stroke when symptoms go away on their own in less than:
   A. half an hour
   B. 1 hour
   C. 12 hours
   D. 24 hours

_____ **10.** Patients with a decreased level of consciousness:
   A. should not be given anything by mouth
   B. should be given glucose regardless of the underlying condition
   C. do not require medical care
   D. require immediate assessment of their pupils

_____ **11.** Hypoglycemia can mimic conditions such as:
   A. cystic fibrosis
   B. myocardial infarction
   C. high fevers
   D. stroke

_____ **12.** When assessing a patient with a history of seizure activity, it is important to:
   A. determine whether this episode differs from any previous ones
   B. ask if the patient has had any recent surgeries
   C. assess whether the patient has swallowed his or her tongue
   D. ask whether anyone else in the household has had a seizure

_____ **13.** Signs and symptoms of possible seizure activity include all the following EXCEPT:
   A. altered mental status
   B. incontinence
   C. muscle rigidity and twitching
   D. petechiae

_____ **14.** Common causes of altered mental status include all of the following EXCEPT:
   A. body temperature abnormalities
   B. hypoxia
   C. unequal pupils
   D. hypoglycemia

_____ **15.** The principal difference between a patient who has had a stroke and a patient with hypoglycemia almost always has to do with the:
   A. papillary response
   B. mental status
   C. communication
   D. capillary refill time

_____ **16.** Consider the possibility of _____ in a patient who has had a seizure.
   A. hyperkalemia
   B. hyperglycemia
   C. hypoglycemia
   D. hypertension

_____ **17.** _____ headaches are thought to be caused by changes in blood vessel size in the base of the brain.
   A. Sinus
   B. Tension
   C. Migraine
   D. Compression

_____ **18.** Headache, vomiting, altered mental status, and seizures are all considered early signs of:
   A. increased intracranial pressure
   B. decreased intracranial pressure
   C. increased extracranial pressure
   D. decreased extracranial pressure

_____ **19.** People with _____ have a higher risk of hemorrhagic stroke.
   A. uncontrolled hyperglycemia
   B. uncontrolled hypertension
   C. high fevers
   D. meningitis

_____ **20.** Headaches caused by muscle contractions in the head and neck are typically associated with:
- **A.** sinus headaches
- **B.** migraine headaches
- **C.** compression headaches
- **D.** tension headaches

_____ **21.** The following conditions may simulate a stroke EXCEPT:
- **A.** hyperglycemia
- **B.** a postictal state
- **C.** hypoglycemia
- **D.** subdural bleeding

_____ **22.** When assessing a patient with a possible cerebrovascular accident (CVA), you should check the _____ first.
- **A.** pulse
- **B.** airway
- **C.** pupils
- **D.** blood pressure

_____ **23.** A _____ is usually a warning sign that a larger, significant stroke may occur in the future.
- **A.** heart attack
- **B.** seizure
- **C.** transient ischemic attack
- **D.** migraine headache

_____ **24.** Which mnemonic is used to check a patient's mental status?
- **A.** OPQRST
- **B.** SAMPLE
- **C.** AVPU
- **D.** PEARRL

Questions 25–29 are derived from the following scenario: You are called to a home and find a 56-year-old woman supine in her bed. She appears alert but has slurred speech. Her family tells you she has a history of TIAs and hypertension. Her vital signs are as follows: blood pressure 174/116, heart rate 112 beats/minute, respiratory rate 16 breaths/minute, SpO_2 95%, and blood glucose 97 mg/dL.

_____ **25.** How would you best determine the probability of this patient having a stroke?
- **A.** By using AVPU
- **B.** By using the Cincinnati Prehospital Stroke Scale
- **C.** By using the Glasgow Coma Scale
- **D.** By assessing her blood glucose

_____ **26.** Which of the following would NOT be pertinent information regarding her condition?
- **A.** Knowing the time of onset of symptoms
- **B.** Gathering a list of patient medications
- **C.** Determining if the patient has a facial droop
- **D.** Asking the patient about childhood illnesses

_____ **27.** You ask the patient, "What day is it today?" Her reply is "butterfly." Which area of the brain is likely affected?
- **A.** Occipital lobe
- **B.** Left hemisphere
- **C.** Cerebellum
- **D.** Right hemisphere

28. If the receiving facility told you the cause of her stroke was due to a buildup of calcium and cholesterol, forming a plaque inside the walls of her blood vessels, you would know that this patient has:

A. atherosclerosis

B. multiple sclerosis

C. polyarteritis

D. liver dysfunction

29. Treatment for this patient should include all of the following EXCEPT:

A. providing oxygen to maintain SpO_2 of at least 94%

B. providing rapid transport

C. continuously talking to the patient

D. providing oral glucose

True/False

If you believe the statement to be more true than false, write the letter "T" in the space provided. If you believe the statement to be more false than true, write the letter "F."

1. Longer and more severe seizures will usually result in a longer postictal period.

2. A low oxygen level can affect the entire brain, often causing anxiety, restlessness, and confusion.

3. Febrile seizures result from sudden high fevers and are generally well tolerated by children.

4. Hemiparesis is the inability to speak or understand speech.

5. Patients with migraine headaches are sometimes sensitive to light and sound.

6. Right-sided facial droop is most likely an indication of a problem in the right cerebral hemisphere.

7. Serious conditions that include headache as a symptom are hemorrhagic stroke, brain tumors, and meningitis.

8. A cerebral embolism is an obstruction of a cerebral artery caused by a clot that was formed somewhere else and traveled to the brain.

9. Hemorrhagic stroke is the most common type of stroke.

10. Patients with a stroke affecting the right hemisphere of the brain can usually understand language, but their speech may be slurred.

11. A patient who has bleeding in the brain may have very low blood pressure.

12. All seizures involve muscle twitching and general convulsions.

13. A patient having a seizure may become cyanotic from a lack of oxygen.

14. Patients with a decreased level of consciousness should not be given anything by mouth.

15. Hypoglycemia should be considered in a patient following a motor vehicle collision (MVC) with an altered mental status.

16. Psychological problems and complications of medications can cause altered mental status.

17. Patients who have had a stroke can lose their airway or stop breathing without warning.

18. You should wait until you get an accurate pulse oximeter reading on a seizure patient before administering oxygen.

19. Letting the hospital know the specifics regarding the patient's neurologic symptoms is generally not important.

20. A key piece of information to document is the time of onset of the patient's signs and symptoms.

Fill-in-the-Blank

Read each item carefully and then complete the statement by filling in the missing words.

1. There are _____ cranial nerves.

2. Playing the piano is coordinated by the _____.

3. The two main types of strokes are _____ and _____.

4. The brain is most sensitive to _____, _____, and _____ levels.

5. An incident in which you have more than one patient complaining of a headache may indicate _____ _____ _____.

6. A(n) _____-_____ _____ seizure may cause twitching of the extremity muscles that may spread slowly to another body part.

7. Each hemisphere of the cerebrum controls activities on the _____ side of the body.

8. Focal-onset, impaired-awareness seizures result from abnormal discharges from the _____ lobe of the brain.

9. _____ is a loss of bowel and bladder control and can be due to a generalized seizure.

10. Dilantin and Tegretol are medicines used to control _____ _____.

11. A period following a seizure in which the muscles relax and the breathing becomes labored is called a(n) _____ _____.

12. Weakness on one side of the body is known as _____.

13. A person who was eating prior to having a seizure may have a(n) _____ _____ _____.

14. All patients with an altered mental status should have a(n) _____ _____ _____ score calculated.

15. _____ _____ may reverse stroke symptoms and even stop the stroke if given within 3 to 6 hours of the onset of symptoms.

Labeling

Label the following diagrams with the correct terms.

1. Brain

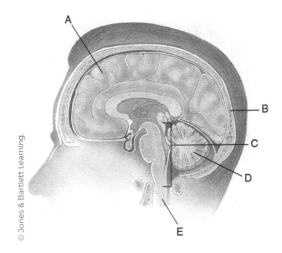

A. _____

B. _____

C. _____

D. _____

E. _____

2. Spinal Cord

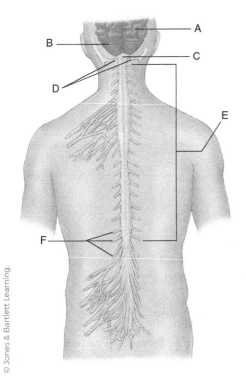

A. _____

B. _____

C. _____

D. _____

E. _____

F. _____

Critical Thinking

Short Answer

Complete this section with short written answers using the space provided.

1. Discuss the Cincinnati Prehospital Stroke Scale, including normal and abnormal findings.

_____

_____

_____

2. Why is prompt transport of stroke patients critical?

_____

_____

_____

3. Describe the characteristics of a postictal state.

_____

_____

_____

4. What is the difference between a focal-onset aware and a focal-onset, impaired-awareness seizure?

_____

_____

_____

5. List three conditions that may simulate stroke.

_____

_____

_____

6. Determine the Glasgow Coma Scale score for the following patients.

_____ **A.** You respond to the scene of a 45-year-old woman with hypoglycemia. As you walk into the room, the patient looks at you and smiles. The patient is oriented to place but does not know the day of the week or the year. When you ask the patient to raise her arms, she smiles at you. When you pinch her hand, she pushes your hand away and says, "Ouch."

_____ **B.** You are at a nursing home where an 84-year-old man was found on the floor next to his bed, having a seizure. The patient is now postictal and opens his eyes when you pinch his hand. When you ask the patient whether he remembers what happened, he responds with garbled speech. The patient is unable to follow your commands but pulls away when you pinch his hand.

_____ **C.** You respond to the scene of an MVC. On arrival, you find a 25-year-old man who was ejected from his vehicle as it rolled down an embankment. The patient fails to open his eyes to any external stimuli. The bystanders state that he has been unresponsive since the crash and has not moved. You place an oral airway into the patient and continue to manage his airway and provide cervical spine immobilization. You attempt multiple times to elicit a painful response; however, the patient does not move his extremities or open his eyes.

_____ **D.** You and your partner are eating at a local restaurant when your server tells you the manager is not feeling well. As you approach the manager, he apologizes to you for interrupting your meal. The patient tells you that he has not felt right since he opened the restaurant this morning. The manager is able to tell you the daily specials on the menu and is able to roll up his sleeves so that you can take his blood pressure.

Ambulance Calls

The following case scenarios provide an opportunity to explore the concerns associated with patient management and to enhance critical-thinking skills. Read each scenario and answer each question to the best of your ability.

1. You are dispatched to a private residence for a "confused man." You arrive to find an older man sitting in a recliner. As you begin your assessment, you notice that he has right-sided weakness and does not seem to understand your questions. He is alone in the home, and it appears that no one lives with him in the residence.

   How would you best manage this patient?

   _____

   _____

   _____

2. You are dispatched to a 36-year-old man who had seizure activity at least an hour ago. The patient is incontinent, cold, clammy, and unresponsive. His friends tell you that the "shaking" stopped and he has not woken up. They thought he might just be tired until they discovered they could not wake him. He has no history of seizure activity. He has diabetes, for which he takes medication.

   How would you best manage this patient?

   _____

   _____

   _____

3. You are dispatched to a local business for "woman with severe headache." The 55-year-old patient states that she has had headaches in the past, but this headache is the worst she has ever had in her life. She feels like the room is spinning around, she is seeing "double," and she feels sick to her stomach. She has a history of hypertension. She tells you that she stopped taking her blood pressure medicine about 6 to 8 months ago because she could no longer afford it.

   How would you best manage this patient?

   _____

   _____

   _____

4. You are dispatched to a local shopping center for a 42-year-old woman who is having a seizure. On arrival, you find your patient alert and sitting in a chair. The patient has a Glasgow Coma Scale score of 15 and states that it has been a few months since she has had a seizure. The patient states that she feels fine and does not want to go to the hospital.

How would you manage this situation?

_____

_____

_____

_____

Skills

Assessment Review

Answer the following questions pertaining to the types of emergencies discussed in this chapter.

Questions 1–4 are derived from the following scenario: You are dispatched to a local residence for a change in mental status. On arrival, you find a 67-year-old man sitting at his kitchen table. The patient seems to be having trouble speaking and is leaning to his left. The patient's wife called 9-1-1 because she thought her husband was having a stroke.

_____ **1.** Which of the following is NOT part of the Cincinnati Prehospital Stroke Scale criteria?

    A. Facial droop

    B. Speech

    C. Gait

    D. Arm drift

_____ **2.** The patient's wife tells you the patient has a history of hypertension, myocardial infarction, renal failure, diabetes, and gastroesophageal reflux disease (GERD). Based on the patient's history, what are possible conditions that could explain his symptoms?

    A. Heart attack

    B. Hypoglycemia

    C. Hyperglycemia

    D. Hyperkalemia

_____ **3.** As you are packaging the patient, the wife says she called 9-1-1 right away because she read about how time was an important factor with stroke patients. With regard to thrombolytic therapy at the hospital, what is the timeline that will allow this therapy to be most effective?

    A. Given within 3 hours of symptom onset

    B. Given within 12 hours of symptom onset

    C. Given within the first 24 hours of symptom onset

    D. There is no optimal time requirement for this treatment.

_____ **4.** While transporting the patient to the hospital, his left-sided weakness and speech improve. By the time you reach the hospital, the patient appears almost normal. Which of the following is most likely to be the underlying cause of the patient's condition?

    A. Hemorrhagic stroke

    B. Ischemic stroke

    C. Transient ischemic attack

    D. Partial simple seizure

Gastrointestinal and Urologic Emergencies

General Knowledge

Matching

Match each of the items in the left column to the appropriate definition in the right column.

_____ **1.** Aneurysm

_____ **2.** Cholecystitis

_____ **3.** Retroperitoneal

_____ **4.** Ulcer

_____ **5.** Hernia

_____ **6.** Ileus

_____ **7.** Guarding

_____ **8.** Uremia

_____ **9.** Emesis

_____ **10.** Referred pain

_____ **11.** Acute abdomen

_____ **12.** Cystitis

_____ **13.** Strangulation

_____ **14.** Peritonitis

_____ **15.** Peritoneum

A. Paralysis of the bowel

B. Pain felt in an area of the body other than the actual source

C. Protective, involuntary abdominal muscle contractions

D. Inflammation of the gallbladder

E. Behind the peritoneum

F. Vomiting

G. A condition of sudden onset of pain within the abdomen

H. A membrane lining the abdomen

I. Swelling or enlargement of a weakened arterial wall

J. A buildup of waste products in the blood as a result of kidney failure

K. A protrusion of a loop of an organ or tissue through an abnormal body opening

L. An obstruction of blood circulation resulting from compression or entrapment of organ tissue

M. Erosion of the stomach or small intestinal lining

N. Inflammation of the bladder

O. Inflammation of the peritoneum

Match the condition in the left column with the appropriate localization of pain in the right column.

_____ **16.** Appendicitis

_____ **17.** Cholecystitis

_____ **18.** Ulcer

_____ **19.** Diverticulitis

_____ **20.** Abdominal aortic aneurysm

_____ **21.** Cystitis

_____ **22.** Kidney infection

_____ **23.** Kidney stone

_____ **24.** Pancreatitis

_____ **25.** Peritonitis

A. Lower midabdomen (retropubic)

B. Right upper quadrant (direct); right shoulder (referred)

C. Upper abdomen (both quadrants); back

D. Costovertebral angle

E. Low part of back and lower quadrants

F. Right lower quadrant (direct); around navel (referred); rebounding pain

G. Anywhere in the abdominal area

H. Right or left flank, radiating to genitalia

I. Left lower quadrant

J. Upper midabdomen or upper part of back

Multiple Choice

Read each item carefully and then select the one best response.

_____ **1.** Peritonitis, with associated fluid loss, is the result of:

    A. abnormal shift of fluid from body tissue into the bloodstream

    B. abnormal shift of fluid from the bloodstream into body tissue

    C. normal shift of fluid from body tissue into the bloodstream

    D. normal shift of fluid from the bloodstream into body tissue

_____ **2.** Distention of the abdomen is gauged by:

    A. visualization

    B. auscultation

    C. palpation

    D. the patient's complaint of pain around the umbilicus

_____ **3.** A hernia that returns to its proper body cavity is said to be:

    A. reducible

    B. extractable

    C. incarcerated

    D. replaceable

_____ **4.** A patient who presents with vomiting, signs of shock, and history of eating disorder is likely to be suffering from:

    A. diverticulitis

    B. Mallory-Weiss syndrome

    C. appendicitis

    D. cholecystitis

_____ **5.** When an organ of the abdomen is enlarged, rough palpation may cause _____ of the organ.

    A. distention

    B. nausea

    C. swelling

    D. rupture

_____ **6.** Severe back pain may be associated with which of the following conditions?

    A. Abdominal aortic aneurysm

    B. Pelvic inflammatory disease (PID)

    C. Appendicitis

    D. Mittelschmerz

_____ **7.** The _____ are found in the retroperitoneal space.

    A. stomach and gallbladder

    B. kidneys, ovaries, and pancreas

    C. liver and pancreas

    D. adrenal glands and uterus

_____ **8.** _____ can be caused by an obstructing gallstone, alcohol abuse, and other diseases.

    A. Appendicitis

    B. A peptic ulcer

    C. Pancreatitis

    D. Diverticulitis

_____ **9.** _____ commonly produces symptoms about 30 minutes after a particularly fatty meal and usually at night.

    A. A peptic ulcer

    B. Cholecystitis

    C. Appendicitis

    D. Pancreatitis

_____ **10.** Which of the following is NOT a common disease that produces signs of an acute abdomen?
   A. Diverticulitis
   B. Cholecystitis
   C. Acute appendicitis
   D. Glomerulonephritis

_____ **11.** _____ occur(s) when there is excess pressure within the portal system and surrounding vessel; it may lead to life-threatening bleeding.
   A. Esophageal rupture
   B. Esophageal varices
   C. Esophageal ulcers
   D. Esophageal reflux

Questions 12–16 are derived from the following scenario: You have been dispatched to the home of a 52-year-old woman with severe flank pain.

_____ **12.** Which of the following would NOT be pertinent regarding the pain?
   A. Do you have a headache?
   B. Do you feel nauseous?
   C. Is the pain constant or intermittent?
   D. Have you been urinating more or less?

_____ **13.** The patient tells you that she has right flank pain that radiates into her groin. What is the most likely cause of her condition?
   A. Cholecystitis
   B. Ileus
   C. Appendicitis
   D. Kidney stone

_____ **14.** In addition to the patient's presentation, which of the following would NOT be an additional expected sign or symptom?
   A. Diarrhea
   B. Hematuria
   C. Nausea
   D. Vomiting

_____ **15.** You should transport her:
   A. in a position of comfort
   B. supine
   C. left lateral recumbent
   D. in the recovery position

_____ **16.** Which of the following is NOT a function of the liver?
   A. It filters toxic substances.
   B. It creates glucose stores.
   C. It acts as a reservoir for bile.
   D. It produces substances for blood clotting.

_____ **17.** A patient presents with lower quadrant abdominal pain, tenderness above the pubic bone, and frequent urination with urgency. What is the most likely underlying condition?
   A. Cholecystitis
   B. Cystitis
   C. Gastroenteritis
   D. Diverticulitis

_____ **18.** Infected pouches in the lining of the colon are described as:
  A. cholecystitis
  B. cystitis
  C. gastroenteritis
  D. diverticulitis

_____ **19.** Pregnancy, straining at stool, and chronic constipation cause increased pressure that could result in:
  A. Mallory-Weiss syndrome
  B. diverticulitis
  C. hemorrhoids
  D. gallstones

_____ **20.** Diarrhea is the principal symptom in:
  A. gastroenteritis
  B. esophagitis
  C. pancreatitis
  D. peptic ulcers

_____ **21.** Bowel inflammation, diverticulitis, and hemorrhoids are common causes of bleeding in the:
  A. upper gastrointestinal (GI) tract
  B. middle GI tract
  C. lower GI tract
  D. urinary tract

_____ **22.** A patient complains of heartburn, pain with swallowing, and feeling like an object is stuck in the throat. Which of the following is the most likely cause?
  A. Esophageal varices
  B. Esophagitis
  C. Peptic ulcer
  D. Gastroenteritis

_____ **23.** Pain that initially starts in the umbilical area and then later moves to the lower right quadrant is typically associated with:
  A. gastroenteritis
  B. pancreatitis
  C. appendicitis
  D. diverticulitis

24. When the abdominal muscles become rigid in an effort to protect the abdomen from further irritation,
_____ this is referred to as:
  A. guarding
  B. tenderness
  C. rebound tenderness
  D. referred pain

_____ **25.** If a patient misses a dialysis treatment, weakness and _____ can be the first in a series of conditions that can become progressively more serious.
  A. diarrhea
  B. rhinorrhea
  C. hearing loss
  D. edema

_____ **26.** _____ regulates the amount of glucose in the bloodstream.
  A. Bicarbonate
  B. Amylase
  C. Insulin
  D. Bile

_____ **27.** Regulation of acidity and blood pressure is largely attributed to the:

    A. liver

    B. kidneys

    C. gallbladder

    D. pancreas

_____ **28.** Which of the following organs is part of the lymphatic system and plays a role in the regulation of red blood cells and the immune system?

    A. Bladder

    B. Liver

    C. Spleen

    D. Pancreas

_____ **29.** Which of the following is NOT part of the male reproductive system?

    A. Epididymis

    B. Prostate gland

    C. Seminal vesicles

    D. Fallopian tubes

_____ **30.** _____ is responsible for the breakdown of starches into sugar.

    A. Insulin

    B. Bile

    C. Amylase

    D. Bicarbonate

True/False

If you believe the statement to be more true than false, write the letter "T" in the space provided. If you believe the statement to be more false than true, write the letter "F."

_____ **1.** Referred pain is a result of the connection between ligaments in the abdominal and chest cavities.

_____ **2.** The adverse effects of dialysis include hypotension, muscle cramps, nausea and vomiting, and hemorrhage and infection at the access site.

_____ **3.** Questioning about bowel habits and flatulence is not necessary and considered unprofessional.

_____ **4.** If a female is of childbearing age, you should question her about her last menstrual period.

_____ **5.** The parietal peritoneum lines the walls of the abdominal cavity.

_____ **6.** Peritonitis is associated with a loss of blood from the abdominal cavity.

_____ **7.** When palpating the abdomen, always start with the quadrant where the patient complains of the most severe pain.

_____ **8.** Massive hemorrhaging is associated with rupture of an abdominal aortic aneurysm.

_____ **9.** Peptic ulcer disease affects both men and women equally.

_____ **10.** Patients with abdominal pain should be transported in a position of comfort.

Labeling

Label the following diagrams with the correct terms.

1. Solid Organs

A. _____

B. _____

C. _____

D. _____

E. _____

F. _____

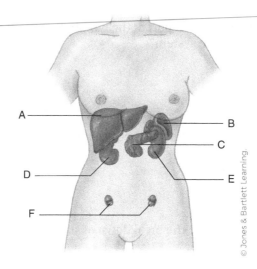

2. Hollow Organs

A. _____

B. _____

C. _____

D. _____

E. _____

F. _____

G. _____

H. _____

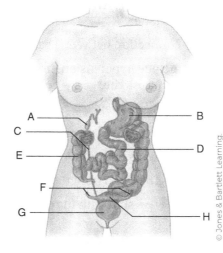

3. Urinary System

A. _____

B. _____

C. _____

D. _____

E. _____

F. _____

G. _____

H. _____

Critical Thinking

Short Answer

Complete this section with short written answers using the space provided.

1. Explain the phenomenon of referred pain.

_____

_____

_____

2. List questions to ask yourself when reassessing a patient with abdominal pain.

_____

_____

_____

3. Why does abdominal distention accompany ileus?

_____

_____

_____

4. Explain the steps used to physically assess the abdomen.

_____

_____

_____

Ambulance Calls

The following case scenarios provide an opportunity to explore the concerns associated with patient management and to enhance critical-thinking skills. Read each scenario and answer each question to the best of your ability.

1. You are called to the local high school nurse's office for a 16-year-old girl complaining of fever and abdominal pain that started around the umbilicus but now is localized to the right lower quadrant. The patient also complains of nausea and vomiting.

How would you best manage this patient?

_____

_____

_____

2. You are dispatched to a long-term care facility for a geriatric man with abdominal pain. On arrival, a staff member tells you that this patient has been bedridden and taking pain medications for the past few weeks. Recently, he's had problems passing a normal bowel movement. He now has a distended, tender abdomen with nausea, vomiting, and tachycardia.

How would you best manage this patient?

_____

_____

_____

3. You are dispatched to the home of another responder for "severe back pain." You arrive to find your coworker writhing in pain on the floor. He tells you that when he tried to urinate (unsuccessfully), he immediately experienced a sharp, cramping sensation in his right side. As you are talking to him, he vomits. After vomiting, he tells you the pain is worse and is now spreading to his groin.

How would you best manage this patient?

_____

_____

_____

Skills

Assessment Review

Answer the following questions pertaining to the assessment of the types of emergencies discussed in this chapter.

Questions 1–5 are derived from the following scenario: You respond to the home of a 46-year-old male complaining of severe back pain. You find the patient in the fetal position in obvious pain. He tells you that his pain is along his right flank and radiates to his groin.

_____ **1.** What will you NOT be able to determine during the primary assessment?
- **A.** The priority of care
- **B.** The patient's level of consciousness
- **C.** Finding and treating any life threats
- **D.** Patient history

_____ **2.** Your partner obtains a SAMPLE history. Which question(s) should she ask?
- **A.** "Do you know what medications you are currently taking?"
- **B.** "Where is your wife?"
- **C.** "Have you traveled out of the country recently?"
- **D.** "Rate your pain on a scale from 1 to 10."

_____ **3.** Which of the following questions would be appropriate given the patient's presentation?
- **A.** "Do you have a headache?"
- **B.** "Do you have pain when you urinate?"
- **C.** "How long have you lived here?"
- **D.** "When was your last tetanus shot?"

_____ **4.** On examination of the abdomen, you should:
- **A.** expose the abdomen and visually assess it
- **B.** palpate the painful area first
- **C.** place the patient in a semi-Fowler's position
- **D.** palpate without watching the patient's face

_____ **5.** During your reassessment, you should do all of the following EXCEPT:
- **A.** repeat the primary assessment
- **B.** repeat the secondary assessment
- **C.** reassure the patient
- **D.** make your initial transport decision

CHAPTER

20 Endocrine and Hematologic Emergencies

General Knowledge

Matching

Match each of the items in the left column to the appropriate definition in the right column.

_____	**1.** Hormone	**A.** Inherited disease that affects red blood cells
_____	**2.** Sickle cell disease	**B.** The study of blood-related diseases
_____	**3.** Type 1 diabetes	**C.** Diabetes caused by autoimmune destruction of pancreatic beta cells
_____	**4.** Acidosis	**D.** Excessive eating
_____	**5.** Insulin	**E.** Deep, rapid breathing
_____	**6.** Symptomatic hyperglycemia	**F.** Frequent urination
_____	**7.** Polyuria	**G.** A tendency to develop blood clots
_____	**8.** Thrombophilia	**H.** Excessive thirst persisting for a long period of time
_____	**9.** Polyphagia	**I.** Diabetes caused by resistance to insulin
_____	**10.** Hematology	**J.** A chemical produced by a gland that regulates body organs
_____	**11.** Glucose	**K.** A disorder affecting the metabolism of glucose
_____	**12.** Kussmaul respirations	**L.** An extremely high blood glucose level
_____	**13.** Hyperglycemia	**M.** A pathologic condition resulting from the accumulation of acids in the body
_____	**14.** Diabetes mellitus	**N.** A disorder that causes an inability to develop blood clots
_____	**15.** Polydipsia	**O.** A hormone that enables glucose to enter the cells
_____	**16.** Hemophilia	**P.** Primary fuel, along with oxygen, for cellular metabolism
_____	**17.** Type 2 diabetes	**Q.** A state of unconsciousness resulting from several problems, including ketoacidosis, dehydration, and hyperglycemia

Multiple Choice

Read each item carefully and then select the one best response.

_____ **1.** When the body's cells do not receive the glucose they require, the body resorts to burning _____ for energy.

    A. fats

    B. proteins

    C. blood cells

    D. ketones

_____ **2.** Normal blood glucose levels range from _____ mg/dL.

    A. 80 to 120

    B. 90 to 140

    C. 70 to 110

    D. 60 to 100

_____ **3.** A sickle cell–related issue that results in unintentional clot formation is known as a(n):

   A. hemolytic crisis

   B. aplastic crisis

   C. splenic sequestration crisis

   D. vasoocclusive crisis

_____ **4.** Diabetes mellitus is a metabolic disorder in which the hormone _____ is missing or the body has become resistant to it.

   A. estrogen

   B. adrenaline

   C. insulin

   D. epinephrine

_____ **5.** Emergency care of a patient with hematologic disorder includes all of the following EXCEPT:

   A. rapid transport for patients with an altered mental status

   B. providing supportive and symptomatic care

   C. oxygen at 4 L/min for patients with inadequate breathing

   D. placing patients in a position of comfort

_____ **6.** The accumulation of ketones and fatty acids in blood tissue can lead to a dangerous condition in diabetic patients known as:

   A. diabetic ketoacidosis

   B. insulin shock

   C. hyperosmolar hyperglycemic nonketotic coma (HHNC)

   D. hypoglycemia

_____ **7.** The term for excessive eating as a result of cellular "hunger" is:

   A. polyuria

   B. polydipsia

   C. polyphagia

   D. polyphony

_____ **8.** Insulin is produced by the:

   A. adrenal glands

   B. hypothalamus

   C. spleen

   D. pancreas

_____ **9.** The patient with diabetic ketoacidosis (DKA) will generally have a fingerstick glucose level higher than:

   A. 100 mg/dL

   B. 200 mg/dL

   C. 300 mg/dL

   D. 400 mg/dL

_____ **10.** Where is glycogen stored in the body?

   A. Liver

   B. Brain

   C. Pancreas

   D. Heart

_____ **11.** A sweet or fruity odor on the breath of a patient is commonly found in what condition?

   A. Hypoglycemia

   B. Hyperglycemia

   C. Hemophilia

   D. Thrombophilia

_____ **12.** What condition increases a patient's risk for developing thrombophilia?
   A. Diabetes
   B. Sickle cell disease
   C. Cirrhosis of the liver
   D. Cancer

_____ **13.** Oral diabetic medications do NOT include:
   A. Micronase
   B. Glucotrol
   C. Januvia
   D. insulin

_____ **14.** Which of the following is a contraindication to the administration of oral glucose?
   A. Inability to swallow
   B. History of diabetic ketoacidosis
   C. Active infection
   D. Recent abdominal surgery

_____ **15.** _____ is the hormone that is normally produced by the pancreas that enables glucose to enter the cells.
   A. Insulin
   B. Adrenaline
   C. Estrogen
   D. Epinephrine

_____ **16.** The term for excessive urination is:
   A. polyuria
   B. polydipsia
   C. polyphagia
   D. polyphony

_____ **17.** When fat is used as an immediate energy source, _____ and fatty acids are formed as waste products.
   A. dextrose
   B. sucrose
   C. ketones
   D. bicarbonate

_____ **18.** An African American patient complaining of severe, generalized pain may have undiagnosed:
   A. sickle cell disease
   B. type 1 diabetes
   C. thrombopenia
   D. hemophilia

_____ **19.** The onset of hypoglycemia can occur within:
   A. seconds
   B. minutes
   C. hours
   D. days

_____ **20.** Without _____, or with very low levels, brain cells rapidly suffer permanent damage.
   A. epinephrine
   B. ketones
   C. bicarbonate
   D. glucose

_____ 21. _____ is/are a potentially life-threatening complication of hypoglycemia.
- **A.** Kussmaul respirations
- **B.** Hypotension
- **C.** Seizures
- **D.** Polydipsia

_____ 22. Diabetic ketoacidosis may develop as a result of:
- **A.** too little insulin
- **B.** too much insulin
- **C.** overhydration
- **D.** metabolic alkalosis

_____ 23. Always suspect hypoglycemia in any patient with:
- **A.** Kussmaul respirations
- **B.** an altered mental status
- **C.** nausea and vomiting
- **D.** stridor

_____ 24. The most important step in caring for the unresponsive diabetic patient is to:
- **A.** give oral glucose immediately
- **B.** perform a focused assessment
- **C.** open the airway
- **D.** obtain a SAMPLE history

_____ 25. Determination of hyperglycemia or hypoglycemia should be:
- **A.** made before transport of the patient
- **B.** made before administration of oral glucose
- **C.** determined by a urine glucose test
- **D.** based on your knowledge of the signs and symptoms of each condition

_____ 26. When obtaining the medical history of a patient experiencing a sickle cell crisis, you should:
- **A.** determine the patient's level of consciousness
- **B.** ask the patient about recent illnesses or stress
- **C.** take the patient's vital signs
- **D.** avoid asking about previous sickle cell crises

_____ 27. A deep vein thrombosis (DVT) is a worrisome risk for patients who have had:
- **A.** gallbladder surgery
- **B.** alcoholism
- **C.** pneumonia
- **D.** joint replacement surgery

_____ 28. When reassessing the diabetic patient after administration of oral glucose, watch for all of the following EXCEPT:
- **A.** airway problems
- **B.** seizures
- **C.** sudden loss of consciousness
- **D.** joint pain

_____ 29. Signs and symptoms associated with hypoglycemia include:
- **A.** warm, dry skin
- **B.** slow pulse
- **C.** Kussmaul respirations
- **D.** anxious or combative behavior

_____ **30.** Hospital interventions for hemophilia may include all of the following EXCEPT:
    A. blood transfusions
    B. analgesics for pain
    C. intravenous (IV) therapy
    D. decontamination

_____ **31.** Because hyperglycemia is a complex metabolic condition that usually develops over time and involves all of the tissues of the body, correcting this condition may:
    A. be accomplished quickly through the use of oral glucose
    B. require rapid infusion of IV fluid to prevent permanent brain damage
    C. take many hours in a hospital setting
    D. include a reduction in the amount of insulin normally taken by the patient

_____ **32.** A patient with hypoglycemia or hyperglycemia may appear to be:
    A. having a heart attack
    B. perfectly normal
    C. intoxicated
    D. having a stroke

True/False

If you believe the statement to be more true than false, write the letter "T" in the space provided. If you believe the statement to be more false than true, write the letter "F."

_____ **1.** When patients use fat for energy, the fat waste products increase the amount of acid in the blood and tissue.

_____ **2.** The life span of a normal red blood cell is approximately 50 to 75 days.

_____ **3.** If blood glucose levels remain low, a patient may lose consciousness or have permanent brain damage.

_____ **4.** Higher glucose levels in the blood cause the excretion of glucose in urine.

_____ **5.** People with hemophilia A have an increased ability to create a clot after an injury.

_____ **6.** Diabetic emergencies can occur when a patient's blood glucose level gets too high or drops too low.

_____ **7.** Diabetic patients may require insulin to control their blood glucose.

_____ **8.** Insulin is one of the basic sugars essential for cell metabolism in humans.

_____ **9.** A clot that forms deep in a vein is called an aplastic crisis.

_____ **10.** Diabetes can cause kidney failure, blindness, and damage to blood vessels.

_____ **11.** Most children with diabetes are insulin dependent

_____ **12.** Within the red blood cells, leukocytes are responsible for carrying oxygen.

_____ **13.** Many adults with diabetes can control their blood glucose levels with diet alone.

Fill-in-the-Blank

Read each item carefully and then complete the statement by filling in the missing words.

1. The full name of diabetes is _____ _____.

2. _____ is a general term for many different conditions that result in the blood clotting more easily than normal.

3. Type 1 diabetes is considered to be a(n) _____ problem, in which the body becomes allergic to its own tissues and literally destroys them.

4. An African American patient or any patient of _____ descent who complains of severe pain may have undiagnosed _____ _____ disease.

5. Diabetes is defined as a lack of or _____ action of insulin.

6. In _____, the patient cannot drink enough fluid to keep up with the exceedingly high glucose levels in the blood.

7. _____ is the study and prevention of blood-_____ diseases.

8. A patient with hypoglycemia needs _____ immediately, and a patient with hyperglycemia needs _____ and IV fluid therapy.

Fill-in-the-Table

	Hyperglycemia	Hypoglycemia
History		
Onset		
Skin		
Infection		
Gastrointestinal Tract		
Thirst		
Hunger		
Vomiting/abdominal pain		
Respiratory System		
Breathing		
Odor of breath		
Cardiovascular System		
Blood pressure		
Pulse		
Nervous System		
Consciousness		
Treatment		
Response		

Critical Thinking

Multiple Choice

Read each critical-thinking item carefully and then select the one best response.

Questions 1–4 are derived from the following scenario: A 54-year-old golfer collapsed on the 17th green at the golf course. His friend said he wasn't feeling well after the eighth hole but insisted on walking and finishing out the game. His skin is pale, cool, and diaphoretic, and he provides incoherent answers to your questions.

_____ 1. During your rapid full-body scan, you discover a medical alert necklace around his neck that reads "Type 1 Diabetic." This tells you that he most likely:
- **A.** developed diabetes later in life
- **B.** produces inadequate amounts of insulin
- **C.** takes noninsulin-type oral medications
- **D.** will develop HHNS

_____ 2. His blood glucose level is 65 mg/dL. You:
- **A.** do not suspect hypoglycemia and begin to think that his condition is cardiac in nature
- **B.** suspect hyperglycemia and proceed to give oral glucose
- **C.** suspect hypoglycemia and proceed to give oral glucose
- **D.** suspect hypoglycemia, but oral glucose is contraindicated for him

_____ 3. The patient loses consciousness, and a second blood glucose level reads 48 mg/dL. You should do all of the following EXCEPT:
- **A.** call for, or rendezvous with, an ALS unit
- **B.** ensure a patent airway
- **C.** provide high-flow oxygen
- **D.** give oral glucose

_____ 4. Because the patient is unconscious and his blood glucose level is 48 mg/dL, how should the glucose be delivered?
- **A.** Between the cheek and gum
- **B.** Placed on the back of the tongue
- **C.** Placed on the tip of the tongue
- **D.** You should not deliver oral glucose.

Short Answer

Complete this section with short written answers using the space provided.

1. What is insulin, and what is its role in metabolism?

_____

_____

_____

2. What are the preparations of commercially available oral glucose?

_____

_____

_____

3. What two basic complications are caused by the shape of the red blood cells in people with sickle cell disease?

_____

_____

_____

4. When should you not give oral glucose to a patient experiencing a suspected diabetic emergency?

_____

_____

_____

5. How can thrombophilia lead to a pulmonary embolism?

_____

_____

_____

6. List at least four key signs and symptoms of HHNS.

_____

_____

_____

7. When taking a history on a patient with known diabetes, what questions should be asked?

_____

_____

_____

8. If a diabetic patient was "fine" 2 hours ago and now is unconscious and unresponsive, which diabetes-related condition would you suspect and why?

_____

_____

_____

Ambulance Calls

The following case scenarios provide an opportunity to explore the concerns associated with patient management and to enhance critical-thinking skills. Read each scenario and answer each question to the best of your ability.

1. You are called to a local residence where you find a 22-year-old woman supine in bed, unresponsive to your attempts to rouse her. She is cold and clammy, with gurgling respirations. Her mother tells you that her only history is diabetes, which she has had since she was a small child.

   How would you best manage this patient?

   _____

   _____

   _____

2. You are requested to respond to a local convenience store for an unknown medical problem. On arrival, you find a young African American man sitting on the curb, clutching his torso, and crying. He tells you that he is in severe pain and has a history of sickle cell disease.

   How would you best manage this patient?

   _____

   _____

   _____

3. You are dispatched to assist with a diabetic patient well known in your department for being noncompliant with his medications and diet. You have responded numerous times to his residence, all for instances of low blood sugar. Family members greet you at the door and say, "It's Jon again. Just give him some sugar like you usually do." You walk into the patient's bedroom to discover him unconscious, with snoring respirations.

   How would you best manage this patient?

   _____

   _____

   _____

Fill-in-the-Patient Care Report

Read the incident scenario and then complete the following patient care report (PCR).

"Truck Nine, trauma emergency," the dispatcher's voice bursts from the radio on your hip, drawing glances from several people around you in the grocery store.

"Go ahead to Nine," your partner, Jerry, responds over the radio from somewhere else in the store.

"Truck Nine, trauma emergency at 12556 Old Lake House Drive, for a laceration with uncontrolled bleeding. Showing you dispatched at 1752."

Within 3 minutes, both of you converge on the ambulance parked outside under a line of spruce trees and are en route through rush-hour traffic to the subdivision on the east end of the town lake.

"Central, Truck Nine, we are on scene," you say quickly into the mic before opening your door and climbing from the truck.

"Showing you on scene at 1803," comes the muffled reply from the cab radio.

You are quickly ushered into the home and led by a frantic woman to an upstairs bedroom. As you pass through the door, you see a 14-year-old boy holding a blood-soaked T-shirt against his forearm. In front of him on a desk is a half-completed wooden model of an old pirate ship, now sprinkled with darkening blood.

"The blade slipped, and he cut his arm," the boy's mother says rapidly. "Oh, please help him; he's got hemophilia!" You gently move the soaked T-shirt and see a 1-inch (3-cm) laceration that is bleeding profusely, running steadily down his arm and onto the carpet. You immediately apply pressure to the wound and direct Jerry to start high-flow oxygen therapy. You position the patient onto the stair chair and move him down to the wheeled stretcher in the living room, happy that he weighs only 132 pounds (60 kg).

Once on the gurney, you and Jerry cover the boy with a blanket and load him into the ambulance. You look at your watch (1813) and ask Jerry to get a quick blood pressure on the patient while you continue holding pressure on the wound.

"108 over 60," he says, before closing you in with the patient and climbing into the cab of the truck while you check his pulse and count 98 beats/min, get a respiratory rate of 16 breaths/min with good tidal volume, and get a pulse oximetry reading of 96%. While en route to the hospital, you realize that the bleeding is just not going to stop with pressure, so you apply a tourniquet on the patient's arm and clearly document the time.

At 1819, Jerry backs into the trauma center's ambulance parking bay, and you both roll the patient into the waiting trauma bay, where you turn him over to the waiting team and provide a verbal report.

Fill-in-the-Patient Care Report

EMS Patient Care Report (PCR)				
Date:	Incident No.:	Nature of Call:		Location:
Dispatched:	En Route:	At Scene:	Transport:	At Hospital:	In Service:

Patient Information

Age: Sex: Weight (in kg [lb]):	Allergies: Medications: Past Medical History: Chief Complaint:

Vital Signs

Time:	BP:	Pulse:	Respirations:	SpO$_2$:
Time:	BP:	Pulse:	Respirations:	SpO$_2$:
Time:	BP:	Pulse:	Respirations:	SpO$_2$:

EMS Treatment
(circle all that apply)

Oxygen @ ___ L/min via (circle one): NC NRM BVM	Assisted Ventilation	Airway Adjunct	CPR
Defibrillation	Bleeding Control	Bandaging	Splinting	Other:

Narrative

CHAPTER

21

Allergy and Anaphylaxis

General Knowledge

Matching

Match each of the items in the left column to the appropriate definition in the right column.

_____ **1.** Allergic reaction

_____ **2.** Leukotrienes

_____ **3.** Wheezing

_____ **4.** Urticaria

_____ **5.** Stridor

_____ **6.** Allergen

_____ **7.** Wheal

_____ **8.** Toxin

A. A substance made by the body; released in anaphylaxis

B. A harsh, high-pitched inspiratory sound, usually resulting from upper airway obstruction

C. A raised, swollen area on the skin resulting from an insect bite or allergic reaction

D. An exaggerated immune response to any substance

E. Raised areas on the skin that itch or burn, sometimes called hives

F. A poison or harmful substance

G. A substance that causes an allergic reaction

H. High-pitched, whistling breath sound usually resulting from bronchospasm or bronchoconstriction, usually heard on exhalation

Multiple Choice

Read each item carefully and then select the one best response.

_____ **1.** Steps for assisting a patient with administration of an EpiPen include:

    A. shaking the injector to mix the medication

    B. placing the tip of the auto-injector against the lateral part of the patient's thigh

    C. recapping the injector before placing it in the trash

    D. holding the injector in place for 30 seconds

_____ **2.** Which of the following is NOT one of the five common allergen categories?

    A. Food

    B. Insect bites

    C. Plants

    D. Environments

_____ **3.** One commonly observed sign of anaphylaxis includes:

    A. burning with urination

    B. angioedema

    C. diarrhea

    D. anosmia

_____ **4.** Signs and symptoms of insect stings or bites include all of the following EXCEPT:

    A. swelling

    B. ecchymosis

    C. localized heat

    D. wheals

_____   **5.** All of the following are true regarding allergic reactions EXCEPT:

   A. Mild reactions will usually only require supportive care.

   B. A stiff card should be used to remove an insect stinger if necessary.

   C. All allergic reactions will require epinephrine administration.

   D. Deterioration can be extremely rapid when anaphylaxis is present.

_____   **6.** Speed is essential because in severe cases of anaphylaxis, _____ can occur rapidly.

   A. urticaria

   B. compensation

   C. death

   D. recovery

_____   **7.** Questions to ask when obtaining a history from a patient appearing to have an allergic reaction include:

   A. whether the patient has recently traveled

   B. what the patient ate yesterday

   C. asking bystanders if anyone else is ill

   D. how the patient was exposed

_____   **8.** The dosage of epinephrine in an adult EpiPen is:

   A. 0.10 mg

   B. 0.15 mg

   C. 0.30 mg

   D. 0.50 mg

_____   **9.** Epinephrine, whether made by the body or by a drug manufacturer, works rapidly to:

   A. decrease the pulse rate and blood pressure

   B. increase an allergic reaction

   C. increase wheezing

   D. relieve bronchospasm

_____   **10.** Because the stinger of the honeybee is barbed and remains in the wound, it can continue to inject venom for up to:

   A. 1 minute

   B. 15 minutes

   C. 20 minutes

   D. several hours

_____   **11.** You should not use tweezers or forceps to remove an embedded stinger because:

   A. squeezing may cause the stinger to inject more venom into the wound

   B. the stinger may break off in the wound

   C. the tweezers are not sterile and may cause infection

   D. removing the stinger may cause bleeding

_____   **12.** Your assessment of the patient experiencing an allergic reaction should include evaluations of all of the following EXCEPT the:

   A. respiratory system

   B. circulatory system

   C. skin

   D. reproductive system

_____   **13.** Allergic reactions to certain foods, such as shellfish or nuts, may take up to _____ minutes before a reaction appears.

   A. 10

   B. 20

   C. 30

   D. 60

_____ **14.** Wheezing occurs because excessive _____ and mucus are secreted into the bronchial passages.
- **A.** fluid
- **B.** carbon dioxide
- **C.** blood
- **D.** oxygen

True/False

If you believe the statement to be more true than false, write the letter "T" in the space provided. If you believe the statement to be more false than true, write the letter "F."

_____ **1.** Allergic reactions can occur in response to almost any substance.

_____ **2.** An allergic reaction occurs when the body has an immune response to a substance.

_____ **3.** Wheezing is a low-pitched breath sound, usually resulting from blockage of the airway, and is heard on expiration.

_____ **4.** For a patient appearing to have an allergic reaction with respiratory distress, give high-flow oxygen.

Fill-in-the-Blank

Read each item carefully and then complete the statement by filling in the missing words.

1. Wheezing, a high-pitched, whistling breath sound, is typically heard on _____.

2. Small areas of generalized itching or burning that appear as multiple, small, raised areas on the skin are called _____.

3. The stinger of the honeybee is _____, so the bee cannot withdraw it.

4. An allergic reaction involving multiple body systems is called _____.

5. The presence of _____ _____ or respiratory distress indicates that the patient is having a severe enough allergic reaction to lead to death.

6. Epinephrine reverses hypotension by constricting the _____ _____.

Critical Thinking

Multiple Choice

Read each critical-thinking item carefully and then select the one best response.

You have been called to a park where a local church is holding a potluck dinner. As you exit your ambulance, a woman approaches you holding her 7-year-old son, who is wheezing and having difficulty breathing. She informs you that he had inadvertently eaten a brownie with nuts, and he is allergic to nuts.

_____ **1.** You lift the child's shirt and find small, raised areas that he is trying to scratch. They are likely to be:
- **A.** leukotrienes
- **B.** histamines
- **C.** urticaria
- **D.** toxins

_____ **2.** Why is this patient wheezing?

  A. He has had an envenomation.

  B. His bronchioles are constricting.

  C. His bronchioles are dilating.

  D. His uvula has swollen.

_____ **3.** The child's mother has an EpiPen that contains the appropriate dose of epinephrine for a child. What dose would that be?

  A. 0.8 mg

  B. 0.5 mg

  C. 0.4 mg

  D. 0.15 mg

_____ **4.** When assisting with an auto-injector, how long should you hold the pen against the thigh?

  A. 3 seconds

  B. 5 seconds

  C. 10 seconds

  D. 30 seconds

_____ **5.** After removing the auto-injector from the child's thigh, you should do all of the following EXCEPT:

  A. record the time

  B. record the dose

  C. reassess his vital signs

  D. place ice over the injection site

Short Answer

Complete this section with short written answers using the space provided.

1. List the common side effects of epinephrine.

_____

_____

_____

2. What are the five general categories that most often cause allergic reactions?

_____

_____

_____

3. What are the steps for administering or assisting with the administration of an EpiPen?

_____

_____

_____

4. What are the common respiratory and cardiovascular signs and symptoms of an allergic reaction?

_____

_____

_____

Ambulance Calls

The following case scenarios provide an opportunity to explore the concerns associated with patient management and to enhance critical-thinking skills. Read each scenario and answer each question to the best of your ability.

1. You are dispatched to assist a 12-year-old child who was climbing a tree and apparently disturbed a wasp nest. When you arrive, the child is lying under the tree, and the nest is on the ground next to her.

How would you best manage this patient?

_____

_____

_____

2. You are dispatched to a local seafood restaurant for a person who is having difficulty breathing. On arrival, you find a 22-year-old woman with facial edema, cyanosis around the lips, audible wheezing, and urticaria on her face and upper body. Her boyfriend tells you she ate shrimp and she is allergic to them. He also tells you she has some medicine in her purse and hands you an EpiPen prescribed to her.

How would you best manage this patient?

_____

_____

_____

Fill-in-the-Patient Care Report

Read the incident scenario and then complete the following patient care report (PCR).

"Unit six-twelve, emergency assignment, you're headed to Crab Town Restaurant at 231 Seaside Parkway for an allergic reaction. Showing you dispatched at 1734."

Your partner, Ed, confirms the dispatch over the radio as you activate the lights and sirens and steer toward Seaside Parkway.

"Six-twelve is on scene," Ed says, snapping the microphone back into its holder as you shift the ambulance into park and pull on a pair of exam gloves.

"Unit six-twelve, copying you on scene at 1742."

As you roll the gurney into the restaurant, you are met by a frantic waitress who leads you to a small table at the rear of the bustling restaurant. A 37-year-old man is holding the edge of the table so tightly that his knuckles are white as he struggles to breathe. His face, neck, and hands are obviously swollen; bright hives are visible just above the collar of his shirt; and there is a bluish tinge to his lips and fingernails.

"Get some oxygen on him, Ed, and get the bag-mask device ready," you say, pulling the portable radio from your belt. "I'm going to call for an ALS crew."

As Ed places a nonrebreathing mask onto the patient with 15 L/min of oxygen, you request an ALS rendezvous and then turn to the small group of terrified diners who were sitting with the patient. "Does he have an EpiPen or anything for this allergy?"

"No," a woman says, tears smearing the mascara down her cheeks. "He's my husband, and I've never seen him react like this to anything."

"Let's load him, Ed!" You pull the gurney over, and the two of you help the 63-kg (138-lb) patient onto it as he sucks noisily on the oxygen. About 6 minutes after arriving, Ed is pulling the ambulance out of the parking lot while you get a baseline set of vitals on the patient.

His blood pressure is 100/64 mm Hg, pulse is 116 beats/min, and you note that it is strong and rapid. His respirations are 26 breaths/min and becoming more labored by the minute, coupled with an obvious anxiety; the patient is becoming very restless. The digital pulse oximeter screen shows 92%.

"Okay, sir, I'm going to help you to breathe." You grab the bag-mask device and show it to him. "I'm going to help your breathing with this. Try to relax, although I know that's tough right now."

You remove the nonrebreathing mask and attach the bag-mask device to the truck oxygen supply and begin gently forcing air into the patient with every inhalation. He is beginning to panic, so you have to reassure him loudly and constantly every time that you squeeze the bag.

The back door suddenly pops open, and a paramedic whom you know climbs aboard with his jump kit. You feel the ambulance start rolling again.

"Great job, my friend," he says to you. "Keep it up while I get my stuff together." The paramedic quickly assembles a syringe and jabs it into the patient's upper arm and then begins to monitor his pulse and breathing. Within a few minutes, you can see that the swelling is reversing, and the patient starts to take deeper breaths, exhaling in relieved yells. You look at your watch (1755) and get another set of vitals while the paramedic talks calmly to the patient. His blood pressure is now 140/94 mm Hg, pulse rate is 128 beats/min, and breathing is 18 breaths/min and much less labored. The SpO$_2$ is showing 96%, and you reconnect the nonrebreathing mask and place it on the patient.

You call in a quick but thorough verbal report to the receiving facility and provide the ETA given by Ed.

At 1801, you arrive at the hospital, followed closely by the ALS ambulance that the paramedic had come from, and wheel the deeply breathing patient through the emergency department doors. You and the paramedic provide verbal reports to the physician, and he assumes care of the quickly recovering patient.

At 1814, your unit goes back into service.

Fill-in-the-Patient Care Report

EMS Patient Care Report (PCR)					
Date:	Incident No.:		Nature of Call:		Location:
Dispatched:	En Route:	At Scene:	Transport:	At Hospital:	In Service:
Patient Information					
Age: Sex: Weight (in kg [lb]):			Allergies: Medications: Past Medical History: Chief Complaint:		
Vital Signs					
Time:	BP:		Pulse:	Respirations:	SpO$_2$:
Time:	BP:		Pulse:	Respirations:	SpO$_2$:
Time:	BP:		Pulse:	Respirations:	SpO$_2$:
EMS Treatment (circle all that apply)					
Oxygen @ ____ L/min via (circle one): NC NRM BVM		Assisted Ventilation	Airway Adjunct		CPR
Defibrillation	Bleeding Control	Bandaging	Splinting		Other:
Narrative					

Skills

Skill Drill

Test your knowledge of this skill by filling in the correct words in the photo captions.

Skill Drill 21-1: Using an EpiPen Auto-Injector

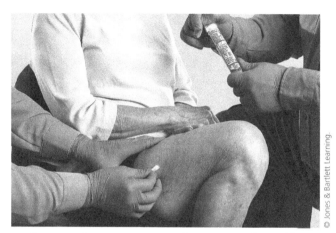

© Jones & Bartlett Learning.

1. Remove the _____ safety cap, and quickly wipe the thigh with _____, if possible.

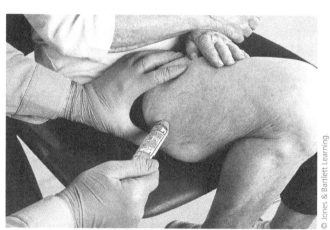

© Jones & Bartlett Learning.

2. Place the _____ of the auto-injector against the _____ part of the thigh. Push the auto-injector _____ against the thigh until a(n) _____ is heard. Hold it in place until all the _____ has been injected (3 seconds).

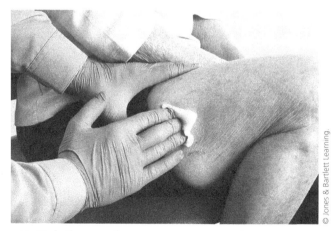

© Jones & Bartlett Learning.

3. Rub the area for _____ seconds.

Assessment Review

Answer the following questions pertaining to the assessment of the types of emergencies discussed in this chapter.

_____ 1. As you begin to assess a patient suspected of anaphylactic shock, which of these steps would be done first?

    A. Assess and treat for life threats.

    B. Assess lung sounds.

    C. Provide high-flow oxygen.

    D. Obtain a pulse oximetry reading.

_____ 2. After assisting with an EpiPen, what is the first thing that should be done?

    A. Make sure the medication is not expired.

    B. Take a set of vital signs.

    C. Place the used EpiPen in a biohazard container.

    D. Rub the area for 10 seconds.

_____ 3. When using the EpiPen auto-injector, do all of the following EXCEPT:

    A. remove the safety cap

    B. wipe the thigh with antiseptic

    C. push the auto-injector firmly against the thigh for about 3 seconds

    D. place ice over the injection site

CHAPTER

22 | Toxicology

General Knowledge

Matching

Match each of the items in the left column to the appropriate definition in the right column.

_____ **1.** Poison

_____ **2.** Substance abuse

_____ **3.** Antidote

_____ **4.** Tolerance

_____ **5.** Cholinergic

_____ **6.** Ingestion

_____ **7.** Hematemesis

_____ **8.** Stimulant

_____ **9.** Opioid

_____ **10.** Sedative

_____ **11.** Anticholinergic

A. A substance that decreases activity and excitement

B. A type of narcotic medication used to relieve pain

C. Atropine, Benadryl, some cyclic antidepressants

D. A need for increasing amounts of a drug to obtain the same effect

E. An agent that produces an excited state

F. A substance whose chemical action can damage body structures or impair body functions

G. A substance that will counteract the effects of a particular poison

H. Misuse of any substance to produce a desired effect

I. Taking a substance by mouth

J. Overstimulates body functions controlled by parasympathetic nerves

K. Vomiting blood

Multiple Choice

Read each item carefully and then select the one best response.

_____ **1.** Activated charcoal is in the form of a(n):

 A. elixir

 B. suspension

 C. syrup

 D. emulsion

_____ **2.** The presence of burning of the mucous membranes around the mouth suggests:

 A. ingestion of depressants

 B. ingestion of poison

 C. overdose of heroin

 D. that the patient may be a heavy smoker

_____ **3.** Treatment for ingestion of poisonous plants includes all of the following EXCEPT:

 A. assessing the patient's airway and vital signs

 B. taking the plant to the emergency department

 C. administering activated charcoal

 D. prompt transport

_____ 4. The most important consideration in caring for a patient who has been exposed to an organophosphate insecticide or some other cholinergic agent is to:
   A. maintain the airway
   B. apply high-flow oxygen
   C. avoid exposure yourself
   D. initiate CPR

_____ 5. Which of the following would NOT provide clues to the nature of the poison?
   A. Patient age
   B. Scattered pills
   C. Chemicals
   D. A needle or syringe

_____ 6. Which of the following is TRUE regarding injected poisons?
   A. Injected poisons cannot be diluted after injection.
   B. Injected poisons can be easily removed from the body.
   C. Injected poisons are absorbed over time.
   D. Injected poisons only include intravenous drugs.

_____ 7. The major side effect of ingesting activated charcoal is:
   A. depressed respirations
   B. overproduction of stomach acid
   C. constipation
   D. increased blood pressure

_____ 8. Alcohol is a powerful central nervous system depressant. It:
   A. sharpens the sense of awareness
   B. slows reflexes
   C. increases reaction time
   D. increases reflexes

_____ 9. Which of the following is NOT a narcotic?
   A. Heroin
   B. Morphine
   C. Ativan
   D. Codeine

_____ 10. Which of the following is NOT part of the treatment of patients who have overdosed with sedative-hypnotics and have respiratory depression?
   A. Provide airway clearance.
   B. Provide ventilatory assistance.
   C. Provide prompt transport.
   D. Induce vomiting.

_____ 11. Anticholinergic medications have properties that block the _____ nerves.
   A. parasympathetic
   B. sympathetic
   C. adrenergic
   D. parasympatholytic

_____ 12. _____ crack produces the most rapid means of absorption and therefore the most potent effect.
   A. Injected
   B. Absorbed
   C. Smoked
   D. Ingested

_____ **13.** Cholinergic agents overstimulate normal body functions that are controlled by parasympathetic nerves, causing:

    A. increased salivation

    B. pupil dilation

    C. decreased urination

    D. decreased lacrimation

_____ **14.** Signs and symptoms of staphylococcal food poisoning include:

    A. difficulty speaking

    B. nausea, vomiting, and diarrhea

    C. skin boils or abscesses

    D. respiratory distress

_____ **15.** Inhalant effects range from mild drowsiness to coma, but unlike most other sedative-hypnotics, these agents may often cause:

    A. seizures

    B. vomiting

    C. swelling of the tongue

    D. rashes

_____ **16.** Cocaine is called all of the following EXCEPT:

    A. lady

    B. snow

    C. blow

    D. weed

_____ **17.** The effects of bath salts can last as long as:

    A. 12 hours

    B. 24 hours

    C. 48 hours

    D. 72 hours

_____ **18.** The ingestion of marijuana can lead to cannabinoid hyperemesis syndrome, resulting in extreme nausea and vomiting. How are these symptoms typically relieved?

    A. Hot showers

    B. Oxygen therapy

    C. Activated charcoal

    D. Massaging the feet

_____ **19.** Sympathomimetics are central nervous system stimulants that frequently cause:

    A. hypotension

    B. tachycardia

    C. pinpoint pupils

    D. muscle weakness

_____ **20.** Characteristics of carbon monoxide include all of the following EXCEPT:

    A. is odorless

    B. produces severe hypoxia

    C. does not damage or irritate the lungs

    D. smells like rotten eggs

_____ **21.** Chlorine:

    A. is odorless

    B. does not damage or irritate the lungs

    C. causes pulmonary edema

    D. does not cause sore throat or hoarseness

_____ **22.** Localized signs and symptoms of absorbed poisoning include:

    A. a history of exposure

    B. burns and irritation of the skin

    C. dyspnea

    D. muscle weakness

_____ **23.** Which of the following statements regarding injected poisons is FALSE?

    A. They may result in dizziness, fever, and chills.

    B. They are frequently the cause of drug overdoses.

    C. They are easily diluted once in the bloodstream.

    D. You should remove rings, watches, and bracelets in areas of swelling.

_____ **24.** _____ is a highly toxic, colorless, and flammable gas with a distinctive rotten-egg odor.

    A. Carbon monoxide

    B. Hexane

    C. Chlorine

    D. Hydrogen sulfide

_____ **25.** Injected poisons are impossible to dilute or remove because they are usually _____ or cause intense local tissue destruction.

    A. absorbed quickly into the body

    B. bound to hemoglobin

    C. large compounds

    D. combined with the cerebrospinal fluid

_____ **26.** Medical problems that may cause the patient to present as intoxicated include all of the following EXCEPT:

    A. head trauma

    B. diarrhea

    C. uncontrolled diabetes

    D. toxic reactions

_____ **27.** Which of the following is NOT considered a sign or symptom of alcohol withdrawal?

    A. Agitation and restlessness

    B. Fever and sweating

    C. Seizures

    D. Chest pain

_____ **28.** Treatments for inhaled poisons include:

    A. removing the patient from the exposure

    B. applying a self-contained (SCBA) to the patient

    C. covering the patient to prevent spread of the poison

    D. considering continuous positive airway pressure (CPAP) application

_____ **29.** Signs and symptoms of chlorine exposure include all of the following EXCEPT:

    A. cough

    B. chest pain

    C. rales

    D. wheezing

_____ **30.** Which of the following is NOT a typically ingested poison?

    A. Aerosol propellants

    B. Household cleaners

    C. Plants

    D. Contaminated food

_____ **31.** Naloxone (Narcan) should only be used in a patient with a suspected opiate or opioid overdose who has:
   A. an altered mental status
   B. dilation of the pupils
   C. carpopedal spasms
   D. agonal respirations or apnea

_____ **32.** Inhaled poisons include:
   A. chlorine
   B. venom
   C. _Dieffenbachia_
   D. _Salmonella_

_____ **33.** Which of the following is NOT considered a typical route of administration for naloxone?
   A. Intravenous
   B. Intranasal
   C. Intramuscular
   D. Intradermal

Questions 34–38 are derived from the following scenario: You have responded to the home of a 26-year-old woman who has reportedly taken a large number of pills in an attempt to commit suicide. As you enter the living room, you see her unresponsive in a chair, with several empty alcohol bottles. She is breathing heavily.

_____ **34.** You are able to arouse her consciousness for a short period of time. Which course of action takes priority?
   A. Administer syrup of ipecac.
   B. Cover her with a blanket to maintain body temperature.
   C. Ensure scene safety.
   D. Attempt to administer naloxone.

_____ **35.** You have decided to give her activated charcoal. How much should you give her?
   A. Half a glass
   B. 12.5 to 25 g
   C. 30 to 100 g
   D. 30 to 100 mL

_____ **36.** What would be the desired goal of giving her activated charcoal?
   A. To vomit the drugs and alcohol
   B. To bind the toxin and prevent absorption
   C. To teach her a lesson
   D. To prevent excretion

_____ **37.** If she does not want to take the activated charcoal, you should:
   A. restrain her, pinch her nose, and make her drink it
   B. have her sign a patient refusal form
   C. attempt to persuade her
   D. leave the scene

_____ **38.** Side effects of ingesting activated charcoal include all of the following EXCEPT:
   A. constipation
   B. hematemesis
   C. vomiting
   D. black stools

_____ **39.** Which of the following is NOT commonly associated with an overdose from a cardiac medication?
   A. Cardiac arrhythmia
   B. Bleeding
   C. Unconsciousness
   D. Urinary incontinence

_____ **40.** Ringing in the ears is associated with an overdose of:
   A. acetaminophen
   B. aspirin
   C. ethylene alcohol
   D. methyl alcohol

True/False
If you believe the statement to be more true than false, write the letter "T" in the space provided. If you believe the statement to be more false than true, write the letter "F."

_____ **1.** The usual adult dose of activated charcoal is 30 to 100 g.

_____ **2.** The general treatment of a poisoned patient is to induce vomiting.

_____ **3.** Activated charcoal is a standard of care in all ingestions.

_____ **4.** Inhaled chlorine may produce pulmonary edema and lung irritation.

_____ **5.** Shaking activated charcoal decreases its effectiveness.

_____ **6.** Opioid overdose typically presents with pinpoint pupils.

_____ **7.** Cholinergics include nerve gases used in chemical warfare and organophosphate insecticides.

_____ **8.** Alcohol is a stimulant.

_____ **9.** Dilaudid and Vicodin are examples of opioids.

_____ **10.** Cocaine is classically inhaled through the nose and absorbed in the nasal mucosa.

_____ **11.** Alcohol can result in significant respiratory depression.

_____ **12.** Ingestion of the plant _Dieffenbachia_ can cause irritation of the upper airway.

Fill-in-the-Blank
Read each item carefully and then complete the statement by filling in the missing words.

1. The most severe form of toxin ingestion from food poisoning is _____.

2. _____ _____ produce euphoria, increased mental clarity, and sexual arousal.

3. _____ _____ is the misuse of any substance to produce a desired effect.

4. If the patient has a liquid chemical agent on the skin, you should flood the affected part for _____ to _____ minutes.

5. Opioid analgesics are central nervous system depressants and can cause severe _____ _____.

6. Severe acute alcohol ingestion may cause _____.

7. Your primary responsibility to the patient who has been poisoned is to _____ that a poisoning occurred.

8. The usual dosage for activated charcoal for an adult or child is _____ _____ of activated charcoal per _____ of body weight.

9. As you irrigate the eyes, make sure that the fluid runs from the bridge of the nose _____.

10. Approximately 80% of all poisoning is by _____, including plants, contaminated food, and most drugs.

11. Patients experiencing alcohol withdrawal may develop _____ _____ if they no longer have their daily source of alcohol.

12. The _____ _____ is a single auto-injector containing 2 mg of atropine and 600 mg of pralidoxime.

13. A person with a(n) _____ has an overwhelming desire or need to continue using the substance, at whatever cost, with a tendency to increase the dose.

14. _____ may develop from sweating, fluid loss, insufficient fluid intake, or vomiting associated with delirium tremens.

Fill-in-the-Table

Fill in the missing parts of the table.

Table 22-1 Typical Signs and Symptoms of Specific Overdoses

Agent	Signs and Symptoms
Opiates (Examples: morphine, codeine) Opioids (Examples: heroin, fentanyl, methadone, oxycodone)	• Hypoventilation or respiratory arrest • _____ • Sedation or coma • _____
_____ (Examples: epinephrine, albuterol, cocaine, methamphetamine)	• Hypertension • _____ • Dilated pupils • Agitation or seizures • _____
Sedative-hypnotics (Examples: diazepam, secobarbital, flunitrazepam, midazolam)	• _____ • Sedation or coma • Hypoventilation • _____
_____ (Examples: atropine, diphenhydramine, chlorpheniramine, doxylamine, *Datura stramonium* [jimson weed])	• _____ • _____ • Hypertension • Dilated pupils • _____ • Sedation, agitation, seizures, coma, or delirium • _____

Agent	Signs and Symptoms
_____ (Examples: organophosphates, pilocarpine, nerve gas)	• Airway compromise • SLUDGEM • S_____ • L_____ • U_____ • D_____ • G_____ • E_____ • M_____

Critical Thinking

Short Answer

Complete this section with short written answers using the space provided.

1. How does activated charcoal work to counteract ingested poison?

2. What are four routes of contact for poisoning?

3. List the typical signs and symptoms of an overdose of sympathomimetics.

4. What are the two main types of food poisoning?

5. Why is it that accidental acetaminophen overdose may in some ways be worse than intentional overdose? What does this mean to the prehospital caregiver?

6. What condition do the mnemonics DUMBELS and SLUDGEM pertain to, and what do they mean?

_____

_____

_____

_____

7. List at least five questions should you ask a possible poisoning victim.

_____

_____

_____

_____

Ambulance Calls

The following case scenarios provide an opportunity to explore the concerns associated with patient management and to enhance critical-thinking skills. Read each scenario and answer each question to the best of your ability.

1. You are dispatched to a private residence for "accidental ingestion." You arrive to find a 3-year-old whose parents tell you he "got into some rat poison." The child is alert, crying, and responding appropriately to his parents and environmental stimuli.

How would you best manage this patient?

_____

_____

_____

2. You are dispatched to the sidewalk in front of a small business for "an intoxicated man." You arrive to find a 60-year-old man sitting on the curb, holding a bottle inside a paper bag. He is not fully alert and can only tell you that his name is Andy. He allows you to take his blood pressure, and as you roll up his sleeve, you notice needle marks along his veins.

How would you best manage this patient?

_____

_____

_____

3. You are called to a possible suicide attempt. You arrive on the scene to find police and a neighbor in the home of a 25-year-old woman who is unresponsive, supine on her bed. The neighbor tells you that the patient recently broke up with her boyfriend and has been very distraught. There is an empty pill bottle on the nightstand. When you look at the label, you see that the prescription was filled yesterday and that 30 tablets were dispensed. An empty liquor bottle is on the floor.

How would you best manage this patient?

_____

_____

_____

Skills

Assessment Review

Answer the following questions pertaining to the assessment of the types of emergencies discussed in this chapter.

_____ **1.** Which of the following would NOT be an appropriate question to ask regarding an ingested poison?

   A. What is the substance?

   B. How much did the patient ingest?

   C. Why have you not gotten help for your addiction?

   D. Have any interventions been performed?

_____ **2.** "Hot as a hare, blind as a bat, dry as a bone, red as a beet, and mad as a hatter" describes which of the following conditions?

   A. Cholinergic poisoning

   B. Anticholinergic poisoning

   C. Delirium tremens

   D. Sympathomimetic poisoning

_____ **3.** _Shigella, Campylobacter,_ and _Enterococcus_ are associated with what type of poisoning?

   A. Plant

   B. Food

   C. Hallucinogen

   D. Sympathomimetic

_____ **4.** Ice, crank, speed, uppers, and meth are all street names for which type of drug?

   A. Hallucinogens

   B. Sympathomimetics

   C. Sedative-hypnotics

   D. Anticholinergics

_____ **5.** When would you NOT give activated charcoal?

   A. If the patient drank methanol

   B. If the patient overdosed on aspirin

   C. If the patient overdosed on antidepressants

   D. If the patient overdosed on opiates

CHAPTER

23 | Psychiatric Emergencies

General Knowledge

Matching

Match each of the items in the left column to the appropriate definition in the right column.

_____ **1.** Psychosis

_____ **2.** Schizophrenia

_____ **3.** Delirium

_____ **4.** Depression

_____ **5.** Psychiatric disorder

_____ **6.** Behavior

_____ **7.** Functional disorder

_____ **8.** Behavioral health emergency

_____ **9.** Behavioral crisis

_____ **10.** Organic brain syndrome

A. What you can see of a person's response to the environment; his or her actions

B. A temporary or permanent dysfunction of the brain caused by a disturbance in brain tissue function

C. Similar to a behavioral health emergency but typically less serious

D. A persistent feeling of sadness or despair

E. Abnormal operation of an organ that cannot be traced to an obvious change in the structure or physiology of the organ

F. A complex disorder that can involve delusions, hallucinations, a lack of interest in pleasure, and erratic speech

G. An illness with psychological or behavioral symptoms that may result in impaired functioning

H. When a patient shows agitation or violence and becomes a threat to themselves or others

I. A state of delusion in which the person is out of touch with reality

J. Condition of impairment in cognitive function that can present with disorientation, hallucinations, or delusions

Multiple Choice

Read each item carefully and then select the one best response.

_____ **1.** Which of the following is NOT typically linked to a psychological or behavioral crisis?

    A. Mind-altering substances

    B. An underlying medical problem

    C. History of smoking

    D. Stress

_____ **2.** Which of the following is a normal reaction to a crisis situation?

    A. Being sad the majority of days for weeks on end

    B. Feeling blue after the breakup of a long-term relationship

    C. Feeling depressed week after week with no discernible cause

    D. Thoughts of suicide

_____ **3.** Which of the following statements is FALSE?

    A. You may be able to predict whether a person will become violent.

    B. Scene safety is always your primary concern.

    C. Behavior problems may be the result of drug or alcohol abuse.

    D. Most people with a mental illness are dangerous.

_____ **4.** Learning to adapt to a variety of situations in daily life, including stresses and strains, is called:
   A. disruption
   B. coping
   C. behavior
   D. functional

_____ **5.** If a patient becomes agitated, violent, or uncooperative and may become a danger to themselves or others, it is considered a _____ crisis.
   A. mental health
   B. functional
   C. behavioral
   D. psychogenic

_____ **6.** Patients may show agitation or violence or become a threat to themselves or others when they experience a(n) _____ emergency.
   A. psychiatric
   B. behavioral
   C. functional
   D. adjustment

_____ **7.** Which of the following is NOT considered a possible cause of a psychiatric disorder?
   A. Social disturbance
   B. Chemical disturbance
   C. Biologic disturbance
   D. Emotional disturbance

_____ **8.** An altered mental status may arise from:
   A. an oxygen saturation of 98%
   B. moderate temperatures
   C. inadequate blood flow to the brain
   D. adequate glucose levels in the blood

_____ **9.** Organic brain syndrome may be caused by:
   A. daily stress
   B. seizure disorders
   C. myocardial infarction
   D. thoracic spinal cord injury

_____ **10.** All of the following are examples of a functional disorder EXCEPT:
   A. anxiety
   B. depression
   C. organic brain syndrome
   D. schizophrenia

_____ **11.** When documenting abnormal behavior, it is important to:
   A. document restraints only when leather restraints are used
   B. document everything that happened on the call
   C. avoid quoting the patient's own words
   D. interject your interpretations of the patient's thoughts

_____ **12.** Safety guidelines for behavioral emergencies include all of the following EXCEPT:
   A. assessing the scene
   B. being prepared to spend extra time
   C. encouraging purposeful movement
   D. determining the underlying psychiatric disorder

_____   **13.** In evaluating a situation that is considered a behavioral emergency, the first things to consider are:
    A. airway and breathing
    B. scene safety and patient response
    C. history of medications
    D. respiratory and circulatory status

_____   **14.** _____ is a behavior that is characterized by restlessness and irregular physical activity.
    A. Agitation
    B. Aggression
    C. Anxiety
    D. Apathy

_____   **15.** Which of the following is NOT considered a risk factor for suicide?
    A. Alcohol abuse
    B. Recent marriage
    C. Family history of suicide
    D. Depression

_____   **16.** Which of the following is NOT a risk factor to consider when assessing a suicidal patient?
    A. Does the patient appear to be well groomed?
    B. Is the environment unsafe?
    C. Is there an imminent threat to the patient or others?
    D. Is there evidence of self-destructive behavior?

_____   **17.** Signs and symptoms of agitated delirium include all of the following EXCEPT:
    A. diarrhea
    B. tachycardia
    C. vivid hallucinations
    D. dilated pupils

_____   **18.** You should request the assistance of a _____ when a mentally impaired patient refuses to go to the hospital.
    A. physician
    B. court order
    C. law enforcement officer
    D. psychologist

_____   **19.** When restraining a patient without an appropriate order, legal actions may involve charges of:
    A. abandonment
    B. negligence
    C. battery
    D. breach of duty

_____   **20.** When restraining a patient on a stretcher, it is necessary to constantly reassess the patient's:
    A. level of consciousness
    B. respiration and circulation status
    C. emotional status
    D. pain status

Questions 21–24 are derived from the following scenario: Dean, a man in his 50s, is acting irrationally. His wife states that he thinks he is the dictator of a small country, and he is wearing nothing but a baseball cap and a belt with a small handgun attached to it.

_____   **21.** What is your best course of action?
    A. Call ALS.
    B. Assess Dean from a distance.
    C. Have his wife take the gun from him.
    D. Call for police backup.

_____ **22.** The scene is safe. Dean now tells you he is "God" and can do anything he wants to. Which of the following should you NOT consider?

    A. He is probably not a threat to you.

    B. He may have a history of psychiatric problems.

    C. He could be suffering from an underlying medical problem.

    D. Alcohol or drugs could be a factor in his behavior.

_____ **23.** What are some tactics you can use to have Dean cooperate with your assessment?

    A. Reflective listening

    B. Threatening him with restraints

    C. Aggressive communication

    D. Passive listening

_____ **24.** Dean becomes agitated and states, "You'll never take me alive." A decision is made to restrain Dean. How many people should ideally be present to restrain Dean?

    A. Two

    B. Five

    C. Six

    D. Eight

True/False

If you believe the statement to be more true than false, write the letter "T" in the space provided. If you believe the statement to be more false than true, write the letter "F."

_____ **1.** Depression lasting 8 months after being fired from a job is a normal mental health response.

_____ **2.** Low blood glucose or lack of oxygen to the brain may cause behavioral changes to the degree that a psychiatric emergency could exist.

_____ **3.** A disturbed patient should always be transported with restraints.

_____ **4.** It is sometimes helpful to allow a patient with a behavioral emergency some time alone to calm down and collect his or her thoughts.

_____ **5.** It is important to maintain eye contact with the patient when dealing with a behavioral crisis.

_____ **6.** A patient should never be asked if he or she is considering suicide.

_____ **7.** Urinary tract infections can cause behavioral changes in elderly patients.

_____ **8.** All individuals with mental health disorders are dangerous, violent, or otherwise unmanageable.

_____ **9.** When completing the documentation, it is important to record the reasons why you restrained a patient.

_____ **10.** When restraining a patient, at least three people should ideally be present to carry out the restraint.

_____ **11.** A patient should be placed facedown when being restrained to a litter.

_____ **12.** Reassessment of respiratory and circulatory status in restrained patients should take place continuously.

_____ **13.** Tears, sweating, and blushing may be significant indicators of state of mind, such as sadness, nervousness, or embarrassment.

_____ **14.** Most medical or trauma situations will include a behavioral component.

_____ **15.** Military personnel who experienced combat have a low incidence of posttraumatic stress disorder (PTSD).

_____ **16.** Flashbacks are uncontrolled events triggered by sound, sight, or smell.

_____ **17.** A competent adult may not refuse treatment when life-saving treatment is needed.

Fill-in-the-Blank

Read each item carefully and then complete the statement by filling in the missing words.

1. _____ is what you can see of a person's response to the environment, such as his or her actions.

2. A(n) _____ _____ _____ or crisis is any reaction to events that interferes with the activities of daily living or has become unacceptable to the patient, family, or community.

3. Chronic _____, or a persistent feeling of sadness or despair, may be a symptom of an underlying health disorder.

4. _____ _____ _____ is a temporary or permanent dysfunction of the brain caused by a disturbance in the physical or physiologic functioning of the brain.

5. Any time you encounter an emotionally depressed patient, you must consider the possibility of _____.

6. People with _____ may experience symptoms including delusions, hallucinations, a lack of interest in pleasure, and erratic speech.

7. Violent or dangerous people should be managed by _____ _____ before emergency care is rendered.

8. When a patient is not mentally competent to grant consent, the law assumes that there is _____ _____.

9. _____ _____ occurs when the person attempts to find an escape from constant internal distress or a particularly disturbing event.

10. In subduing a disturbed patient, use the _____ force necessary.

Critical Thinking

Short Answer

Complete this section with short written answers using the space provided.

1. What three major areas should be considered when evaluating the history of a patient experiencing a behavioral crisis or emergency?

   _____

   _____

   _____

2. What are three factors to consider in determining the level of force required to restrain a patient?

   _____

   _____

   _____

3. List at least 10 safety guidelines for dealing with behavioral emergencies.

_____

_____

_____

4. List at least 10 risk factors for suicide.

_____

_____

_____

5. Explain the process for reflective listening.

_____

_____

_____

6. List five risk factors to consider when dealing with a potentially violent patient.

_____

_____

_____

Ambulance Calls

The following case scenarios provide an opportunity to explore the concerns associated with patient management and to enhance critical-thinking skills. Read each scenario and answer each question to the best of your ability.

1. You are dispatched to a nonemergency transport of a girl from a local hospital emergency department to a care facility that provides treatment for emotionally disturbed teenagers. She became violent in the emergency department and was placed in four-point restraints. As you begin transporting the patient, she begins to cry and asks you to remove the restraints.

How would you best manage this patient?

_____

_____

_____

2. You are dispatched to a "suicide attempt" at a private residence. When you arrive on scene, you are greeted by a calm, middle-aged man who appears to have been crying. He tells you that he was on the phone with his sister who lives out of state and that she must have called for the ambulance. The patient tells you that he was just upset, but he's fine now. Dispatch informed you via cell phone that this man recently lost his wife of 15 years to breast cancer.

How would you best manage this patient?

_____

_____

_____

3. You are dispatched to the residence of a 40-year-old woman who is upset over the loss of her mother 5 weeks ago. She tells you that she has no family and has cared for her elderly mother for the past 7 years. She has not eaten for several days and is severely depressed.

How would you best manage this patient?

_____

_____

_____

Skills

Assessment Review

Answer the following questions pertaining to the assessment of the types of emergencies discussed in this chapter. These questions are based on risk factors in assessing the level of danger in a behavior call.

_____ **1.** When assessing the history, all of the following are past behaviors you want to know if the patient has exhibited EXCEPT:

    A. hostile behavior

    B. overly aggressive behavior

    C. violent behavior

    D. cooperative behavior

_____ **2.** Physical tension is often a warning signal of impending hostility. What sign might warn you of physical tension?

    A. Posture

    B. Eye movement

    C. Facial expression

    D. Laughter

_____ **3.** What warning signs can be detected from the scene?

    A. Hunting magazines on the table

    B. Known weapons in the outside shed

    C. Guns or knives near the patient

    D. Photos of hunting trips on the wall

_____ **4.** What kind of speech may be an indicator of emotional distress?

    A. Quiet speech

    B. Obscene speech

    C. Rational speech

    D. Organized speech

_____ **5.** What type of physical activity may be an indicator of risk to the EMT?

    A. Tense muscles

    B. Continuous stretching

    C. Lying down

    D. Vigorous exercise

Gynecologic Emergencies

General Knowledge

Matching

Match each of the items in the left column to the appropriate definition in the right column.

_____ **1.** Ovaries

_____ **2.** Fallopian tubes

_____ **3.** Uterus

_____ **4.** Cervix

_____ **5.** Vagina

_____ **6.** Labia

_____ **7.** Perineum

_____ **8.** Chlamydia

_____ **9.** Pelvic inflammatory disease (PID)

_____ **10.** Bacterial vaginosis

_____ **11.** Gonorrhea

A. Folds of tissue that surround the urethral and vaginal openings

B. The narrowest portion of the uterus; opens to the vagina

C. A disease causing lower abdominal and back pain, nausea, fever, pain during intercourse, and/or bleeding between menstrual cycles

D. The area of skin between the vagina and the anus

E. Connect(s) each ovary with the uterus

F. Infection of the uterus, ovaries, and fallopian tubes

G. The primary female reproductive organ(s), produce(s) an ovum, or an egg

H. The outermost cavity of a woman's reproductive system; forms the lower part of the birth canal

I. A condition in which bacteria can grow and multiply rapidly in the reproductive tract, mouth, throat, eyes, and anus

J. A condition in which normal bacteria is replaced by an overgrowth of other bacterial forms

K. A muscular organ where the fetus grows

Multiple Choice

Read each item carefully and then select the one best response.

_____ **1.** Possible causes of vaginal bleeding include all of the following EXCEPT:

    A. ectopic pregnancy

    B. cervical polyps

    C. vaginal trauma

    D. peptic ulcer

_____ **2.** Painful urination associated with burning and a yellowish discharge is associated with:

    A. chlamydia

    B. gonorrhea

    C. endometriosis

    D. syphilis

_____ **3.** Which of the following statements is FALSE regarding the assessment and treatment of a woman who was the victim of sexual assault?

   A. You may be called to testify in court regarding the incident.

   B. You should question the victim thoroughly about the assaulter in case the police missed any details.

   C. The patient should be given the option of being treated by a female responder.

   D. The patient should be discouraged from urinating or changing her clothes prior to examination at the hospital.

_____ **4.** The onset of menstruation usually occurs between the ages of:

   A. 8 and 10 years

   B. 11 and 16 years

   C. 16 and 18 years

   D. 17 and 20 years

_____ **5.** What is the most common presenting sign or symptom of PID?

   A. Vaginal discharge

   B. Fever

   C. Nausea and vomiting

   D. Lower abdominal pain

_____ **6.** In rare cases, _____ causes arthritis that may be accompanied by skin lesions and inflammation of the eyes and urethra.

   A. chlamydia

   B. gonorrhea

   C. PID

   D. vaginal bleeding

_____ **7.** Left untreated, _____ can lead to premature birth or low birth weight in pregnant women.

   A. chlamydia

   B. gonorrhea

   C. bacterial vaginosis

   D. vaginal bleeding

_____ **8.** If a patient with vaginal bleeding presents with a rapid pulse and pale or cool skin, you should:

   A. attempt to locate the source of bleeding and correct it

   B. place the patient in a supine position

   C. consider this to be a normal sign in a menstruating woman

   D. inquire about recent problems with urination

_____ **9.** When taking a history on a patient experiencing a gynecologic emergency, you should consider asking all of the following EXCEPT:

   A. Are you taking birth control?

   B. When was your last menstrual period?

   C. How many sexual partners have you had in the past?

   D. Do you have any history of sexually transmitted diseases?

_____ **10.** A shuffling gait with diffuse lower abdominal pain may indicate which of the following conditions?

   A. Pelvic inflammatory disease

   B. Bacterial vaginosis

   C. Chlamydia

   D. Gonorrhea

_____ **11.** EMTs treating a victim of a sexual assault may not only be dealing with medical issues but with _____ issues as well.

   A. psychological

   B. physiological

   C. educational

   D. sociological

_____ **12.** When performing a physical exam on a victim of sexual assault, you should:

    A. always expose and evaluate the patient's vaginal area

    B. allow multiple people to observe the examination in case you have to testify

    C. limit your examination to a brief survey for life-threatening injuries

    D. place the patient's clothes into a plastic evidence bag

_____ **13.** Rape is considered to be a _____ diagnosis, not a medical diagnosis.

    A. psychological

    B. surgical

    C. sociological

    D. legal

_____ **14.** Often the most important intervention for a sexual assault patient is _____ and transport to a facility with a staff specially trained to deal with this scenario.

    A. comforting reassurance

    B. excellent assessment skills

    C. bandaging skills

    D. promising legal justice

_____ **15.** Your _____ is the best tool to gain the patient's confidence to seek medical help.

    A. confidence

    B. content knowledge

    C. compassion

    D. empathy

Questions 16–18 are derived from the following scenario: You are called to the scene of a possible assault. On arrival, you are directed by police to a dark room, where you find a 22-year-old woman who says she was sexually assaulted by a coworker this afternoon.

_____ **16.** Your first course of action should be to:

    A. determine whether the patient is physically injured

    B. establish the exact events of what took place

    C. allow the patient to use the restroom

    D. let the police question the patient before conducting a primary assessment

_____ **17.** The second course of action involves the psychological care of the patient. You should avoid:

    A. making attempts to get a female EMT to examine the patient

    B. examination of the vaginal canal, even if active bleeding is taking place

    C. attempting to gather information to assist the police

    D. granting the patient's wishes for refusing care and transport

_____ **18.** The patient tells you that she would really like to be transported to the hospital but refuses a physical examination. You should:

    A. explain to her that she cannot be transported without a physical exam

    B. have the police take the patient into custody in order to legally force a physical exam

    C. explain to her that this is a criminal case and that she must be examined

    D. follow your system's policy and respect the patient's wishes without judgment

True/False

If you believe the statement to be more true than false, write the letter "T" in the space provided. If you believe the statement to be more false than true, write the letter "F."

_____ **1.** Chlamydial infection of the cervix can spread to the rectum, leading to rectal pain, discharge, or bleeding.

_____ **2.** If gonorrhea is not treated, the bacteria may enter the bloodstream and spread to other parts of the body, including the brain.

_____ **3.** Because menstrual bleeding is a monthly occurrence, it is not necessary to assess for other causes of vaginal bleeding.

_____ **4.** Obtaining an accurate and detailed patient assessment is critical when dealing with gynecologic issues.

_____ **5.** Most cases of gynecologic emergencies are not life threatening.

_____ **6.** Gynecologic emergencies are typically not embarrassing for women.

_____ **7.** When taking a history of a woman with a gynecologic complaint, you should inquire about the possibility of pregnancy and exposure to sexually transmitted diseases.

_____ **8.** Most presentations of tachycardia and hypotension are related to anxiety.

_____ **9.** Any report of syncope in a woman complaining of vaginal bleeding is considered significant.

_____ **10.** It is acceptable to place dressings into the vaginal canal to stop significant bleeding.

_____ **11.** When examining a female, you should limit the number of people involved.

_____ **12.** Gynecologic emergencies can occur at any age during a woman's lifetime.

_____ **13.** Injuries to the external genitals are typically not painful due to the very sparse nerve supply.

_____ **14.** When completing documentation of a sexual assault incident, adding your personal thoughts can help with the investigation.

_____ **15.** Determining the cause of vaginal bleeding should be of less importance than treating for shock and transporting the patient to an appropriate facility.

Fill-in-the-Blank

Read each item carefully and then complete the statement by filling in the missing words.

1. The _____ are located on each side of the lower abdomen and produce the ovum, or egg.

2. When a female reaches _____, she begins to ovulate and experience menstruation.

3. _____ _____ _____ is an infection of the upper female reproductive organs.

4. _____ _____ can be very messy, sometimes involving large amounts of blood and bodily fluids.

5. _____ _____ and _____ _____ are two conditions that can cause vaginal bleeding in women who do not appear to be pregnant and who may not realize they are pregnant.

6. Make sure to use _____ _____ when attempting to control vaginal bleeding.

7. _____ _____ can cause significant blood loss and lead to hypovolemia.

8. You will need to work together with _____ _____ when dealing with a victim of sexual assault.

9. Symptoms of _____ appear approximately 2 to 10 days after exposure.

10. Women will continue to experience menstruation until they reach _____.

Labeling

Label the following diagrams with the correct terms.

1. Female Reproductive System

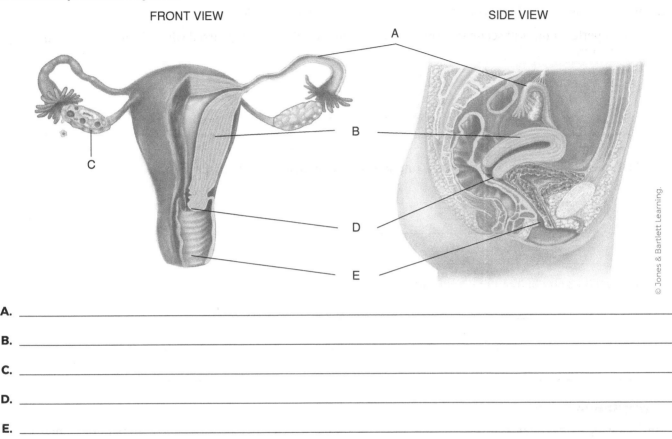

FRONT VIEW   SIDE VIEW

A. _____

B. _____

C. _____

D. _____

E. _____

2. External Genitalia

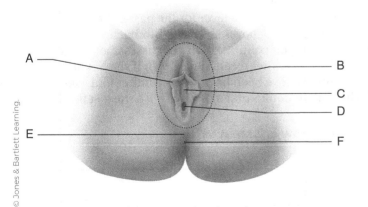

A. _____

B. _____

C. _____

D. _____

E. _____

F. _____

Critical Thinking

Short Answer

Complete this section with short written answers using the space provided.

1. When performing your scene size-up, what questions should you ask yourself when dealing with a gynecologic emergency?

_____

_____

_____

2. List at least five signs and symptoms commonly found with a gonorrhea infection.

_____

_____

_____

3. Explain the general treatment strategies for vaginal bleeding.

_____

_____

_____

Ambulance Calls

The following case scenarios provide an opportunity to explore the concerns associated with patient management and to enhance critical-thinking skills. Read each scenario and answer each question to the best of your ability.

1. You are dispatched to a local college campus for a 21-year-old woman with abdominal pain. The dispatcher tells you that the patient has lower abdominal pain, fever, nausea, and vomiting. When you arrive on the campus, you are directed by campus police to the health center. There you find your patient lying supine on a bed. The patient tells you that she has had lower abdominal pain and a fever for the past 24 hours. She describes the pain as "achy" and says it gets worse with walking. She believes she has a "stomach virus" due to the fever and vomiting. Your partner obtains vital signs as you continue with your assessment. After finishing your SAMPLE history, you casually ask if she has had any other recent illnesses or if she has any other complaints. The patient says, "Well, since you mentioned it, I've been having some rather foul vaginal discharge lately. But I just thought it would go away." The patient denies pregnancy because she just finished her menstrual period last week.

What is the likely cause of this patient's condition, and how is it treated?

_____

_____

_____

2. You are dispatched to an apartment complex at 538 N. 10th Street, Apartment 4-C, for an assault. You look at your watch and note the time as 2101. On the way to the unit, your partner remarks, "Six hundred and eighty-ninth call for the year so far. No doubt we'll hit 700 before the end of the night." You make note of the incident number at 011689 and mark responding 2 minutes after dispatch. The additional information states this is for a 32-year-old woman who was sexually assaulted.

You arrive on scene 8 minutes after the initial dispatch and notice the apartment is very well kept and is not cluttered. The police lead you to the back bedroom, where you find your patient sitting up on the side of the bed, speaking to the investigator. The patient appears alert, and you notice bleeding from the nose along with bruises to the patient's face. The patient tells you that she was raped by a maintenance worker at the apartment complex. She complains of pain to the nose, face, and groin. The patient says she is not sure whether she wants to go to the hospital, but she definitely wants to take a shower and change her clothes.

Explain the key issues to consider when treating a victim of sexual assault.

_____

_____

_____

Fill-in-the-Patient Care Report

Using the previous case (Ambulance Call 2) and the additional information provided, complete the patient care report (PCR) for this incident.

You explain to the patient that she should refrain from changing her clothes or washing because she could disrupt any potential evidence. The police agree with your statement.

As the police continue with some questions, you complete an initial assessment while your partner obtains the following vital signs at 2114: pulse, 102 beats/min; respirations, 22 breaths/min; blood pressure, 144/98 mm Hg; pulse oximetry, 98%.

You ask the patient if she would be more comfortable with a female EMT. Her response is a simple "No." The patient appears withdrawn and emotionally traumatized. You notice no obvious life-threatening injuries and ask the patient if she has bleeding anywhere. Her response is, "No." The only visible external injuries you can find are multiple contusions to the face.

The patient does not make eye contact with you while questioning her medical history (diabetes), medications (lispro, Lantus, lisinopril), and allergies (none). When you ask her if she would like to tell you "what happened," she responds by saying, "Can't we just get going to the hospital? I would rather speak to the doctor."

You smile and say, "Absolutely."

Your partner applies oxygen at 2 L/min via nasal cannula. The patient is packaged on the litter and is loaded into the unit. Your partner verifies the hospital destination with the police so that they can continue with their investigation. You note that you were on scene for a total of 11 minutes.

During transport, you notice that it has been 11 minutes since the vitals were assessed and ask the patient if she is having any pain. Her response is, "No." You reassess the patient's vital signs: pulse, 108 beats/min; respirations, 20 breaths/min; blood pressure, 148/92 mm Hg; pulse oximetry, 97%.

Instead of calling in a report to the hospital, your partner calls in a basic update from the front of the cab so that the patient does not relive the experience.

You arrive at the hospital about 6 minutes after you reassessed the vitals. Care is transferred to the hospital staff, with no change in the patient's status. The nurse asks for a report, and you motion for her to leave the room with you. You give the report to the nurse away from the patient and any potentially unnecessary personnel.

You and your partner don't have much to say to one another. The unit is cleaned and restocked, and you put yourself back in service at 2147.

Fill-in-the-Patient Care Report

EMS Patient Care Report (PCR)					
Date:	Incident No.:		Nature of Call:		Location:
Dispatched:	En Route:	At Scene:	Transport:	At Hospital:	In Service:
Patient Information					
Age: Sex: Weight (in kg [lb]):			Allergies: Medications: Past Medical History: Chief Complaint:		
Vital Signs					
Time:	BP:	Pulse:		Respirations:	SpO$_2$:
Time:	BP:	Pulse:		Respirations:	SpO$_2$:
Time:	BP:	Pulse:		Respirations:	SpO$_2$:
EMS Treatment (circle all that apply)					
Oxygen @ ___ L/min via (circle one): NC NRM BVM		Assisted Ventilation		Airway Adjunct	CPR
Defibrillation	Bleeding Control	Bandaging		Splinting	Other:
Narrative					

CHAPTER

25

Trauma Overview

General Knowledge

Matching

Match each of the items in the left column to the appropriate definition in the right column.

_____ **1.** Cavitation

_____ **2.** Multisystem trauma

_____ **3.** Kinetic energy

_____ **4.** Mechanism of injury (MOI)

_____ **5.** Potential energy

_____ **6.** Blunt trauma

_____ **7.** Penetrating trauma

_____ **8.** Work

A. The result of force to the body that causes injury but does not penetrate soft tissue or internal organs and cavities

B. The force acting over a distance

C. The product of mass, gravity, and height

D. An injury caused by objects that pierce the surface of the body

E. How trauma occurs

F. The energy of a moving object

G. A significant MOI that causes injuries to more than one body system

H. Speed causes a bullet to generate pressure waves, which cause damage distant from the bullet's path

Multiple Choice

Read each item carefully and then select the one best response.

_____ **1.** Your awareness of and concern for potentially serious obvious and underlying injuries is referred to as the:

    A. mechanism of injury

    B. index of suspicion

    C. scene size-up

    D. general impression

_____ **2.** The energy of a moving object is called:

    A. potential energy

    B. thermal energy

    C. kinetic energy

    D. work

_____ **3.** Energy can be:

    A. created

    B. destroyed

    C. converted

    D. lost

_____ 4. The amount of kinetic energy that is converted to do work on the body dictates the _____ of the injury.

    A. location

    B. severity

    C. cause

    D. speed

_____ 5. All of the following are considered types of motorcycle impacts EXCEPT:

    A. head-on collision

    B. angular collision

    C. controlled collision

    D. rear collision

_____ 6. Which of the following is considered a type of impact from a motor vehicle collision?

    A. Ejection

    B. Rollover

    C. Crush

    D. Penetration

_____ 7. The three collisions in a frontal impact include all of the following EXCEPT:

    A. car striking object

    B. passenger striking vehicle

    C. airbag striking passenger

    D. internal organs striking solid structures of the body

_____ 8. Which of the following is NOT considered appropriate use of air medical services?

    A. The distance to a trauma center is greater than 25 miles.

    B. Traffic/road conditions make it unlikely to get the patient to the hospital in a timely manner.

    C. There is a mass-casualty incident.

    D. The closest trauma center is 10 minutes away by ground transport.

_____ 9. Medium-velocity penetrating injuries may be caused by a:

    A. knife

    B. military assault rifle

    C. handgun

    D. slingshot

_____ 10. In a motor vehicle collision, as the passenger's head hits the windshield, the brain continues to move forward until it strikes the inside of the skull, resulting in a _____ injury.

    A. compression

    B. laceration

    C. lateral

    D. motion

_____ 11. Your quick primary assessment of the patient and evaluation of the _____ can help to direct life-saving care and provide critical information to the hospital staff.

    A. environment

    B. index of suspicion

    C. mechanism of injury

    D. abdominal area

_____ 12. A contusion to a patient's forehead along with a spider-webbed windshield suggests possible injury to the:

    A. nose

    B. brain

    C. face

    D. heart

_____ **13.** Which of the following is the most common cause of death from a blast injury?

    A. Amputation

    B. Burns

    C. Chest trauma

    D. Head trauma

_____ **14.** Significant clues to the possibility of severe injuries in motor vehicle collisions include:

    A. death of an occupant

    B. a blown-out tire

    C. broken glass

    D. a deployed airbag

_____ **15.** Damage to the body that resulted from a pressure wave generated by an explosion is found in what type of blast injury?

    A. Primary

    B. Secondary

    C. Tertiary

    D. Miscellaneous

_____ **16.** Airbags decrease injury to all of the following EXCEPT:

    A. chest

    B. heart

    C. face

    D. head

_____ **17.** Optimally, the on-scene time for critically injured patients should be less than _____ minutes.

    A. 5

    B. 10

    C. 15

    D. 20

_____ **18.** _____ impacts are commonly referred to as T-bone crashes.

    A. Frontal

    B. Lateral

    C. Rear-end

    D. Rollover

_____ **19.** The most common life-threatening event in a rollover is _____ or partial ejection of the passenger from the vehicle.

    A. vehicle intrusion

    B. centrifugal force

    C. ejection

    D. spinal cord injury

_____ **20.** A fall from more than _____ is considered to be significant.

    A. 10 feet

    B. 20 feet

    C. 30 feet

    D. 40 feet

Questions 21–24 are derived from the following scenario: A young boy was riding his bicycle down the street when he hit a parked car.

_____ **21.** How many collisions took place?

    A. One

    B. Two

    C. Three

    D. Four

_____ **22.** What was the first collision?
   A. The bike hitting the car
   B. The bike rider hitting his bike or the car
   C. The bike rider's internal organs against the solid structures of the body
   D. The bike rider striking the pavement

_____ **23.** What was the second collision?
   A. The bike hitting the car
   B. The bike rider hitting his bike or the car
   C. The bike rider's internal organs against the solid structures of the body
   D. The bike rider striking the pavement

_____ **24.** What will raise your index of suspicion for this collision?
   A. The mechanism of injury
   B. The type of bike
   C. How loudly he's crying
   D. A quick visual assessment

_____ **25.** "For every action, there is an equal and opposite reaction" is:
   A. Newton's first law
   B. Newton's second law
   C. Newton's third law
   D. a false statement

_____ **26.** "A comprehensive regional resource capable of providing every aspect of trauma care, from prevention through rehabilitation" is the definition of a _____ trauma center.
   A. Level I
   B. Level II
   C. Level III
   D. Level IV

_____ **27.** Which of the following is NOT considered a type of impact associated with a motorcycle crash?
   A. Head-on
   B. Rotational
   C. Controlled
   D. Ejection

_____ **28.** Burns from hot gases and respiratory injuries from inhaling toxic gas are associated with which type of blast injury?
   A. Primary
   B. Secondary
   C. Tertiary
   D. Quaternary

_____ **29.** A patient complaining of chest tightness, coughing up blood, and subcutaneous emphysema following an explosion may be suffering from a:
   A. myocardial blast injury
   B. ruptured tympanic membrane
   C. ruptured peritoneal cavity
   D. pulmonary blast injury

_____ **30.** Patients suffering from an open wound to the neck may experience all of the following EXCEPT:
   A. significant bleeding
   B. air embolism
   C. tension pneumothorax
   D. subcutaneous crepitation

True/False

If you believe the statement to be more true than false, write the letter "T" in the space provided. If you believe the statement to be more false than true, write the letter "F."

_____ **1.** *Work* is defined as force acting over distance.

_____ **2.** Energy can be both created and destroyed.

_____ **3.** The energy of a moving object is called potential energy.

_____ **4.** Rear-end collisions often cause whiplash injuries.

_____ **5.** Penetration or perforation to the chest wall is called an open chest wound.

_____ **6.** The injury potential of a fall is related to the height from which the patient fell.

_____ **7.** In the United States, traumatic injuries are the leading cause of death for people younger than 44 years.

_____ **8.** Rapid transport of an unstable trauma patient takes priority over assessing and managing the ABCs.

_____ **9.** Injuries to the aorta are relatively common in lateral impacts from a motor vehicle collision.

_____ **10.** Headrests are the major cause of whiplash-type injuries in rear-impact collisions.

_____ **11.** In car-versus-pedestrian collisions, the speed of the vehicle should be the first step in determining the mechanism of injury.

_____ **12.** Helmets are reliable in protecting against cervical spine injuries.

_____ **13.** Tertiary blast injuries result from flying debris, such as glass or shrapnel, striking the patient.

_____ **14.** You should perform frequent neurologic assessments in patients with a presumed head injury.

_____ **15.** All patients with chest trauma, regardless of the injury, should be reassessed every 5 minutes.

Fill-in-the-Blank

Read each item carefully and then complete the statement by filling in the missing words.

1. Energy that is available to cause injury _____ when an object's weight doubles but _____ when its

speed doubles.

2. _____ _____ causes injury by objects that pierce the surface of the body and cause damage to soft

tissues, internal organs, and body cavities.

3. A compression injury to the anterior portion of the brain and stretching of the posterior portion is called a(n)

_____ brain injury.

4. The formula for calculating kinetic energy is _____.

5. Whiplash-type injuries are typically caused by _____ impacts.

6. Airbags provide the final capture point of the passengers and decrease the severity of _____ injuries.

7. _____ trauma is a term that describes a person who has been subjected to multiple traumatic injuries

involving more than one body system.

8. A T-bone collision typically refers to a(n) _____ impact.

9. The most common life-threatening event in a rollover collision is _____.

10. The liver, spleen, pancreas, and kidneys are all considered _____ organs in the abdomen.

11. The _____ _____ Scale uses eye opening, verbal response, and motor response to rate a patient's level of consciousness.

12. Air collecting between the lung tissue and the chest wall is commonly referred to as a(n) _____.

13. _____ _____ describes the limited on-scene time for patients with multisystem trauma.

14. _____ _____ _____ states that an object at rest tends to stay at rest, and an object in motion tends to stay in motion, unless acted on by some force.

15. A(n) _____ emergency occurs when the patient has an illness or condition that is not caused by an outside force.

Fill-in-the-Table

Fill in the missing parts of the table.

Table 25-1 Recognizing Developing Problems in Trauma Patients

Mechanism of Injury	Signs and Symptoms	Index of Suspicion
Blunt or penetrating trauma to the neck	• • • • • • • •	• Significant bleeding or foreign bodies in the upper or lower airway, causing obstruction • Be alert for airway compromise.
Significant chest wall trauma from motor vehicle, car-versus-pedestrian, and other crashes; penetrating trauma to the chest wall	• • • • • • • • • •	• Cardiac or pulmonary contusion • Pneumothorax or hemothorax • Broken ribs, causing breathing compromise

Any significant blunt-force trauma from motor vehicle crashes or penetrating injury	• • • • • • • •	• Injuries in these regions may tear and cause damage to the large blood vessels located in these body areas, resulting in significant internal and external bleeding. • Be alert to the possibility of bruising to the brain and bleeding in and around the brain tissue, which may cause the development of excess pressure inside the skull around the brain.
Any significant blunt-force trauma, falls from a significant height, or penetrating trauma	• • •	• Injuries to the bones of the spinal column or to the spinal cord

Critical Thinking

Short Answer

Complete this section with short written answers using the space provided.

1. Describe potential energy.

_____

_____

_____

2. List the series of collisions typical with motor vehicles.

_____

_____

_____

3. List the three factors to consider when evaluating a fall.

_____

_____

_____

4. Describe the phenomenon of cavitation as it relates to an injury from a bullet.

_____

_____

_____

5. Why is it important to try to determine the type of gun and ammunition used when you are caring for a gunshot victim?

_____

_____

_____

6. What type of injuries can you expect from a motor vehicle collision with a lateral impact and substantial intrusion?

_____

_____

_____

7. List the information you should gather when determining the MOI of a motorcycle crash.

_____

_____

_____

8. What is the definition of a Level I trauma center?

_____

_____

_____

Ambulance Calls

The following case scenarios provide an opportunity to explore the concerns associated with patient management and to enhance critical-thinking skills. Read each scenario and answer each question to the best of your ability.

1. You are dispatched to a one-car crash. As you arrive, you notice that the car hit a large deer, which is lying in the road, dead. Highway speed limits on this road are 65 mph (105 kph). The driver was restrained with a lap belt only, and his vehicle was not equipped with airbags. He is complaining of head and neck pain and tells you that he doesn't remember what happened.

How would you best manage this patient?

_____

_____

_____

2. You are dispatched to assist a man who fell from a ladder as he was repairing shingles on the roof of his two-story home. You arrive to find an unconscious middle-aged man lying on the ground. He is breathing and has a pulse. The call to 9-1-1 was placed after the man was found by a neighbor.

How would you best manage this patient?

_____

_____

_____

3. You are called to the residence of a 19-year-old man who was stabbed in the abdomen with an ice pick. The scene is safe, and the patient is lying on the floor with the ice pick impaled in his left lower quadrant. Bystanders tell you that he did not fall. He is alert and complaining of severe pain.

How would you best manage this patient?

_____

_____

_____

4. You are called to the scene of a pedestrian struck by a motor vehicle in a residential neighborhood. As you approach the scene, you notice a vehicle pulled off to the side with damage to its bumper and hood and what appears to be a person lying unresponsive in the roadway.

What factors do you need to consider when determining the mechanism of injury?

_____

_____

_____

CHAPTER

26 Bleeding

General Knowledge

Matching

Match each of the items in the left column to the appropriate definition in the right column.

_____ **1.** Pulmonary artery

_____ **2.** Heart

_____ **3.** Ventricle

_____ **4.** Aorta

_____ **5.** Atrium

_____ **6.** Pulmonary vein

_____ **7.** Coagulation

_____ **8.** Ecchymosis

_____ **9.** Epistaxis

_____ **10.** Hematoma

_____ **11.** Hemophilia

_____ **12.** Hemorrhage

_____ **13.** Hypovolemic shock

A. A mass of blood in the soft tissues beneath the skin

B. The formation of a clot to plug an opening in an injured blood vessel, stopping blood flow

C. The upper chamber

D. A congenital condition in which a patient lacks one or more of the blood's normal clotting factors

E. Works as two paired pumps

F. The largest artery in the body

G. A condition in which low blood volume results in inadequate perfusion

H. Returns oxygen-rich blood from the lungs to the left atrium

I. Bruising

J. Blood flow to the left and right lungs

K. The lower chamber

L. Bleeding

M. A nosebleed

Multiple Choice

Read each item carefully and then select the one best response.

_____ **1.** The function of the blood is to _____ all of the body's cells and tissues.

   A. remove oxygen from

   B. deliver nutrients to

   C. carry waste products to

   D. hydrate

_____ **2.** The cardiovascular system consists of all of the following EXCEPT:

   A. a pump

   B. a container

   C. fluid

   D. a battery

_____ **3.** Blood leaves each chamber of a normal heart through a(n):

   A. vein

   B. artery

   C. one-way valve

   D. capillary

_____ 4. Blood enters the right atrium from the:
    A. coronary arteries
    B. lungs
    C. vena cava
    D. coronary veins

_____ 5. Blood enters the left atrium from the:
    A. coronary arteries
    B. pulmonary veins
    C. vena cava
    D. coronary veins

_____ 6. Which of the following is NOT a factor in the formation of blood clots?
    A. Pumping function of the heart
    B. Blood stasis
    C. Ability of blood to clot
    D. Changes to the walls of blood vessels

_____ 7. The _____ link(s) the arterioles and the venules.
    A. aorta
    B. capillaries
    C. vena cava
    D. valves

_____ 8. _____ are the key to the formation of blood clots.
    A. Capillaries
    B. White blood cells
    C. Red blood cells
    D. Platelets

_____ 9. Blood contains all of the following EXCEPT:
    A. white blood cells
    B. plasma
    C. cerebrospinal fluid
    D. platelets

_____ 10. _____ is the circulation of blood within an organ or tissue in adequate amounts to meet the cells' current needs for oxygen, nutrients, and waste removal.
    A. Anatomy
    B. Perfusion
    C. Physiology
    D. Conduction

_____ 11. The _____ only require(s) a minimal blood supply when at rest.
    A. brain
    B. kidneys
    C. skeletal muscles
    D. heart

_____ 12. What part of the human body helps the cardiovascular system adapt to changes in order to maintain homeostasis?
    A. Respiratory system
    B. Central nervous system
    C. Autonomic nervous system
    D. Musculoskeletal system

_____ **13.** _____ is inadequate tissue perfusion.

    A. Shock

    B. Hyperperfusion

    C. Hypertension

    D. Contraction

_____ **14.** The brain and spinal cord usually cannot go for more than _____ minutes without perfusion, or the nerve cells will be permanently damaged.

    A. 30 to 45

    B. 12 to 20

    C. 8 to 10

    D. 4 to 6

_____ **15.** Keeping the patient _____ is an important aspect of bleeding and trauma management.

    A. warm

    B. cold

    C. hypotensive

    D. hypertensive

_____ **16.** The body will not tolerate an acute blood loss of greater than _____ of blood volume.

    A. 10%

    B. 20%

    C. 30%

    D. 40%

_____ **17.** If the typical adult loses more than 1 L of blood, significant changes in vital signs, such as _____, will occur.

    A. decreased heart rate

    B. increased respiratory rate

    C. increased blood pressure

    D. improved capillary refill time

_____ **18.** _____ shock is a condition in which low blood volume results in inadequate perfusion or even death.

    A. Hypovolemic

    B. Metabolic

    C. Septic

    D. Psychogenic

_____ **19.** Life-threatening external bleeding demands your immediate attention, even before the _____ has been managed.

    A. fracture

    B. extrication

    C. airway

    D. scene

_____ **20.** The process of blood clotting and plugging the hole is called:

    A. conglomeration

    B. configuration

    C. coagulation

    D. coalition

_____ **21.** Which of the following inhibits the body's ability to control bleeding?

    A. Medications that interfere with normal clotting

    B. Wounds that are extremely small in size

    C. Increased constriction of the blood vessels

    D. Shifting of blood to protect organs

_____ 22. A lack of one or more of the blood's clotting factors is called:
  A. a deficiency
  B. hemophilia
  C. platelet anomaly
  D. anemia

_____ 23. You respond to a 25-year-old man who has cut his arm with a circular saw. The bleeding appears to be bright red and spurting. The patient is alert and oriented and converses with you freely. He appears to be stable at this point. What is your first step in controlling his bleeding?
  A. Direct pressure
  B. Maintaining the airway
  C. Standard precautions
  D. Elevation

_____ 24. When applying a bandage to hold a dressing in place, stretch the bandage tight enough to control the bleeding. You should still be able to _____ after the bandage is secure.
  A. palpate a distal pulse
  B. see bleeding through the dressing
  C. examine the wound
  D. remove the dressing

_____ 25. If bleeding continues after applying a pressure dressing, you should do all of the following EXCEPT:
  A. remove the dressing and apply another sterile dressing
  B. apply manual pressure through the dressing
  C. add more gauze pads over the first dressing
  D. secure both dressings tighter with a roller bandage

_____ 26. When using an air splint to control bleeding in a fractured extremity, you should reassess the _____ frequently.
  A. airway
  B. breathing
  C. circulation in the injured extremity
  D. fracture site

_____ 27. When treating a patient with signs and symptoms of hypovolemic shock and no outward signs of bleeding, always consider the possibility of bleeding into the:
  A. thoracic cavity
  B. abdomen
  C. skull
  D. chest

_____ 28. Which of the following is NOT a cause of nontraumatic internal bleeding?
  A. Ulcer
  B. Ruptured ectopic pregnancy
  C. Aneurysm
  D. Laceration

_____ 29. The most common symptom of internal abdominal bleeding is:
  A. bruising around the abdomen
  B. distention of the abdomen
  C. rigidity of the abdomen
  D. acute abdominal pain

_____ 30. Signs and symptoms of internal bleeding in both trauma and medical patients include:
  A. hematemesis
  B. abrasions
  C. lacerations
  D. avulsions

_____   **31.** The first sign of hypovolemic shock is a change in:
  A. respirations
  B. heart rate
  C. mental status
  D. blood pressure

True/False

If you believe the statement to be more true than false, write the letter "T" in the space provided. If you believe the statement to be more false than true, write the letter "F."

_____   **1.** Venous blood tends to spurt and is difficult to control.

_____   **2.** The human body is tolerant of blood losses of greater than 20% of blood volume.

_____   **3.** The first step in controlling external bleeding is applying pressure to the proximal artery.

_____   **4.** The first step in preparing to treat a bleeding patient is standard precautions.

_____   **5.** A properly applied tourniquet should be loosened by the EMT every 10 minutes.

_____   **6.** You should only loosen a tourniquet if instructed to do so by medical control.

_____   **7.** If a wound continues to bleed after it is bandaged, you should remove the bandage and start over again.

_____   **8.** A tourniquet is always required for massive, spurting blood loss.

_____   **9.** You should provide high-flow oxygen whenever you suspect internal bleeding and signs of shock are present.

Fill-in-the-Blank

Read each item carefully and then complete the statement by filling in the missing words.

1. The _____ side of the heart circulates blood from the body to the lungs.

2. _____ is the circulation of blood within an organ or tissue in adequate amounts to meet the cells' current needs for oxygen, nutrients, and waste removal.

3. A(n) _____ is also called a contusion.

4. _____ bleeding is any bleeding in a cavity or space inside the body.

5. A systolic blood pressure of less than _____ mm Hg with a weak, rapid pulse suggests the presence of hypoperfusion in a patient who may have significant bleeding.

6. _____ is vomited blood.

7. _____ blood is dark red and oozes from a wound steadily but slowly.

8. The _____ _____ system monitors the body's needs from moment to moment and adjusts blood flow by changing the vascular tone, as needed.

9. _____ are small tubes that are about the same diameter as a single red blood cell.

10. All organs depend on the _____ to provide a rich blood supply.

Labeling

Label the following diagrams with the correct terms.

1. The Left and Right Sides of the Heart

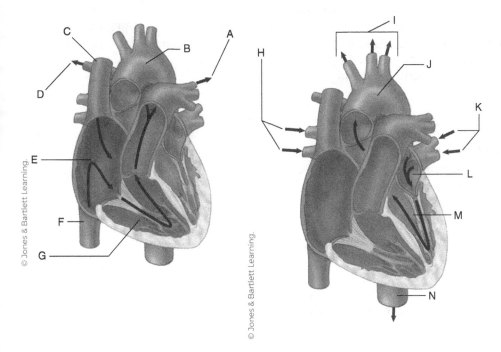

A. _____

B. _____

C. _____

D. _____

E. _____

F. _____

G. _____

H. _____

I. _____

J. _____

K. _____

L. _____

M. _____

N. _____

2. Perfusion

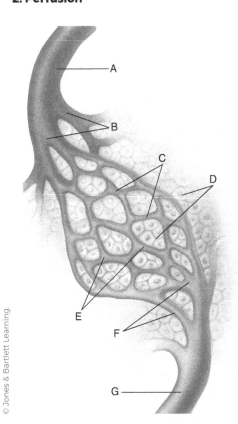

A. _____

B. _____

C. _____

D. _____

E. _____

F. _____

G. _____

Critical Thinking

Multiple Choice

Read each critical-thinking item carefully and then select the one best response.

_____ **1.** You and your partner respond to a patient who has had his hand nearly severed by a drill press. As you approach, you note that the patient is pale, and there appears to be a lot of blood on the floor. The wound continues to bleed copiously. After applying a tourniquet, you write _____ on a piece of adhesive tape and apply it to the patient's forehead.

   A. the patient's name

   B. your last name

   C. the exact time applied

   D. estimated amount of blood loss

_____ **2.** In Question 1, when applying the tourniquet, you must be sure to:

   A. use the narrowest bandage possible to minimize the area restricted

   B. cover the tourniquet with a bandage

   C. never pad underneath the tourniquet

   D. not loosen the tourniquet after you have applied it

_____ **3.** You are called to a playground for an 8-year-old girl who has an uncontrolled nosebleed. The child is crying and will not talk to you. The babysitter and other children present did not witness any trauma, but there is a bump on the temporal portion of the girl's head. The babysitter does state that the girl has had a cold for several days but can give you no further information on her medical history. What could NOT be the possible cause of the bleeding?

   A. A skull fracture

   B. Sinusitis

   C. Coagulation disorder

   D. A temper tantrum

_____ **4.** You respond to a 33-year-old man who was hit in the ear by a line drive during a softball game. He is complaining of a severe headache, ringing in his ears, and dizziness. He has blood draining from his ear. Why would you NOT apply pressure to control bleeding?

   A. It should be collected to be reinfused at the hospital.

   B. It could collect within the head and increase the pressure on the brain.

   C. It is contaminated.

   D. You could fracture the skull with the pressure needed to staunch the flow of blood.

_____ **5.** You are dispatched to a store in the downtown mall for an arm injury. When you arrive, you are directed to a small stockroom where you find a teenage girl holding a blood-soaked cloth tightly on her left forearm. You notice blood droplets high up the wall and on the floor several feet from where she is sitting. "I was opening a shipment with a box cutter," she says, her skin noticeably pale. "And it slipped and cut my arm. The blood spurted everywhere." What type of bleeding should you anticipate?

   A. You should suspect heavy venous bleeding.

   B. She most likely has arterial bleeding.

   C. Internal bleeding is probably causing her skin to appear pale.

   D. Very sharp blades usually only cause capillary bleeding.

Short Answer

Complete this section with short written answers using the space provided.

1. Describe how the autonomic nervous system responds to severe bleeding.

   _____

   _____

   _____

2. Describe the characteristics of bleeding from each type of vessel (artery, vein, capillary).

   _____

   _____

   _____

3. List, in the proper sequence, the methods by which an EMT should attempt to control the external bleeding of an extremity.

   _____

   _____

   _____

4. List at least 10 signs and symptoms of hypovolemic shock.

   _____

   _____

   _____

5. List, in the proper sequence, the general EMT emergency care for patients with internal bleeding.

   _____

   _____

   _____

Ambulance Calls

The following case scenarios provide an opportunity to explore the concerns associated with patient management and to enhance critical-thinking skills. Read each scenario and answer each question to the best of your ability.

1. You arrive at a local school playground for a 9-year-old boy with a minor laceration on his left wrist. The teacher, who is holding a blood-soaked dressing on the boy's wound, tells you that she cannot stop the bleeding and that the boy has a history of hemophilia. The blood is steady, but not spurting, and dark in color.

   How would you best manage this patient?

   _____

   _____

   _____

2. You are dispatched to a local lumberyard for a machinery accident. When you arrive, you observe a man sitting on the ground, surrounded by coworkers. The very pale foreman runs up to you as you get out of the truck and says, "His shirt got caught in a chop saw. His arm got cut off just below the elbow." As you approach, you see that the man is holding a blood-soaked towel to the shortened end of his right arm.

   How would you best manage this patient?

   _____

   _____

   _____

3. Your team is called to the local jail for an inmate who has injured his arm with a ballpoint pen. You find that he is bleeding continuously from a wound that is in the area of the antecubital vein of his left arm.

   How would you best manage this patient?

   _____

   _____

   _____

Fill-in-the-Patient Care Report

Read the incident scenario and then complete the following patient care report (PCR).

You and your partner are posted at the corner of Seventh Street and Brogan Avenue, completing the paperwork for a recent respiratory distress call, when emergency tones burst from the radio:

"Two-fifty-three, priority traffic," the dispatcher says immediately. "Go ahead two-fifty-three," you respond.

"Two-fifty-three, code-three call to 1467 Abner Lane for a leg laceration. Show your time of dispatch at 1653."

You copy the assignment and slowly roll out into traffic after activating the lights and siren, proceeding to the address about six blocks away.

Five minutes later, you pull up outside of a well-kept home in a newly completed subdivision and are met by a woman frantically waving her arms.

"Please hurry!" she shouts as you open your door. "My husband was chopping wood in the backyard and hit himself with the axe. He's bleeding badly!"

You and your partner grab your bags and walk quickly to the home's backyard. The man, whom you estimate to be about 170 pounds (77 kg), is sitting on the redwood deck, pale and shaking, holding a bloody T-shirt against his lower left leg; a huge circle of blood is soaking into the wood deck under him.

"Sir, we're from the city ambulance service, and we're here to help you," you say, kneeling next to the man. "Can you tell me what happened?"

As the 42-year-old man describes how the axe glanced off a knot in the log that he was chopping, sending it deep into the flesh of his leg, you remove the T-shirt from the wound, observing a jagged laceration approximately 3.5 inches (9 cm) long, and replace it with a wide trauma dressing. Your partner begins assessing vitals.

At 1704, your partner reports the patient's vitals: blood pressure is 136/86 mm Hg; pulse is 88 beats/min, strong and regular; respirations are 16 breaths/min with good tidal volume; pale, cool, and diaphoretic skin; and pulse oximetry is 97%.

About 5 minutes after obtaining vitals, you have stopped the bleeding using a pressure bandage and are loading the patient into the ambulance, keeping him covered with a blanket and placing him in a position of comfort.

His wife tells you that he is allergic to amoxicillin and that he has been taking a cholesterol medication called Crestor ever since he suffered a transient ischemic attack in the spring of last year. You thank her for the information and climb into the patient compartment while your partner jumps into the driver's seat. Within a minute, you are en route to the Southside Medical Center emergency department and taking the patient's vitals again. This time they read as follows: blood pressure is 122/76 mm Hg; pulse is 102 beats/min, weak and regular; respirations are 20 breaths/min and shallow but with adequate tidal volume; skin is still pale, cool, and diaphoretic; and pulse oximetry is 94%.

At 1715, you arrive at the ambulance bay of the Southside Medical Center, quickly move the patient inside, and transfer his care to the emergency department staff. After giving a full report to the receiving nurse and properly cleaning and preparing the ambulance, you and your partner become available again at 1735.

Fill-in-the-Patient Care Report

EMS Patient Care Report (PCR)					
Date:	Incident No.:		Nature of Call:		Location:
Dispatched:	En Route:	At Scene:	Transport:	At Hospital:	In Service:
Patient Information					
Age: Sex: Weight (in kg [lb]):			Allergies: Medications: Past Medical History: Chief Complaint:		
Vital Signs					
Time:	BP:		Pulse:	Respirations:	SpO$_2$:
Time:	BP:		Pulse:	Respirations:	SpO$_2$:
Time:	BP:		Pulse:	Respirations:	SpO$_2$:
EMS Treatment (circle all that apply)					
Oxygen @ ____ L/min via (circle one): NC NRM BVM		Assisted Ventilation	Airway Adjunct		CPR
Defibrillation	Bleeding Control	Bandaging	Splinting		Other:
Narrative					

Skills

Skill Drills

Test your knowledge of these skills by filling in the correct words in the photo captions.

Skill Drill 26-1: Controlling External Bleeding

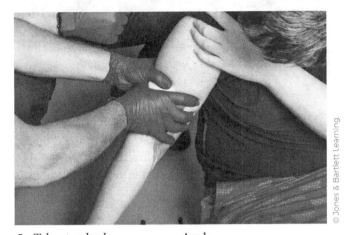

1. Take standard _____. Apply _____ _____ over the wound with a dry, sterile dressing.

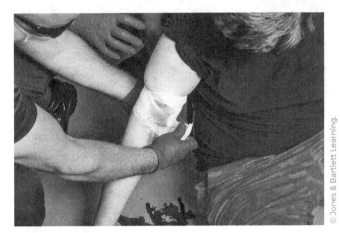

2. Apply a(n) _____ _____.

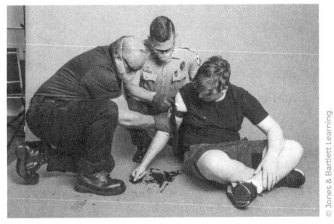

3. If direct pressure with a(n) _____ _____ does not control the bleeding, apply a(n) _____ above the level of the _____.

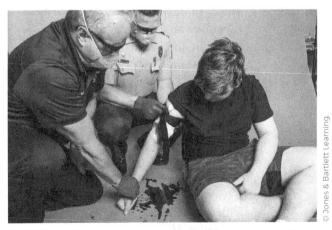

4. Tighten the _____ until bleeding is controlled and _____ are no longer palpable _____ to the tourniquet. Properly position the _____. Apply _____ as necessary. Keep the patient _____. Transport promptly.

Skill Drill 26-3: Applying a MAT Commercial Tourniquet

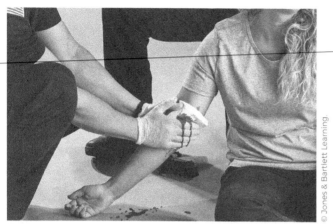

1. Apply _____ over the bleeding site and place the tourniquet _____ to the injury (in the axillary region for upper extremity injuries and at the groin for lower extremity injuries).

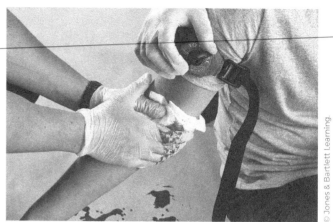

2. Click the buckle into place, pull the strap tight, and turn the tightening dial _____ until pulses are no longer palpable _____ to the tourniquet or until bleeding has been _____.

Assessment Review

Answer the following questions pertaining to the assessment of the types of emergencies discussed in this chapter.

1. When you are performing a scene size-up on a patient with external bleeding, the minimum standard precautions that should be taken are:
   A. gloves and gown
   B. gown and eye protection
   C. gloves and eye protection
   D. gown and face mask

2. For a patient with suspected internal bleeding, you should assess circulation by checking the pulse for:
   A. rate and quality
   B. rate and rhythm
   C. quality and rhythm
   D. presence

3. If you have completed your primary assessment and transport decision on an unresponsive patient with a significant mechanism of injury, what components should be included in the secondary assessment?
   A. Quick check for life-threatening injuries
   B. Detailed, comprehensive exam
   C. Determination of scene safety
   D. A comprehensive reassessment

_____ 4. Your severe external bleeding patient needs a detailed physical exam. When should it be performed?
   A. Immediately after the primary assessment
   B. During the reassessment
   C. When you arrive at the patient's side
   D. En route to the hospital

_____ 5. Why are proper communications to the hospital needed when dealing with a patient with significant bleeding?
   A. Prompts the staff when to schedule breaks
   B. Allows the hospital time to contact the patient's family
   C. Allows the hospital to prepare resources
   D. Encourages good rapport with the staff

CHAPTER 27

Soft-Tissue Injuries

General Knowledge

Matching

Match each of the items in the left column to the appropriate definition in the right column.

_____ 1. Dermis

_____ 2. Sweat glands

_____ 3. Epidermis

_____ 4. Mucous membranes

_____ 5. Sebaceous glands

_____ 6. Abrasion

_____ 7. Laceration

_____ 8. Penetrating wound

_____ 9. Avulsion

_____ 10. Evisceration

A. A puncture caused by an object that pierces, such as a gunshot wound

B. Cool the body by discharging a substance through the pores

C. An injury that separates multiple layers of tissue, tearing them off or leaving a hanging flap

D. A tough external layer forming a watertight covering for the body

E. A jagged cut caused by a sharp object or blunt force that leads to tearing, such as a razor cut

F. Secrete a watery substance that lubricates the openings of the mouth and nose

G. The inner layer of skin that contains the structures that give skin its characteristic appearance

H. Produce oil, which waterproofs the skin and keeps it supple

I. Abdominal wall injury allowing the intestines or other contents to protrude out

J. A wound of the superficial layer of the skin, caused by friction, such as a skinned knee

Multiple Choice

Read each item carefully and then select the one best response.

_____ 1. The _____ is/are our first line of defense against external forces.

    A. extremities

    B. hair

    C. skin

    D. lips

_____ 2. The skin covering the _____ is quite thick.

    A. lips

    B. scalp

    C. ears

    D. eyelids

_____ **3.** As the cells on the surface of the skin are worn away, new cells form in the _____ layer.
  A. dermal
  B. germinal
  C. epidermal
  D. subcutaneous

_____ **4.** The hair follicles, sweat glands, and sebaceous glands are found in the:
  A. dermis
  B. germinal layer
  C. epidermis
  D. subcutaneous layer

_____ **5.** The skin regulates temperature in a cold environment by:
  A. secreting sweat through sweat glands
  B. constricting the blood vessels
  C. dilating the blood vessels
  D. increasing the amount of heat that is radiated from the body's surface

_____ **6.** Closed soft-tissue injuries are characterized by all of the following EXCEPT:
  A. pain at the site of injury
  B. swelling beneath the skin
  C. damage of the protective layer of skin
  D. a history of blunt trauma

_____ **7.** A(n) _____ occurs whenever a blood vessel is damaged and bleeds into the surrounding tissues.
  A. contusion
  B. hematoma
  C. crushing injury
  D. avulsion

_____ **8.** A(n) _____ is usually associated with extensive tissue damage.
  A. contusion
  B. hematoma
  C. crushing injury
  D. avulsion

_____ **9.** _____ develops when edema and swelling result in increased pressure within a closed soft-tissue space.
  A. A hematoma
  B. An avulsion
  C. Compartment syndrome
  D. Ecchymosis

_____ **10.** A(n) _____ occurs when a great amount of force is applied to the body for a long period of time.
  A. contusion
  B. hematoma
  C. crushing injury
  D. avulsion

_____ **11.** More extensive closed injuries may involve significant swelling and bleeding beneath the skin, which could lead to:
  A. compartment syndrome
  B. contamination
  C. obstructive shock
  D. hemothorax

_____ **12.** Open soft-tissue wounds include all of the following EXCEPT:
   A. abrasions
   B. contusions
   C. lacerations
   D. avulsions

_____ **13.** A laceration may be all of the following EXCEPT:
   A. linear
   B. deep
   C. stellate
   D. a scrape

_____ **14.** Because shootings usually end up in court, it is important to factually and completely document:
   A. the statements from witnesses
   B. the suspect's description
   C. the treatment given
   D. the number of shots bystanders say were fired

_____ **15.** All open wounds are assumed to be _____ and present a risk of infection.
   A. contaminated
   B. life threatening
   C. minimal
   D. extensive

_____ **16.** Before you begin caring for a patient with an open wound, you should:
   A. ensure standard precautions
   B. splint potential fractures
   C. notify the hospital
   D. ask about patient medications

_____ **17.** Splinting an extremity, even when there is no fracture, may:
   A. reduce pain
   B. increase damage to an already-injured extremity
   C. make it difficult to move the patient
   D. cause any dressings to move

_____ **18.** Treatment for an abdominal evisceration includes:
   A. pushing the exposed organs back into the abdominal cavity
   B. covering the organs with dry dressings
   C. flexing the knees and legs to relieve pressure on the abdomen
   D. applying moist, adherent dressings

_____ **19.** An open neck injury may result in _____ if enough air is sucked into a blood vessel.
   A. hypovolemic shock
   B. tracheal deviation
   C. an air embolism
   D. an asthma attack

_____ **20.** Burns may result from all of the following EXCEPT:
   A. heat
   B. toxic chemicals
   C. electricity
   D. choking

_____ 21. Which of the following is NOT a factor that can aid in determining the severity of a burn?
   A. The depth of the burn
   B. If the patient is insured
   C. The extent of the burn
   D. Whether critical areas are involved

_____ 22. _____ burns involve only the epidermis.
   A. Full-thickness
   B. Second-degree
   C. Superficial
   D. Third-degree

_____ 23. _____ burns cause intense pain.
   A. First-degree
   B. Second-degree
   C. Superficial
   D. Third-degree

_____ 24. _____ burns may involve the subcutaneous layers, muscle, bone, or internal organs.
   A. Superficial
   B. Partial-thickness
   C. Full-thickness
   D. Second-degree

_____ 25. Significant airway burns may be associated with all of the following EXCEPT:
   A. singeing of the hair within the nostrils
   B. hoarseness
   C. hypoxia
   D. abdominal pain

_____ 26. The most important consideration when dealing with electrical burns is:
   A. standard precautions
   B. scene safety
   C. level of responsiveness
   D. airway

_____ 27. Treatment of electrical burns includes all of the following EXCEPT:
   A. maintaining the airway
   B. monitoring the patient closely for respiratory or cardiac arrest
   C. splinting any suspected injuries
   D. immersion in water

_____ 28. Which of the following should NOT be used as an occlusive dressing?
   A. Gauze pads
   B. Vaseline gauze
   C. Aluminum foil
   D. Plastic wrap

_____ 29. Using elastic bandages to secure dressings may result in _____ if the injury swells or if the bandages are applied improperly.
   A. additional tissue damage
   B. increased edema
   C. increased circulation
   D. further blood loss

_____ **30.** Burns are diffuse soft-tissue injuries created by destructive energy transfers from all of the following sources EXCEPT:

   A. thermal sources

   B. kinetic sources

   C. radiation sources

   D. electrical sources

_____ **31.** _____ is an acute, potentially fatal viral infection of the central nervous system that affects all warm-blooded animals.

   A. Streptococcus

   B. Rabies

   C. Tuberculosis

   D. Emboli

True/False

If you believe the statement to be more true than false, write the letter "T" in the space provided. If you believe the statement to be more false than true, write the letter "F."

_____ **1.** Partial-thickness burns involve the epidermis and some portion of the dermis.

_____ **2.** Blisters are commonly seen with superficial burns.

_____ **3.** Severe burns are usually a combination of superficial, partial-thickness, and full-thickness burns.

_____ **4.** The rule of nines allows you to estimate the percentage of body surface area that has been burned.

_____ **5.** Two factors, depth and extent, are critical in assessing the severity of a burn.

_____ **6.** Your first responsibility with a burn patient is to stop the burning process.

_____ **7.** Burned areas should be immersed in cool water for up to 30 minutes.

_____ **8.** Electrical burns are often more severe than the external signs indicate.

_____ **9.** The hallmark sign of compartment syndrome is severe but painless swelling.

_____ **10.** Occlusive dressings are usually made of Vaseline gauze, aluminum foil, or plastic.

_____ **11.** Gauze pads prevent air and liquids from entering or exiting the wound.

_____ **12.** Elastic bandages should be used to secure dressings.

_____ **13.** Soft roller bandages are slightly elastic, and the layers adhere somewhat to one another.

_____ **14.** Ecchymosis is associated with open wounds.

_____ **15.** A laceration is considered a closed wound.

Fill-in-the-Blank

Read each item carefully and then complete the statement by filling in the missing words.

1. There are three types of ionizing radiation: _____, _____, and _____.

2. A person will sweat in an effort to _____ the body.

3. Nerve endings are located in the _____.

4. When an area of the body is trapped for longer than 4 hours and arterial blood flow is compromised, _____ _____ can develop.

5. In cold weather, blood vessels in the skin will _____.

6. The only exceptions to the rule of not removing an impaled object are an object in the _____ that obstructs breathing and an object in the _____ that interferes with CPR.

7. _____burns can occur when skin is exposed to temperatures higher than _____°F.

8. A(n) _____is an injury in which part of the body is completely severed.

9. The external layer of skin is the _____, and the inner layer is the _____.

10. When the vessels of the skin dilate, heat is _____ from the body.

Labeling

Label the following diagram with the correct terms.

1. Skin

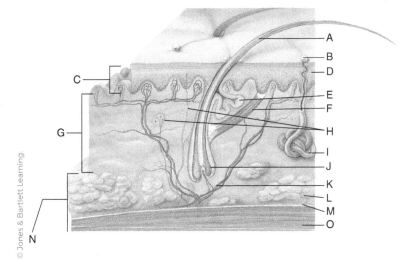

A. _____

B. _____

C. _____

D. _____

E. _____

F. _____

G. _____

H. _____

I. _____

J. _____

K. _____

L. _____

M. _____

N. _____

O. _____

2. Rule of Nines

Label the following diagram with the correct percentage numbers.

A. _____

B. _____

C. _____

D. _____

E. _____

F. _____

G. _____

H. _____

I. _____

J. _____

K. _____

L. _____

M. _____

N. _____

O. _____

P. _____

Q. _____

R. _____

S. _____

T. _____

U. _____

V. _____

W. _____

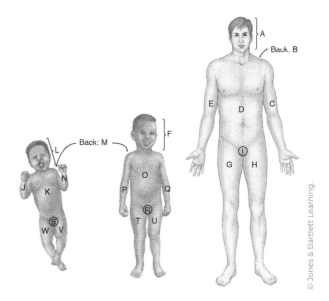

Critical Thinking

Multiple Choice

Read each critical-thinking item carefully and then select the one best response.

_____ 1. You respond to a house fire with the local fire department. They bring a 48-year-old woman out of the house. She is unconscious, but her airway is open. Her breathing is shallow at 30 breaths/min. Her pulse is 110 beats/min, strong and regular. Her blood pressure is 108/72 mm Hg. She has been burned on over 40% of her body. The burned area appears to be dry and leathery. It looks charred and has pieces of fabric embedded in the flesh. You know that this type of burn is considered a:

   A. first-degree burn

   B. second-degree burn

   C. partial-thickness burn

   D. third-degree burn

_____ 2. You respond to a scene where a 24-year-old man has been shot. Law enforcement is on scene, and the scene is safe. As you approach the patient, you notice that he is bleeding from the lower-right abdominal area. He is alert and oriented but seems confused. His airway is open, and he is breathing at a normal rate. His pulse is 120 beats/min, weak and regular. His blood pressure is 98/60 mm Hg. You ask the police officer about the weapon. You need this information because the amount of damage is related to the:

   A. size of the entrance wound

   B. size of the bullet

   C. size of the exit wound

   D. speed of the bullet

_____ 3. You respond to a scene where a 14-year-old girl was playing softball and slid into second base. She states she felt and heard a loud pop. There is no obvious bleeding, but swelling is present. Her pulse is 86 beats/min, and her blood pressure is 114/74 mm Hg. In managing this situation, you decide to use the RICES method of treatment. The "S" stands for:

   A. swelling

   B. soft tissue

   C. splinting

   D. shock

_____ 4. In conducting a more detailed exam on the patient in Question 3, you notice that she has an abrasion on her left knee that she sustained when she slid. The abrasion is covered with dirt and is oozing blood. You know that this injury is classified as:

   A. superficial

   B. deep

   C. full thickness

   D. life-threatening

_____ 5. You decide to manage the injury found in Question 4. You flush the site with sterile water, and it continues to bleed. What would be the best initial way to control the bleeding from this injury?

   A. Elevation

   B. Direct pressure

   C. Tourniquet

   D. Pressure points

Short Answer

Complete this section with short written answers using the space provided.

1. List the three major classifications of depth of burns.

   _____

   _____

   _____

2. List the three general classifications of soft-tissue injuries.

   _____

   _____

   _____

3. Define the acronym RICES.

   R: _____

   I: _____

   C: _____

   E: _____

   S: _____

4. Describe the classification of a severe burn in infants and children.

   _____

   _____

   _____

5. What treatment should be used with a patient who has been burned by a dry chemical?

   _____

   _____

   _____

6. Why are electrical burns particularly dangerous to a patient?

   _____

   _____

   _____

7. Identify the three general types of blast injuries.

   _____

   _____

   _____

8. List the three primary functions of dressings and bandages.

_____

_____

_____

9. List the four types of open soft-tissue injuries.

_____

_____

_____

10. List the five factors used to determine the severity of a burn.

_____

_____

_____

Ambulance Calls

The following case scenarios provide an opportunity to explore the concerns associated with patient management and to enhance critical-thinking skills. Read each scenario and answer each question to the best of your ability.

1. You are dispatched to a residence where a 10-year-old girl fell onto a jagged piece of metal. She has a gaping laceration to the right upper arm that is spurting bright red blood. The mother tried to control the bleeding with a towel, but it kept soaking through.

   How would you best manage this patient?

   _____

   _____

   _____

2. You are dispatched to the home of a 3-year-old boy for an unknown problem. You arrive to find a young mother screaming for your help. She was cooking a meal for her other children when the phone rang. While she was talking, the 3-year-old child grabbed the pot handle, spilling boiling hot water onto his body.

   How would you best manage this patient?

   _____

   _____

   _____

3. You are watching television at the station when a firefighter comes into the room holding his left hand. His wedding ring got caught in a piece of small machinery at the stationhouse, resulting in an avulsion of his ring finger.

   How would you best manage this patient?

   _____

   _____

   _____

Fill-in-the-Patient Care Report

Read the incident scenario and then complete the following patient care report (PCR).

You are just getting back into the ambulance after throwing your lunch bag away when the dispatcher's voice comes across the radio. "Medic Nineteen, priority call, police officer shot at 14th and Berry. Showing you dispatched and responding at 1321."

Your partner, Alicia, fastens her seat belt as you start the truck, and 8 minutes later you arrive at the scene of a traffic stop gone wrong. The intersection is in chaos, police cars block every lane, and you see an obviously dead man hanging from the driver's side door of an old, rusted sedan on the opposite side of the street. You are met by a shaken sergeant who leads you over to a 24-year-old officer who is on the pavement, leaning against the flattened tire of a bullet-riddled patrol car. A motorcycle officer in tall, shining boots is kneeling next to him, holding his hand to the side of the other man's neck; his normally light blue uniform shirt now looks dark purple due to the blood saturation.

"Hang in there, Officer," Alicia says, pulling a nonrebreathing mask from the airway bag and assembling the oxygen cylinder.

You place your gloved hand over the neck wound, and the sergeant has to make the motorcycle officer move away. You use your free hand to fish an occlusive dressing from the jump kit and apply it to the large hole in the officer's neck.

"Am I dying?" the officer asks quietly. His eyes are nearly closed, and his face is pale and sweaty.

"I don't think so," you say as you place a pressure dressing over the occlusive pad while Alicia places the nonrebreathing mask over the man's mouth and nose after setting the flow to 15 L/min. "We're going to do everything that we can for you, though."

Several firefighters on scene help you secure the injured 73-kg (161-lb) officer to a long backboard and load him into the ambulance. You climb into the back, and Alicia slides behind the steering wheel, preparing to drive behind a string of police cars that will be blocking intersections for the entire 9-minute drive to the trauma center.

A quick assessment of the patient shows that he has no injuries other than the apparent gunshot wound to the neck, so you take a baseline set of vital signs as the ambulance begins rolling, a mere 5 minutes after arriving on scene. His blood pressure is 92/60 mm Hg, pulse is 120 beats/min, respirations are 20 breaths/min and shallow, and pulse oximetry is 92%.

"We need to move it, Al," you say to your partner, and you hear the engine grow louder as you cover the officer with blankets and check to make sure that no blood is seeping through the dressing. You then make contact with the trauma center and provide a verbal report and ETA. Four minutes before arriving, you obtain a second set of vital signs and find his blood pressure is 92/58 mm Hg, pulse is 124 beats/min, respirations are still 20 breaths/min and shallow, and pulse oximetry is 94%.

Alicia pulls into the hospital ambulance zone 2 minutes sooner than normal for this transport and unloads the patient. You wheel him into the facility, flanked by grim-faced officers, and pass him to the capable trauma team, providing a brief verbal report to the trauma physician and the charge nurse.

Thirty minutes later, after cleaning and disinfecting the ambulance, you call yourselves available and pull back into the traffic around the downtown medical center.

Fill-in-the-Patient Care Report

EMS Patient Care Report (PCR)					
Date:	Incident No.:		Nature of Call:		Location:
Dispatched:	En Route:	At Scene:	Transport:	At Hospital:	In Service:
Patient Information					
Age: Sex: Weight (in kg [lb]):			Allergies: Medications: Past Medical History: Chief Complaint:		
Vital Signs					
Time:	BP:		Pulse:	Respirations:	SpO₂:
Time:	BP:		Pulse:	Respirations:	SpO₂:
Time:	BP:		Pulse:	Respirations:	SpO₂:
EMS Treatment (circle all that apply)					
Oxygen @ ___ L/min via (circle one): NC NRM BVM		Assisted Ventilation	Airway Adjunct		CPR
Defibrillation	Bleeding Control	Bandaging	Splinting		Other:
Narrative					

Skills

Skill Drills

Test your knowledge of these skills by filling in the correct words in the photo captions.

Skill Drill 27-1: Stabilizing an Impaled Object

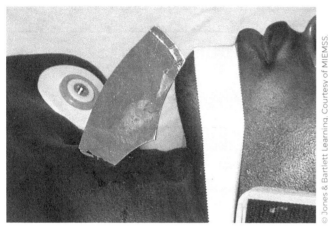

1. Do not attempt to _____ or remove the object. _____ the impaled body part.

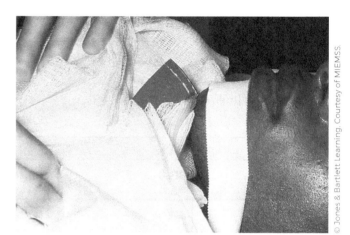

2. Control _____, and stabilize the object in place using _____ _____, gauze, and/or tape.

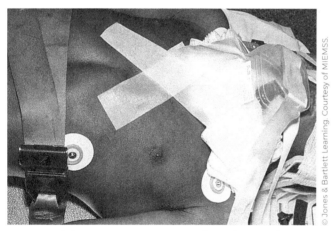

3. Tape a(n) _____ item over the stabilized object to prevent it from _____ during transport.

Skill Drill 27-2: Caring for Burns

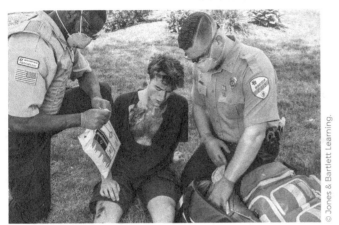

1. Follow _____ precautions to help prevent _____. If safe to do so, remove the _____ from the burning area; extinguish or _____ hot clothing and jewelry as necessary. If the wound is still burning or hot, _____ the hot area in _____, sterile _____, or cover with a wet, cool _____.

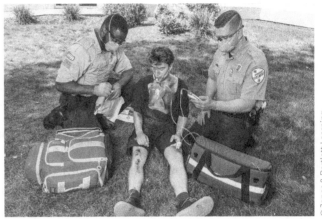

2. Provide high-flow _____, and continue to assess the _____.

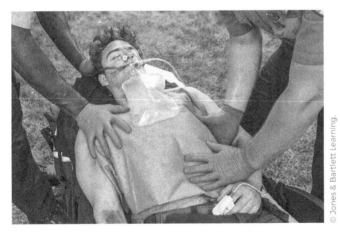

3. Estimate the _____ of the burn, and then cover the area with a(n) _____, sterile dressing or clean _____. Assess and treat the patient for any other _____.

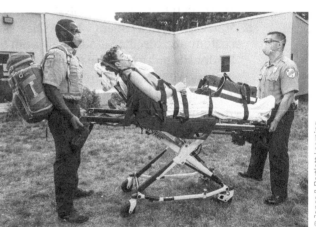

4. Prepare for transport. Treat for _____. Cover the patient with _____ to prevent loss of _____. Transport promptly.

Assessment Review

Answer the following questions pertaining to the assessment of the types of emergencies discussed in this chapter.

_____ 1. During the primary assessment of burns, it is important to remember to:

    A. determine scene safety

    B. obtain vital signs

    C. prevent heat loss

    D. estimate the amount of body surface injuries

_____ 2. You have been dispatched to a residence for a 24-year-old woman who splashed grease on her arm while cooking. As you approach her, she is crying and yelling that it hurts. Her pulse is 130 beats/min and regular. Her blood pressure is 126/86 mm Hg. You decide that she does not require immediate transport. The secondary assessment would include:

    A. proper interventions

    B. an examination of the burned arm

    C. deciding on the patient's priority for transport

    D. an investigation of the chief complaint

_____ 3. During the reassessment of a burn patient with a significant mechanism of injury (MOI), you should:

    A. splint all fractures

    B. determine the transport decision

    C. open all blisters

    D. treat the patient for shock

_____ 4. Your first responsibility in caring for a patient with a burn is to:

    A. stop the burning process

    B. provide complete spinal stabilization

    C. treat for shock

    D. cover burns with moist sterile dressings

_____ 5. You respond to a patient who has been stabbed in the neck. You arrive to find the patient in police custody and bleeding moderately from the neck wound. The patient is alert, oriented, and swearing loudly. His pulse is 120 beats/min. His blood pressure is 124/76 mm Hg. You start to bandage the wound. What type of bandage should you use?

    A. Triangular bandage

    B. Adhesive bandage

    C. Roller bandage

    D. Occlusive bandage

Face and Neck Injuries

General Knowledge

Matching

Match each of the items in the left column to the appropriate definition in the right column.

_____	**1.** Anisocoria	**A.**	Layers of bone within the nasal cavity
_____	**2.** Cornea	**B.**	The light-sensitive area of the eye where images are projected
_____	**3.** Eustachian tube	**C.**	The eyeball
_____	**4.** Globe	**D.**	The eardrum
_____	**5.** Iris	**E.**	The external, visible part of the ear
_____	**6.** Lens	**F.**	The tough, fibrous, white portion of the eye
_____	**7.** Mastoid process	**G.**	Naturally occurring unequal pupils
_____	**8.** Pinna	**H.**	The transparent tissue layer in front of the pupil and iris
_____	**9.** Pupil	**I.**	A bony mass at the base of the skull about 1 inch (2.54 cm) behind the opening to the ear
_____	**10.** Retina	**J.**	Muscle and surrounding tissue behind the cornea that dilate and constrict the pupil
_____	**11.** Sclera	**K.**	The transparent part of the eye through which images are focused on the retina
_____	**12.** Tragus	**L.**	Connects the middle ear to the oropharynx
_____	**13.** Turbinates	**M.**	A small, rounded, fleshy bulge that lies immediately anterior to the ear canal
_____	**14.** Tympanic membrane	**N.**	Cranial nerve that transmits visual information to the brain
_____	**15.** Optic nerve	**O.**	A circular opening in the middle of the iris that admits light to the back of the eye

Multiple Choice

Read each item carefully and then select the one best response.

_____ **1.** As an EMT, your objective when treating patients with face and neck injuries is to do all of the following EXCEPT:

   A. prevent further injury

   B. manage any acute airway problems

   C. control bleeding

   D. disregard the cervical spine

_____ **2.** The head is divided into two parts: the cranium and the:

   A. brain

   B. face

   C. skull

   D. medulla oblongata

_____ 3. The brain connects to the spinal cord through a large opening at the base of the skull known as the:
  A. eustachian tube
  B. spinous process
  C. foramen magnum
  D. vertebral foramina

_____ 4. Approximately _____ of the nose is composed of bone. The remainder is composed of cartilage.
  A. nine-tenths
  B. two-thirds
  C. three-quarters
  D. one-third

_____ 5. Motion of the mandible occurs at the:
  A. temporomandibular joint
  B. mastoid process
  C. chin
  D. mandibular angle

_____ 6. You respond to a 71-year-old woman who is unresponsive. You try to get her to respond but have no success. Her airway is open, and she is breathing at a rate of 14 breaths/min. You know that you can check a pulse on either side of the neck. You know that the jugular veins and several nerves run through the neck next to the trachea. What structure are you trying to locate to take a pulse?
  A. Hypothalamus
  B. Subclavian arteries
  C. Cricoid cartilage
  D. Carotid arteries

_____ 7. The _____ connects the cricoid cartilage and thyroid cartilage.
  A. larynx
  B. cricoid membrane
  C. cricothyroid membrane
  D. thyroid membrane

_____ 8. You respond to a 68-year-old man who was involved in a motor vehicle collision. He is unresponsive, and as you approach, you notice that he is not breathing. He was unrestrained and has massive facial injuries. When you check his airway, it is obstructed. Which of the following is NOT likely to cause an upper airway obstruction in a patient with facial trauma?
  A. Heavy bleeding
  B. Loosened teeth or dentures
  C. Soft-tissue swelling
  D. Inflamed tonsils

_____ 9. You are dispatched to a residential neighborhood for a 6-year-old girl who was bitten by the family pet. The mother meets you at the door with the girl, who is crying uncontrollably and has blood covering the right side of her head. You look at the child and notice that her lower right ear has been completely avulsed. You control the bleeding with direct pressure and bandage the injury. You follow the blood trail back to where the incident occurred and find the avulsed part. How do you manage the avulsed tissue?
  A. Wrap the skin in a sterile dressing, place it in a plastic bag, and keep it cool.
  B. Place the skin in a plastic "biohazard" bag and dispose of it properly.
  C. Place the skin in a plastic bag filled with ice and transport it to the emergency department.
  D. Leave it at the scene to be disposed of later.

_____ 10. The nasal cavity is divided into two chambers by the:
  A. frontal sinus
  B. middle turbinate
  C. zygoma
  D. nasal septum

_____ 11. You are called to the home of a 48-year-old woman who has a history of high blood pressure and now has a major nosebleed. She is alert and oriented and converses freely with you. Her respirations and pulse are within normal limits. Her blood pressure is 194/108 mm Hg. You have been able to rule out trauma. How would you manage the nosebleed?

    A. Apply a sterile dressing.

    B. Pinch the nostrils together.

    C. Place the patient in a supine position.

    D. Have the patient hold ice in her mouth.

_____ 12. The middle ear is connected to the nasal cavity by the:

    A. frontal sinus

    B. zygomatic process

    C. eustachian tube

    D. superior trachea

_____ 13. Which of the following is NOT a sign or symptom of a laryngeal injury?

    A. Hoarseness

    B. Difficulty breathing

    C. Subcutaneous emphysema

    D. Wheezing

_____ 14. Which of the following is NOT a sign of a possible facial fracture?

    A. Bleeding in the mouth

    B. Absent or loose teeth

    C. Bleeding from the forehead

    D. Loose and/or moveable bone fragments

_____ 15. The presence of air in the soft tissues of the neck that produces a crackling sensation is called:

    A. the "Rice Krispies" effect

    B. a pneumothorax

    C. rales

    D. subcutaneous emphysema

_____ 16. Which of the following statements is NOT true regarding the treatment of bleeding from a neck injury?

    A. Apply a circumferential bandage around the neck.

    B. Apply pressure to the bleeding site using a gloved fingertip.

    C. Apply a sterile occlusive dressing.

    D. Use gauze to secure the dressing in place.

_____ 17. What is the main purpose of eye blinking?

    A. Clean the eye

    B. Prevent eye muscle atrophy

    C. Natural reflex to bright light

    D. Refocus the eye

_____ 18. When flushing an eye with saline to remove a foreign object, it is important to remember to:

    A. flush from the outside of the eye in toward the nose

    B. flush from the top of the eye toward the bottom

    C. flush from the nose side of the eye toward the outside

    D. flush only along the bottom of the eye

_____ 19. When stabilizing a large foreign object in the eye, you should first cover the eye with a moist dressing, then:

    A. irrigate the eye with saline

    B. surround the object with a doughnut-shaped collar made from gauze

    C. apply tape around the object and then secure the tape to the forehead

    D. place an ice pack over the eye to reduce swelling

_____ **20.** When a patient has a chemical burn to the eye, you should irrigate the eye for at least 5 minutes; however, if the burn was caused by an alkali or strong acid, you should irrigate for:

A. 10 minutes

B. 15 minutes

C. 20 minutes

D. 25 minutes

True/False

If you believe the statement to be more true than false, write the letter "T" in the space provided. If you believe the statement to be more false than true, write the letter "F."

_____ **1.** Injuries to the face often lead to airway problems.

_____ **2.** Care for facial injuries begins with standard precautions and the ABCs.

_____ **3.** Exposed eye or brain injuries are covered with a dry dressing.

_____ **4.** Clear fluid in the outer ear is normal.

_____ **5.** Any crushing injury of the upper part of the neck likely involves the larynx or the trachea.

_____ **6.** Soft-tissue injuries to the face are common.

_____ **7.** The opening through which the spinal cord leaves the head is called the occiput.

_____ **8.** The muscle that allows movement of the head is the temporomandibular.

_____ **9.** Standard precautions for assessing face and throat injuries should include eye protection and a face mask.

_____ **10.** Stabilization and maintenance of an airway can be difficult in patients with facial injuries.

_____ **11.** Unequal pupil size could possibly indicate a brain injury.

_____ **12.** Gentle irrigation will usually wash out foreign material stuck in the cornea.

_____ **13.** Retinal injuries caused by exposure to extremely bright light are generally painless and may result in permanent damage.

_____ **14.** You should never exert pressure on or manipulate an injured eye in any way.

_____ **15.** Bleeding into the anterior chamber of the eye is commonly called conjunctivitis.

_____ **16.** When dealing with an injured eye, you should always remove contact lenses before treatment.

_____ **17.** Open injuries to the larynx can occur as the result of a stabbing.

_____ **18.** Broken teeth and lacerations to the tongue cause minimal bleeding and are not concerning.

_____ **19.** Oxygen and airway management are important for all patients with face and neck injuries.

Fill-in-the-Blank

Read each item carefully and then complete the statement by filling in the missing words.

1. Pulsations in the neck are felt in the _____ vessels.

2. The _____ vertebrae are in the neck.

3. The _____ regions of the cranium are located on the lateral portion of the head.

4. The _____ connects the oropharynx and the larynx with the main air passages of the lungs.

5. The rings of the trachea are made of _____.

6. The Adam's apple is more prominent in _____ than in _____.

7. The _____ _____ is a large opening at the base of the skull.

8. Blunt trauma that causes fractures to the orbit is commonly called a(n) _____ _____.

9. Trauma to the face and skull that results in the posterior wall of the nasal cavity becoming unstable is caused by

_____ _____ _____.

10. When dealing with an avulsed tooth, handle it by its _____ and not by the _____.

11. A(n) _____ _____ results when an open vein sucks air into it and the air travels to the heart.

Labeling
Label the following diagrams with the correct terms.

1. The Face

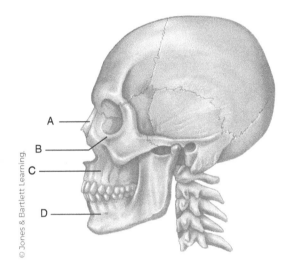

A. _____

B. _____

C. _____

D. _____

2. The Larynx

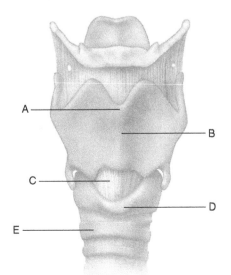

A. _____

B. _____

C. _____

D. _____

E. _____

3. The Eye

A. _____

B. _____

C. _____

D. _____

E. _____

F. _____

G. _____

H. _____

I. _____

J. _____

K. _____

L. _____

M. _____

N. _____

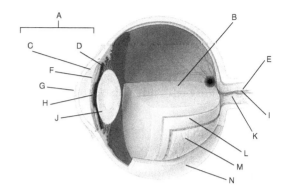

4. The Ear

A. _____

B. _____

C. _____

D. _____

E. _____

F. _____

G. _____

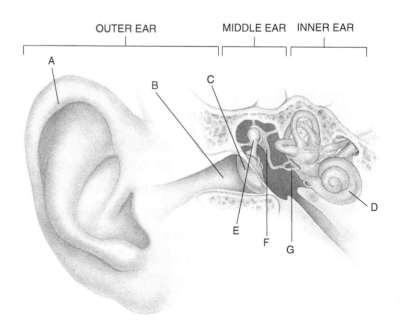

Critical Thinking

Short Answer

Complete this section with short written answers using the space provided.

1. Describe bleeding-control methods for facial injuries.

   _____

   _____

   _____

2. Describe bleeding-control methods for lacerations to veins or arteries in the neck.

   _____

   _____

   _____

3. Explain the physical exam process for evaluation of the eye.

   _____

   _____

   _____

4. List three important guidelines to use when treating an eye laceration.

   _____

   _____

   _____

5. List five eye indications that suggest a closed head injury.

   _____

   _____

   _____

Ambulance Calls

The following case scenarios provide an opportunity to explore the concerns associated with patient management and to enhance critical-thinking skills. Read each scenario and answer each question to the best of your ability.

1. You are dispatched to assist a small child who was attacked by his family's dog. The dog bit the child's face and neck repeatedly, then grabbed him by the neck and shook him violently. The mother found the boy "making funny breathing sounds" and called for help. She has removed the dog from the area.

   How would you best manage this patient?

   _____

   _____

   _____

2. You are dispatched to a 37-year-old man with a large laceration to the right side of his neck. Bleeding is dark and heavy. He is alert but weak.

   How would you best manage this patient?

   _____

   _____

   _____

3. You are dispatched to a Little League baseball game to assist an assault victim. Apparently, emotions were running high when two parents began to argue. You arrive to find a 40-year-old man with a bloody nose.

   How would you best manage this patient?

   _____

   _____

   _____

Skills

Skill Drills

Skill Drill 28-1: Removing a Foreign Object From Under the Upper Eyelid

Test your knowledge of this skill by filling in the correct words in the photo captions.

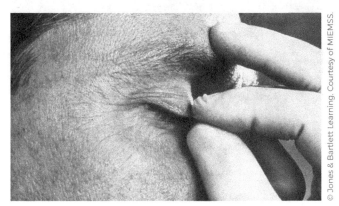

1. Have the patient look _____, grasp the upper _____, and gently pull the _____ away from the eye.

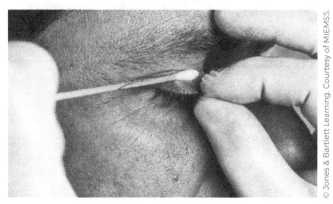

2. Place a cotton-tipped applicator on the _____ surface of the _____ lid.

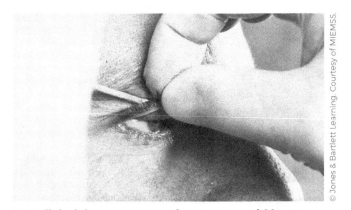

3. Pull the lid _____ and _____, folding it back over the applicator.

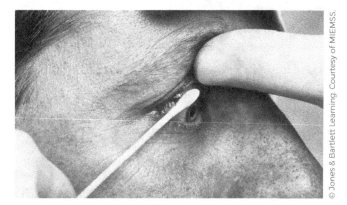

4. Gently remove the foreign object from the eyelid with a moistened, _____, cotton-tipped applicator.

Skill Drill 28-2: Stabilizing a Foreign Object Impaled in the Eye

Test your knowledge of this skill by placing the following photos in the correct order. Number the first step with a "1," the second step with a "2," etc.

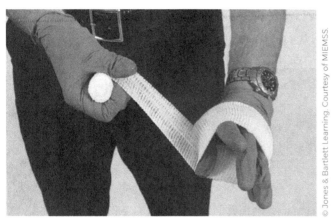

1. _____ Remove the gauze from your hand and wrap the remainder of the gauze roll radially around the ring that you have created.

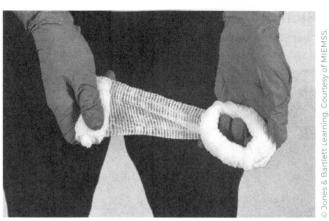

2. _____ Place the dressing over the eye and impaled object to hold the impaled object in place, and then secure it with a roller bandage.

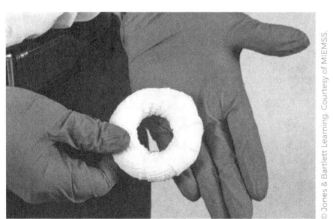

3. _____ To prepare a doughnut ring, wrap a 2-inch roll around your fingers and thumb seven or eight times. Adjust the diameter by spreading your fingers or squeezing them together.

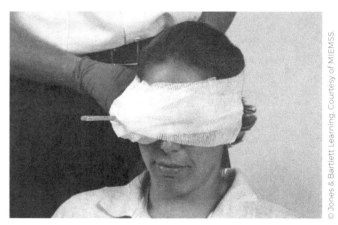

4. _____ Work around the entire ring to form a doughnut.

Assessment Review

Answer the following questions pertaining to the assessment of the types of emergencies discussed in this chapter.

_____ 1. You have responded to a motor vehicle collision and find a 21-year-old man who has massive facial trauma. He is bleeding heavily and is unconscious. The first thing that you do in your treatment of this patient is to:

    A. take cervical spine precautions

    B. open the airway

    C. assess his breathing

    D. take standard precautions

_____ 2. For the patient described in Question 1, how often would you reassess his vitals during your ongoing assessment?

    A. Every 3 minutes

    B. Every 5 minutes

    C. Every 10 minutes

    D. Every 15 minutes

_____ 3. You have a patient who has severe epistaxis. You have been able to rule out trauma. How would you position this patient to help control the bleeding?

    A. Supine

    B. Prone

    C. Sitting leaning back

    D. Sitting leaning forward

_____ 4. You have a patient who has had a tooth knocked out. You find the tooth. How would you transport it to the hospital?

    A. In saline

    B. In dextrose

    C. In ice

    D. In a dry sterile dressing

_____ 5. You respond to a child who has placed a pebble in his ear. He is complaining that his ear hurts. You should:

    A. remove the pebble with a cotton-tipped applicator

    B. have the child try to shake the pebble out

    C. leave the pebble in the ear and transport

    D. not load the patient because this is not an emergency

CHAPTER

29 Head and Spine Injuries

General Knowledge

Matching
Match each of the items in the left column to the appropriate definition in the right column.

_____ 1. Epidural hematoma

_____ 2. Cushing's triad

_____ 3. Subdural hematoma

_____ 4. Retrograde amnesia

_____ 5. Concussion

_____ 6. Anterograde amnesia

_____ 7. Cerebral edema

_____ 8. Connecting nerves

_____ 9. Intervertebral disk

_____ 10. Meninges

A. The temporary loss of the brain's ability to function without actual physical damage

B. Swelling of the brain

C. An inability to remember events after an injury

D. An accumulation of blood between the skull and dura mater

E. Increased blood pressure, decreased pulse, and irregular respirations

F. The three distinct layers of tissue that surround and protect the brain and spinal cord

G. An inability to remember events leading up to a head injury

H. An accumulation of blood beneath the dura mater but outside the brain

I. Located in the brain and spinal cord, these connect the motor and sensory nerves within the skull and spinal canal

J. A cushion that lies between the vertebrae

Multiple Choice
Read each item carefully and then select the one best response.

_____ 1. Which of the following is NOT part of the central nervous system?
   A. The brain
   B. The spinal cord
   C. Cerebrospinal fluid
   D. Cranial nerves

_____ 2. The nervous system is divided into the central nervous system and the:
   A. autonomic nervous system
   B. peripheral nervous system
   C. sympathetic nervous system
   D. somatic nervous system

_____ 3. The brain is divided into the cerebrum, the cerebellum, and the:
   A. foramen magnum
   B. meninges
   C. brainstem
   D. spinal column

_____ **4.** Injury to the head and neck may indicate injury to the:
  A. thoracic spine
  B. lumbar spine
  C. cervical spine
  D. sacral spine

_____ **5.** The _____ is composed of three layers of tissue that suspend the brain and spinal cord within the skull and spinal canal.
  A. meninges
  B. dura mater
  C. pia mater
  D. arachnoid space

_____ **6.** The skull is divided into the cranium and the:
  A. occipital
  B. face
  C. parietal
  D. foramen magnum

_____ **7.** Peripheral nerves include all of the following EXCEPT:
  A. connecting nerves
  B. sensory nerves
  C. motor nerves
  D. the spinal cord

_____ **8.** Which of the following is NOT a function of cerebrospinal fluid?
  A. Acts as a shock absorber
  B. Bathes the brain and spinal cord
  C. Buffers the brain and spinal cord from injury
  D. Provides continuous oxygen to the brain

_____ **9.** The autonomic nervous system is composed of the sympathetic nervous system and the:
  A. peripheral nervous system
  B. central nervous system
  C. parasympathetic nervous system
  D. somatic nervous system

_____ **10.** The most prominent and the most easily palpable spinous process is at the _____ cervical vertebra at the base of the neck.
  A. 7th
  B. 6th
  C. 5th
  D. 4th

_____ **11.** You respond to a 14-year-old boy who fell out of a tree at a local park. He is unresponsive. His airway is open, and respirations are 16 breaths/min and regular. His pulse is strong and regular. Distal pulses are present. You manage the cervical spine. Whom should you NOT ask for help in determining how the injury happened?
  A. First responders
  B. Family members
  C. Bystanders
  D. Curious passersby who did not witness the accident

_____ **12.** Emergency medical care of a patient with a possible spinal injury begins with:
  A. opening the airway
  B. assessing level of consciousness
  C. summoning law enforcement
  D. standard precautions

_____ **13.** The _____ is a tunnel running the length of the spine, which encloses and protects the spinal cord.
  A. foramen magnum
  B. spinal canal
  C. foramen foramina
  D. meninges

_____ **14.** Once the head and neck are manually stabilized, you should assess for:
  A. pulse
  B. motor function
  C. sensation
  D. All of the above

_____ **15.** You are called to a motor vehicle collision where a 27-year-old woman has a bump on her head. You immediately begin manual stabilization of the head. Her airway is open, and respirations are within normal limits. Her pulse is a little fast but strong and regular. Distal pulses are present. You can release manual stabilization when:
  A. the patient's head and torso are in line
  B. the patient is secured to a backboard with the head immobilized
  C. the rigid cervical collar is in place
  D. the patient arrives at the hospital

_____ **16.** One procedure for moving a patient from the ground to the backboard is the:
  A. four-person log roll
  B. lateral slide
  C. four-person lift
  D. push-and-pull maneuver

_____ **17.** You respond to a motor vehicle collision with a 29-year-old woman who struck the rearview mirror and has serious bleeding from the scalp. Her airway is open, and respirations are normal. The pulse is a little rapid but strong and regular. Distal pulses are present, and there is no deformity to the skull. Most bleeding from the scalp can be controlled by:
  A. direct pressure
  B. elevation
  C. pressure point
  D. tourniquet

_____ **18.** Exceptions to using a short spinal extrication device include all of the following EXCEPT:
  A. you or the patient is in danger
  B. the patient is conscious and complaining of lumbar pain
  C. you need to gain immediate access to other patients
  D. the patient's injuries justify immediate removal

_____ **19.** Neck rigidity, bloody cerebrospinal fluid, and headache are associated with what kind of bleeding in the brain?
  A. Epidural hematoma
  B. Subdural hematoma
  C. Intracerebral hematoma
  D. Subarachnoid hemorrhage

_____ **20.** A _____ is a temporary loss or alteration of a part or all of the brain's ability to function without actual physical damage to the brain.
  A. contusion
  B. concussion
  C. hematoma
  D. subdural hematoma

_____ **21.** Which of the following is NOT a symptom of a concussion?

    A. Dizziness

    B. Weakness

    C. Muscle tremors

    D. Visual changes

_____ **22.** Intracranial bleeding outside of the dura mater and under the skull is known as a(n):

    A. concussion

    B. intracerebral hemorrhage

    C. subdural hematoma

    D. epidural hematoma

_____ **23.** The first step in securing a patient to a short backboard is to:

    A. assess pulse, motor function, and sensation

    B. assess the cervical area

    C. provide manual stabilization of the cervical spine

    D. apply an appropriately sized cervical collar

_____ **24.** _____ is the most reliable sign of a head injury.

    A. Vomiting

    B. Decreased level of consciousness

    C. Seizures

    D. Numbness and tingling in extremities

_____ **25.** Hyperventilation should be used with caution in head injury patients and only be attempted when _____ is/are available.

    A. pulse oximetry

    B. capnography

    C. air medical services

    D. noninvasive blood pressure monitoring

_____ **26.** Common causes of head injuries include all of the following EXCEPT:

    A. falls

    B. motor vehicle collisions

    C. seizure activity

    D. sports injuries

_____ **27.** Assessment of mental status is accomplished through the use of the mnemonic:

    A. SAMPLE

    B. OPQRST

    C. AVPU

    D. AEIOU-TIPS

_____ **28.** You respond to a 38-year-old man who fell while rock climbing. He is unconscious, with an open airway. The respiration and pulse rates are within normal limits. His distal pulses are intact. You check his pupils and find that they are unequal. You know this could be a sign of:

    A. brain injury

    B. hypoxia

    C. seizure activity

    D. chronic hypertension

_____ **29.** Which of the following is NOT part of Cushing's triad?

    A. Increased blood pressure

    B. Decreased pulse rate

    C. Decreased pulse oximetry

    D. Irregular respirations

_____ **30.** A cervical collar should be applied to a patient with a possible spinal injury based on:
- **A.** the mechanism of injury
- **B.** the history
- **C.** signs and symptoms
- **D.** All of the above

_____ **31.** Helmets must be removed in all of the following cases EXCEPT:
- **A.** cardiac arrest
- **B.** when the helmet allows for excessive movement
- **C.** when there are no impending airway or breathing problems
- **D.** when a shield cannot be removed for access to the airway

_____ **32.** A vacuum mattress molds to the specific contours of the patient's body and:
- **A.** reduces pressure-point tenderness
- **B.** provides better comfort
- **C.** provides thermal insulation
- **D.** All of the above

True/False

If you believe the statement to be more true than false, write the letter "T" in the space provided. If you believe the statement to be more false than true, write the letter "F."

_____ **1.** An intracerebral hematoma involves bleeding outside the brain tissue.

_____ **2.** If a sensory nerve in the reflex arc detects an irritating stimulus, it will bypass the brain and send a message directly to the motor nerve.

_____ **3.** Voluntary activities are those actions we perform unconsciously.

_____ **4.** The autonomic nervous system is composed of the sympathetic nervous system and the parasympathetic nervous system.

_____ **5.** The parasympathetic nervous system reacts to stress with the fight-or-flight response whenever it is confronted with a threatening situation.

_____ **6.** All patients with suspected head and/or spine injuries should have their heads realigned to an in-line, neutral position when you begin assessing them.

_____ **7.** When assessing a patient for possible spinal injury, you should begin with a full-body scan.

_____ **8.** One procedure for moving a patient from the ground to a backboard is the four-person log roll.

_____ **9.** You should not try to put a patient on a short backboard if the patient is in danger.

_____ **10.** To properly measure a cervical collar, use the manufacturer's specifications.

Fill-in-the-Blank

Read each item carefully and then complete the statement by filling in the missing words.

1. The _____ nerves carry information to the muscles.

2. The dura mater, arachnoid, and pia mater are layers of _____ within the skull and spinal canal.

3. The brain and spinal cord are part of the _____ nervous system.

4. The peripheral nervous system has _____ pairs of spinal nerves.

5. The _____ nerves are the 12 pairs of nerves that emerge from the brainstem and transmit information directly to or from the brain.

6. Vertebrae are separated by cushions called _____ _____.

7. The skull is composed of two groups of bones, the _____ and the _____ bones.

8. The _____ and _____ _____ are the inner two layers of the meninges and are much thinner than the dura mater.

9. The _____ nervous system reacts to stress.

10. The _____ nervous system causes the body to relax.

11. A(n) _____ _____ involves bleeding within the brain tissue itself.

12. A(n) _____ is far more serious than a concussion because it involves physical injury to the brain tissue.

13. When immobilizing a small child, _____ may need to be added to maintain an in-line, neutral position.

14. On completion of spinal immobilization, reassessment of _____, _____, and _____ function in each extremity is necessary.

15. In a patient with a suspected head injury, you should use the _____ method for opening the airway.

Labeling

Label the following diagrams with the correct terms.

1. Brain

A. _____

B. _____

C. _____

D. _____

E. _____

F. _____

G. _____

H. _____

© Jones & Bartlett Learning.

2. Connecting Nerves in the Spinal Cord

A. _____

B. _____

C. _____

D. _____

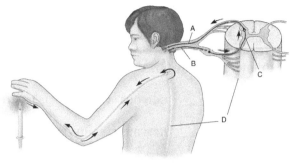

3. Spinal Column

A. _____

B. _____

C. _____

D. _____

E. _____

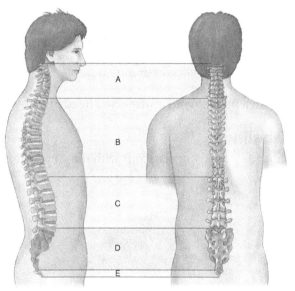

Critical Thinking

Short Answer

Complete this section with short written answers using the space provided.

1. List the 10 mechanisms of injury where you are likely to encounter a head injury.

_____

_____

_____

2. List the reasons for not placing the head and/or spine injury patient's head into a neutral in-line position.

_____

_____

_____

3. What is the difference between a primary brain injury and a secondary brain injury?

_____

_____

_____

4. List at least 10 signs and symptoms of a head injury.

_____

_____

_____

5. List the three general principles for treating a head injury.

_____

_____

_____

6. List the seven questions to ask yourself when deciding whether to remove a helmet.

_____

_____

_____

Ambulance Calls

The following case scenarios provide an opportunity to explore the concerns associated with patient management and to enhance critical-thinking skills. Read each scenario and answer each question to the best of your ability.

1. You are dispatched to a bicycle-versus-car collision. The driver of the car is uninjured, but the bicyclist is reported as "severely injured." You arrive to find the patient lying unconscious in the street and with an apparent head injury. The patient was not wearing a helmet when she was struck by the car. Witnesses say that she was launched into the windshield and then landed in the road.

How would you best manage this patient?

_____

_____

_____

2. You are dispatched to assist a "young child fallen." You arrive to find a frantic parent who tells you that her daughter was playing on the family's trampoline in the backyard. She was bouncing very high and accidentally launched herself off the trampoline, landing facedown on a concrete pad in the neighbor's yard. She responds to painful stimuli and has snoring respirations.

How would you best manage this patient?

_____

_____

_____

3. You are dispatched to a motor vehicle collision with major damage to the patient compartment. Your patient, an 18-month-old boy, is still in his car seat in the center of the back seat. He responds appropriately, and there is no damage to his seat. He has no visible injuries, but a front-seat passenger was killed.

How would you best manage this patient?

_____

_____

_____

Skills

Skill Drills

1. Skill Drill 29-1: Performing Manual In-Line Stabilization

Test your knowledge of this skill by filling in the correct words in the photo captions.

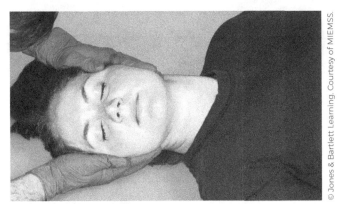

1. Take standard precautions. Kneel behind the patient and firmly place your hands around the _____ of the _____ on either _____.

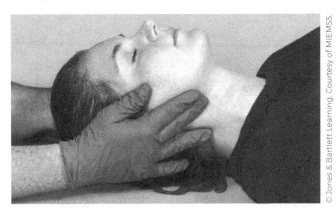

2. Support the lower jaw with your _____ and _____ fingers, and support the head with your _____. Gently lift the head into a(n) _____, _____ position, aligned with the torso. Do not _____ the head or neck excessively, forcefully, or rapidly.

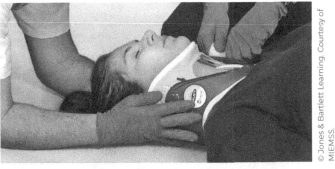

3. Continue to manually _____ the head while your partner places a rigid _____ _____ around the neck. Maintain _____ _____ until you have completely secured the patient to a backboard.

2. Skill Drill 29-3: Securing a Patient to a Long Backboard

Test your knowledge of this skill by placing the following photos in the correct order. Number the first step with a "1," the second step with a "2," etc.

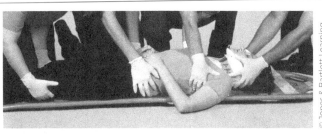

1. _____ Center the patient on the backboard.

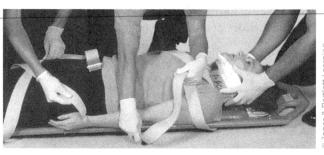

2. _____ Secure the upper torso first.

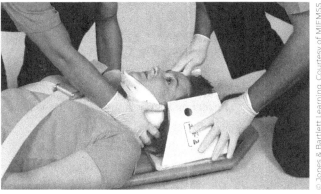

3. _____ Begin to secure the patient's head using a commercial immobilization device or rolled towels.

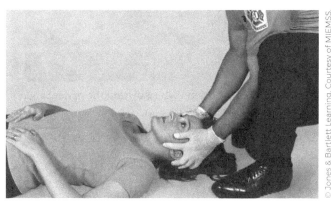

4. _____ Apply and maintain cervical stabilization. Assess distal functions in all extremities.

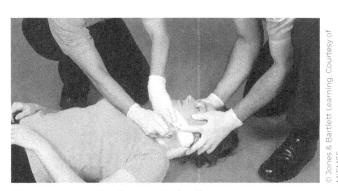

5. _____ Apply a cervical collar.

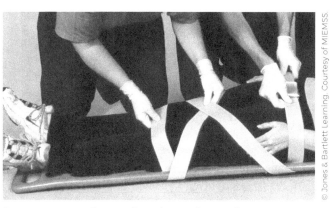

6. _____ Secure the pelvis and upper legs.

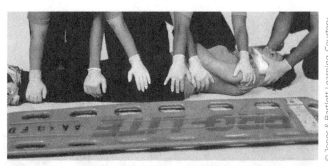

7. _____ Rescuers kneel on one side of the patient and place hands on the far side of the patient.

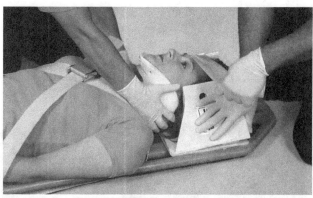

8. _____ Place tape across the patient's forehead to secure the immobilization device.

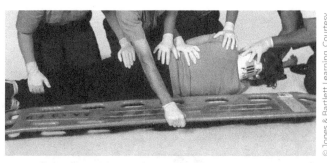

9. _____ On command, rescuers roll the patient toward themselves, quickly examine the back, slide the backboard under the patient, and roll the patient onto the backboard.

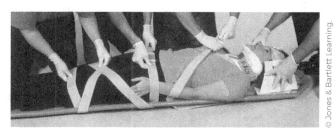

10. _____ Check all straps and readjust as needed. Reassess distal functions in all extremities.

3. Skill Drill 29-5: Securing a Patient Found in a Sitting Position
Test your knowledge of this skill by filling in the correct words in the photo captions.

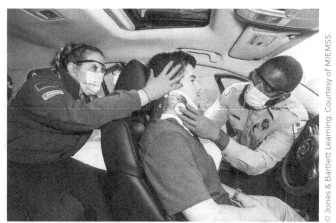

1. Take standard precautions. Stabilize the head and neck in a(n) _____, _____ position. Assess pulse, motor, and sensory function in each extremity. Apply a(n) _____ _____.

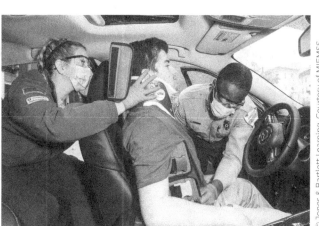

2. Insert an immobilization device between the patient's _____ _____ and the seat.

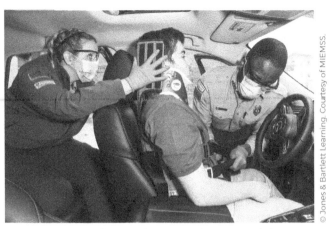

3. Open the side flaps, and position them around the patient's _____, snug around the armpits.

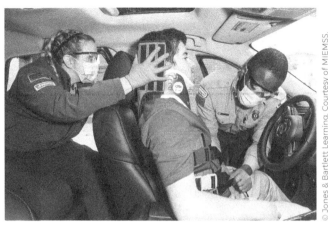

4. _____ Secure the upper torso flaps, then the mid-torso flaps.

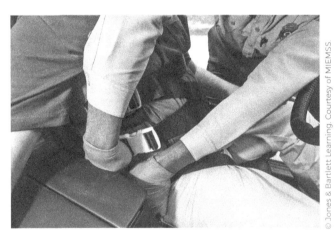

5. Secure the _____ (leg) straps. Check and adjust the _____ straps.

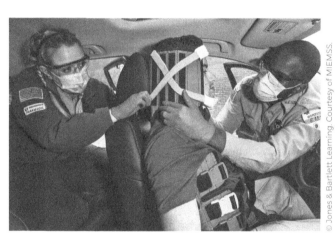

6. _____ between the head and the device as needed. Secure the forehead strap and fasten the _____ head strap around the cervical collar.

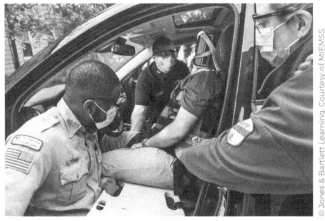

7. Place a long backboard next to the patient's buttocks, _____ to the trunk.

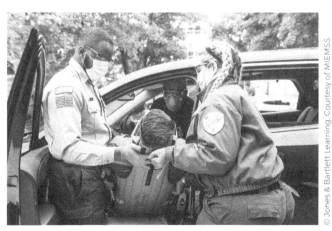

8. Turn and lower the patient onto the long backboard. Lift the _____ and slip the backboard under the immobilization device.

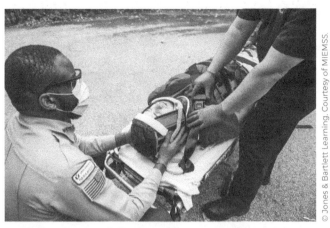

9. Secure the immobilization device and backboard to each other. _____ or _____ the groin straps. Reassess pulse, motor function, and sensory function in each extremity.

4. Skill Drill 29-2: Application of a Cervical Collar
Test your knowledge of this skill by filling in the correct words in the photo captions.

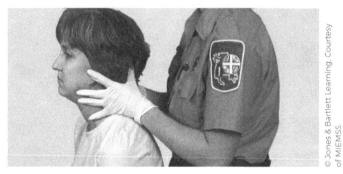

1. Apply in-line _____.

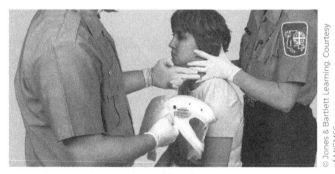

2. Measure the proper _____ _____.

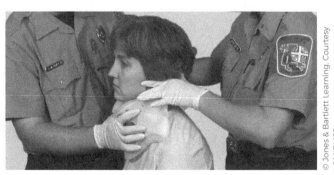

3. Place the _____ _____ first.

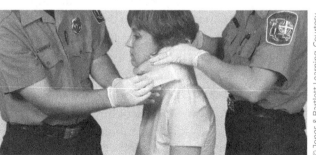

4. _____ the collar around the neck and _____ the collar.

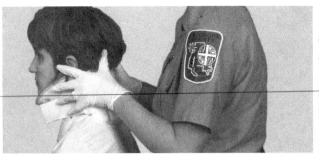

© Jones & Bartlett Learning. Courtesy of MIEMSS.

5. Ensure proper _____ and maintain _____, _____ stabilization until the patient is secured to a(n) _____.

Assessment Review

Answer the following questions pertaining to the assessment of the types of emergencies discussed in this chapter.

_____ **1.** You respond to a patient who was assaulted and is unconscious. On reaching his side, you check his airway, and it is open. Breathing is at 18 breaths/min and regular. Pulse is strong and regular, with distal pulses present. You want to administer oxygen with a nonrebreather mask. At what flow rate would you give it?

    A. 2 L/min

    B. 6 L/min

    C. 10 L/min

    D. 15 L/min

_____ **2.** You and your partner have determined that you need to put the patient from Question 1 in full immobilization. When can your partner release manual stabilization of the head?

    A. When the cervical collar is applied

    B. When the torso is secured to the backboard

    C. When the patient is completely secured to the backboard

    D. When you arrive at the hospital

_____ **3.** You decide to put the patient on a long backboard and use the log-roll technique to accomplish the task. When do you check the patient's back?

    A. After securing the patient to the backboard

    B. As the patient is rolled onto his side

    C. Before any movement is attempted

    D. When you move the patient to the hospital bed

_____ **4.** If you respond to a patient who is in a sitting position and stable, how would you immobilize him or her?

    A. Lay the patient down and perform the log-roll technique.

    B. Use a scoop stretcher.

    C. Use a short backboard.

    D. Have the patient lie down on your backboard.

_____ **5.** You respond to a motorcycle accident. You decide that you need to remove the rider's helmet. What is the minimum number of people required to remove the helmet?

    A. Two

    B. Three

    C. Four

    D. Five

Chest Injuries

General Knowledge

Matching

Match each of the items in the left column to the appropriate definition in the right column.

_____	**1.** Thoracic cage	**A.** Delivering oxygen to the blood by diffusion
_____	**2.** Diaphragm	**B.** The chest
_____	**3.** Ventilation	**C.** The center cavity of the thorax
_____	**4.** Oxygenation	**D.** Separates the chest from the abdomen
_____	**5.** Aorta	**E.** One of the great vessels in the chest; the main artery in the chest
_____	**6.** Closed chest injury	**F.** Usually caused by a penetrating wound
_____	**7.** Hemoptysis	**G.** Rapid respirations
_____	**8.** Pericardium	**H.** Usually caused by blunt trauma
_____	**9.** Open chest injury	**I.** Coughing up blood
_____	**10.** Tachypnea	**J.** The protective membrane around the heart
_____	**11.** Mediastinum	**K.** Moving air in and out of the lungs

Multiple Choice

Read each item carefully and then select the one best response.

_____ **1.** Air is supplied to the lungs via the:

    A. esophagus

    B. trachea

    C. nares

    D. oropharynx

_____ **2.** The _____ separates the thoracic cavity from the abdominal cavity.

    A. diaphragm

    B. mediastinum

    C. xyphoid process

    D. inferior border of the ribs

_____ **3.** On inhalation, which of the following does NOT occur?

    A. The intercostal muscles contract, elevating the rib cage.

    B. The diaphragm contracts.

    C. The pressure inside the chest increases.

    D. Air enters through the nose and mouth.

_____ **4.** You respond to the local rodeo arena for a bull rider. The scene is safe, and the patient is lying unconscious in the middle of the arena. His airway is open, and he is breathing at 20 breaths/min. His pulse is 128 beats/min, and his blood pressure is 110/64 mm Hg. There is no obvious bleeding. Bystanders tell you that he was thrown into the air and landed on the bull's head. He was not wearing a vest. Which of the following injuries is NOT blunt trauma to the chest?

    A. Bruising of the lungs and heart

    B. Fracture of whole areas of the chest wall

    C. Damage to the aorta

    D. Dissection of the carotid arteries

_____ **5.** You respond to a motor vehicle collision and find a 29-year-old woman who is complaining of chest pain. Her chest struck the steering wheel. Her airway is open, she is breathing at 24 breaths/min, and she is coughing up blood. Her pulse is 130 beats/min, rapid and weak, and her blood pressure is 90/58 mm Hg. You notice cyanosis around the lips and note that her fingers are also blue. When you expose the chest, she tells you that it hurts when she takes a breath and points to a bruised spot. Which of the following is a _symptom_ of her chest injury?

    A. Cyanosis around the lips or fingertips

    B. Rapid, weak pulse

    C. Hemoptysis

    D. Pain at the bruised site

_____ **6.** Which of the following is NOT a sign or symptom of a chest injury?

    A. Bruising of the chest wall

    B. Crepitus with palpation of the chest

    C. Clear and equal breath sounds

    D. Unequal expansion of the chest wall

_____ **7.** You respond to an 18-year-old man who has been assaulted with a baseball bat. He was hit once in the chest. He is unresponsive, apneic, and pulseless. This condition is most likely related to:

    A. commotio cordis

    B. cardiac tamponade

    C. pneumothorax

    D. traumatic asphyxia

_____ **8.** Paradoxical motion of the chest refers to:

    A. rib fractures that move with the chest wall during breathing

    B. one segment of the chest wall moving opposite the remainder of the chest

    C. unequal expansion of the chest wall

    D. one segment of the chest wall moving out on inspiration and in on exhalation

_____ **9.** A _____ results when an injury allows air to enter through a hole in the chest wall or the surface of the lung as the patient attempts to breathe, causing the lung on that side to collapse.

    A. tension pneumothorax

    B. hemothorax

    C. hemopneumothorax

    D. pneumothorax

_____ **10.** A sucking chest wound should be treated with:

    A. a standard dressing

    B. taping down of the chest

    C. an occlusive dressing

    D. a sandbag over the wound

_____ 11. You respond to a 20-year-old man who was playing basketball and suddenly developed chest pain and respiratory difficulty. He is alert and oriented and complaining of chest pain. He is breathing at 24 breaths/min. His pulse is 140 beats/min, and his blood pressure is 160/90 mm Hg. When listening to the chest, you notice diminished breath sounds on the left side. This patient is most likely suffering from a(n):

    A. simple pneumothorax

    B. hemothorax

    C. tension pneumothorax

    D. open pneumothorax

_____ 12. Distended jugular veins, a narrowing pulse pressure, and muffled heart sounds are seen in which of the following conditions?

    A. Tension pneumothorax

    B. Cardiac tamponade

    C. Traumatic asphyxia

    D. Commotio cordis

_____ 13. Common signs and symptoms of tension pneumothorax include all of the following EXCEPT:

    A. increasing respiratory distress

    B. distended neck veins

    C. high blood pressure

    D. tracheal deviation away from the injured site

_____ 14. Which of the following statements regarding hemothorax is CORRECT?

    A. It can only be treated by a surgeon.

    B. It results from a collection of air in the pleural space.

    C. Breath sounds tend to be equal.

    D. It is not typically associated with shock.

_____ 15. A _____ is the result of blunt chest trauma and is associated with an irregular pulse and sometimes dangerous cardiac rhythms.

    A. cardiac tamponade

    B. pulmonary contusion

    C. myocardial contusion

    D. traumatic asphyxia

_____ 16. A patient with blunt trauma who is holding the lateral side of his chest and has rapid and shallow respirations is most likely suffering from:

    A. rib fractures

    B. a sternal fracture

    C. a pneumothorax

    D. a pulmonary contusion

_____ 17. Traumatic asphyxia:

    A. is bruising of the lung

    B. occurs when three or more adjacent ribs are fractured in two or more places

    C. is a sudden, severe compression of the chest

    D. results from the pericardial sac filling with blood

_____ 18. _____ can increase intrathoracic pressure, reducing cardiac output and potentially worsening chest injuries such as pneumothorax.

    A. Hypoventilation

    B. Positive pressure ventilation

    C. Hyperventilation

    D. Overventilation

_____ **19.** Which of the following is NOT a pertinent negative to note during your assessment of a patient with chest trauma?

    A. No heart murmurs

    B. No associated shortness of breath

    C. No rapid breathing

    D. No areas of deformity

_____ **20.** Large blood vessels in the chest that can result in massive hemorrhaging include all of the following EXCEPT:

    A. the pulmonary arteries

    B. the femoral arteries

    C. the aorta

    D. the four main pulmonary veins

True/False

If you believe the statement to be more true than false, write the letter "T" in the space provided. If you believe the statement to be more false than true, write the letter "F."

_____ **1.** Dyspnea is difficulty breathing.

_____ **2.** Tachypnea is slow respirations.

_____ **3.** Distended neck veins may be a sign of a tension pneumothorax.

_____ **4.** Rib fractures are especially common in children.

_____ **5.** Narrowing pulse pressure is related to spontaneous pneumothorax.

_____ **6.** Laceration of the large blood vessels in the chest can cause minimal hemorrhage.

_____ **7.** The thoracic cage extends from the lower end of the neck to the umbilicus.

_____ **8.** Patients with spinal cord injuries at C3 or above can lose their ability to breathe.

_____ **9.** A flutter valve is a three-way valve that allows air to leave the chest cavity.

_____ **10.** Open chest injury is caused by penetrating trauma.

_____ **11.** Paradoxical motion can be a sign of a flail segment.

_____ **12.** Because patients with a chest injury have so many risks of mortality, they should be reassessed every 10 minutes.

_____ **13.** You should control external bleeding with direct pressure and a bulky dressing.

_____ **14.** Almost one-third of people who are killed immediately in car crashes die as a result of traumatic rupture of the aorta.

_____ **15.** The right lung contains two lobes, and the left lung contains three lobes.

Fill-in-the-Blank

Read each item carefully and then complete the statement by filling in the missing words.

1. The esophagus is located in the _____ of the chest.

2. During inhalation, the pressure in the chest _____.

3. In the anterior chest, ribs connect to the _____.

4. The trachea divides into the right and left mainstem _____.

5. The _____ nerves supply the diaphragm.

6. Contents of the chest are protected by the _____.

7. The chest extends from the lower end of the neck to the _____.

8. _____ line the area between the lungs and chest wall.

9. An increase in CO_2 in the blood is known as _____.

10. During inhalation, the diaphragm _____.

11. _____ is the body's ability to move air in and out of the chest and lung tissue.

12. The intercostal muscles are innervated from spinal nerves originating in the lower _____ and upper _____ regions of the spinal cord.

13. _____ _____ is the amount of air in mL that is moved into or out of the lungs during a single breath.

14. The _____ _____ may drop as the brain becomes starved for oxygen and overloaded with carbon dioxide and other waste products.

15. A severing of the aorta can occur when the body is exposed to _____ _____.

Labeling

Label the following diagrams with the correct terms.

1. Anterior Aspect of the Chest

A. _____

B. _____

C. _____

D. _____

E. _____

F. _____

G. _____

H. _____

2. Pneumothorax

A. _____

B. _____

C. _____

D. _____

E. _____

F. _____

G. _____

H. _____

© Jones & Bartlett Learning.

Critical Thinking

Short Answer

Complete this section with short written answers using the space provided.

1. List the signs and symptoms associated with a chest injury.

_____

_____

_____

2. Describe the two methods for sealing a sucking chest wound.

_____

_____

_____

3. Describe the method(s) for treating a flail chest segment.

_____

_____

_____

4. Define *traumatic asphyxia* and describe its signs.

_____

_____

_____

5. List the "deadly dozen" chest injuries.

_____

_____

_____

Ambulance Calls

The following case scenarios provide an opportunity to explore the concerns associated with patient management and to enhance critical-thinking skills. Read each scenario and answer each question to the best of your ability.

1. You are dispatched to an area horse ranch for an injury to a rider. You arrive to find that a horse has kicked one of the riders in the chest. The patient is having significant difficulty breathing and appears to be in extreme pain.

How would you best manage this patient?

_____

_____

_____

2. You are dispatched for a man trapped under a car. As you travel to the location, the dispatcher informs you that your patient is now free but is experiencing significant chest and midback pain.

How would you best manage this patient?

_____

_____

_____

3. You are dispatched to a lumberyard where a 27-year-old man was crushed by a piece of heavy equipment. Coworkers pulled the equipment off the patient. He presents with distended neck veins, cyanosis, and bloodshot eyes.

How would you best manage this patient?

_____

_____

_____

Skills

Assessment Review

Answer the following questions pertaining to the assessment of the types of emergencies discussed in this chapter.

_____ **1.** You respond to an accidental shooting of a 37-year-old man. During the primary assessment, you find his airway to be open. His breathing is labored at 24 breaths/min. His pulse is rapid and weak. When exposing the chest, you find a sucking chest wound. Your first priority in caring for this patient should be to:

   A. take a blood pressure reading

   B. seal the wound with an appropriate dressing

   C. continue your assessment

   D. transport the patient immediately

_____ **2.** You respond to a 17-year-old girl who was hit in the chest with a lawn dart. On arrival, she is conscious and able to converse with you. Her airway is open, but her breathing is becoming progressively more difficult. Her pulse is rapid and weak. You can palpate a radial pulse. On examining the chest, you find that she has a penetrating injury to the chest and that there is a sucking sound as she breathes. How do you manage this wound?

   A. Apply oxygen by nasal cannula.

   B. Stabilize the cervical spine.

   C. Use a 4-inch by 4-inch gauze pad.

   D. Use an occlusive dressing.

_____ **3.** When bandaging an open chest wound, what is the minimum number of sides that have to be taped down?

   A. One

   B. Two

   C. Three

   D. Four

_____ **4.** Dispatch sends you to a farm on the edge of town. A 57-year-old man was kicked in the chest by a horse. He walked into his house and collapsed. He is confused and lethargic. His breathing is labored at 28 breaths/min, pulse is rapid and regular, and you are able to palpate a radial pulse. On examining his chest, you notice paradoxical movement on the right chest wall. You should:

   A. provide spinal immobilization

   B. put the patient in a position of comfort

   C. provide oxygen by nasal cannula

   D. provide positive pressure ventilations

_____ **5.** A 16-year-old boy walked into a pipe gate that hit him in the ribs on the left side. On arrival, he is alert and oriented. His breathing is shallow at 22 breaths/min. His pulse is regular and strong. You palpate a radial pulse. You are able to rule out spinal trauma. In which position do you transport him?

   A. Position of comfort

   B. Supine

   C. Prone

   D. Recovery

TRAUMA

Abdominal and Genitourinary Injuries

General Knowledge

Matching

Match each of the items in the left column to the appropriate definition in the right column.

_____ **1.** Closed abdominal injury

_____ **2.** Evisceration

_____ **3.** Flank

_____ **4.** Guarding

_____ **5.** Hollow organs

_____ **6.** Hematuria

_____ **7.** Open abdominal injury

_____ **8.** Peritoneal cavity

_____ **9.** Solid organs

A. Contracting stomach muscles to minimize pain

B. Examples include the liver, pancreas, and spleen

C. Blood in the urine

D. An injury in which a foreign object enters the abdomen and opens the peritoneal cavity to the outside

E. Soft-tissue damage inside the body, but the skin remains intact

F. The posterior region below the margin of the lower rib cage

G. An abdominal cavity

H. Examples include the stomach, small intestine, and ureters

I. Displacement of organs outside the body

Multiple Choice

Read each item carefully and then select the one best response.

_____ **1.** All of the following systems contain organs that make up the contents of the abdominal cavity EXCEPT:

    A. the digestive system

    B. the urinary system

    C. the genitourinary system

    D. the limbic system

_____ **2.** Which of the following is NOT a hollow organ of the abdomen?

    A. Stomach

    B. Liver

    C. Bladder

    D. Ureters

_____ **3.** Which of the following is NOT a solid organ of the abdomen?

    A. Liver

    B. Spleen

    C. Gallbladder

    D. Pancreas

_____ **4.** The first signs of peritonitis include all of the following EXCEPT:

    A. severe abdominal pain

    B. tenderness

    C. muscular spasm

    D. nausea

_____ **5.** Late signs of peritonitis may include:

  A. a soft abdomen

  B. abdominal distention

  C. normal bowel sounds

  D. diarrhea

_____ **6.** _____ take(s) place in the solid organs.

  A. Digestion

  B. Excretion

  C. Endocrine functions

  D. Absorption

_____ **7.** Because solid organs have a rich supply of blood, any injury can result in major:

  A. hemorrhaging

  B. damage

  C. pain

  D. guarding

_____ **8.** The _____ is often injured during motor vehicle collisions, especially in the cases of improperly placed seat belts or impact from the steering wheel, falls from heights or onto sharp objects, and bicycle and motorcycle crashes where the patient hits the handlebars on impact.

  A. pancreas

  B. heart

  C. spleen

  D. colon

_____ **9.** Any air in the peritoneal cavity seeks the most _____ space or void; thus, the location of the air can change with the positioning of the patient.

  A. inferior

  B. superior

  C. distal

  D. proximal

_____ **10.** The abdomen is divided into four:

  A. quadrants

  B. planes

  C. sections

  D. angles

_____ **11.** The largest organ in the abdomen is the:

  A. liver

  B. spleen

  C. pancreas

  D. kidneys

_____ **12.** Open abdominal injuries are also known as:

  A. blunt injuries

  B. collapse injuries

  C. penetrating injuries

  D. peritoneal injuries

_____ **13.** Blunt abdominal injuries may result from:

  A. a stab wound

  B. seat belts

  C. a gunshot wound

  D. an impaled object

_____ **14.** The major complaint of patients with abdominal injury is:

　　A. pain

　　B. tachycardia

　　C. rigidity

　　D. swelling

_____ **15.** A very common early sign of a significant abdominal injury and shock is:

　　A. pain

　　B. tachycardia

　　C. rigidity

　　D. distention

_____ **16.** Late signs of abdominal injury include all of the following EXCEPT:

　　A. distention

　　B. increased blood pressure

　　C. change in mental status

　　D. pale, cool, moist skin

_____ **17.** Your primary concern when dealing with an unresponsive patient with an open abdominal injury is:

　　A. covering the wound with a moist dressing

　　B. maintaining the airway

　　C. controlling the bleeding

　　D. monitoring vital signs

_____ **18.** You respond to an 18-year-old high school football player who was hit in the right flank with a helmet several hours ago. He is complaining of pain in the area. He is alert and oriented. His airway is open, and his respirations are within normal limits. His pulse is rapid and regular. He has a radial pulse. He tells you that he is noticing blood in his urine. Based on this information, the patient is likely to have an injury to the:

　　A. liver

　　B. kidney

　　C. gallbladder

　　D. appendix

_____ **19.** When performing a history on a patient with abdominal trauma, all of the following questions would be appropriate regarding trauma EXCEPT:

　　A. Is there any blood in your stool?

　　B. Does your pain go anywhere?

　　C. Do you have any nausea, vomiting, or diarrhea?

　　D. Are you having trouble with your hearing?

_____ **20.** If the seat belt lies too high, it can do all of the following EXCEPT:

　　A. squeeze abdominal organs

　　B. compress the great vessels

　　C. fracture the lumbar spine

　　D. rupture the appendix

_____ **21.** You are dispatched to a motor vehicle collision. Your patient is a 42-year-old restrained woman. The airbag deployed, and the woman has abrasions on her face. She is complaining of pain to both her chest and abdomen. Her airway is open, and respirations are within normal limits. Her pulse is a little rapid but strong and regular. She has distal pulses. In assessing this patient, which of the following statements is NOT true?

　　A. Bowel sounds may help confirm findings.

　　B. Palpation is typically performed first with light touch.

　　C. If light touch elicits pain, perform deep palpation to assess further injury.

　　D. If you find an entry wound, you should always assess for an exit wound.

_____ **22.** Patients with open abdominal injuries often complain of:

    A. pain

    B. nausea

    C. vomiting

    D. dyspnea

_____ **23.** You are called to the local bar where a fight has taken place. The police department tells you that you have a 36-year-old man who has been stabbed twice in the abdomen. On arrival, the patient is alert and oriented. His airway is open. His respirations are at 24 breaths/min; pulse is rapid, regular, and weak. He has distal pulses. With the penetrating trauma, you should assume that the object has done all of the following EXCEPT:

    A. has penetrated the peritoneum

    B. has entered the abdominal cavity

    C. has possibly injured one or more organs

    D. has damaged only the skin

_____ **24.** When treating a patient with an evisceration, you should:

    A. attempt to replace the abdominal contents

    B. cover the protruding organs with a dry, sterile dressing

    C. cover the protruding organs with adherent dressings

    D. cover the protruding contents with moist, sterile gauze compresses

_____ **25.** The solid organs of the urinary system include the:

    A. kidneys

    B. ureters

    C. bladder

    D. urethra

_____ **26.** All of the following male genitalia lie outside the pelvic cavity EXCEPT:

    A. the urethra

    B. the penis

    C. the seminal vesicles

    D. the testes

_____ **27.** Suspect kidney damage if the patient has a history or physical evidence of all of the following EXCEPT:

    A. an abrasion, laceration, or contusion in the flank

    B. a penetrating wound in the region of the lower rib cage or the upper abdomen

    C. fractures on either side of the lower rib cage

    D. a hematoma in the umbilical region

_____ **28.** Signs of injury to the kidney may include any of the following EXCEPT:

    A. bruises or lacerations on the overlying skin

    B. shock

    C. vomiting

    D. hematuria

_____ **29.** Suspect a possible injury of the urinary bladder in all of the following findings EXCEPT:

    A. bruising to the left upper quadrant

    B. blood at the urethral opening

    C. blood at the tip of the penis or a stain on the patient's underwear

    D. physical signs of trauma on the lower abdomen, pelvis, or perineum

_____ **30.** When treating a patient with an amputation of the penile shaft, your top priority is:

    A. locating the amputated part

    B. controlling bleeding

    C. keeping the remaining tissue dry

    D. delaying transport until bleeding is controlled

_____ **31.** In any case of trauma to a female patient, you should always determine if the patient:
    A. is on birth control
    B. is pregnant
    C. is currently menstruating
    D. has a history of ovarian cysts

_____ **32.** In cases of sexual assault, which of the following is TRUE?
    A. You should always examine the genitalia for any sign of injury.
    B. Advise the patient not to wash, urinate, or defecate.
    C. In addition to recording the facts, it is important to include your personal thoughts.
    D. You should use plastic bags when collecting items such as clothes.

True/False

If you believe the statement to be more true than false, write the letter "T" in the space provided. If you believe the statement to be more false than true, write the letter "F."

_____ **1.** Hollow organs may release free air into the abdomen if injured.

_____ **2.** One of the most common signs of a significant abdominal injury is an elevated pulse rate.

_____ **3.** Patients with abdominal injuries should be kept supine with the head elevated.

_____ **4.** Peritoneal irritation is in response to hollow organ injury.

_____ **5.** Eviscerated organs should be covered with a dry dressing.

_____ **6.** Injuries to the kidneys usually occur in isolation.

_____ **7.** Peritonitis is an inflammation of the peritoneum.

_____ **8.** The abdomen is divided into two quadrants.

_____ **9.** Patients with abdominal pain may want to lie still with their legs drawn up.

Fill-in-the-Blank

Read each item carefully and then complete the statement by filling in the missing words.

1. Severe bleeding may occur with injury to _____ organs.

2. The _____ are filtrations organs and are therefore supplied with large quantities of _____ and prone to bleed heavily when injured.

3. Kidneys are located in the _____ space.

4. A penetrating wound that reaches the kidneys almost always involves _____ _____.

5. When ruptured, the organs of the abdominal cavity can spill their contents into the peritoneal cavity, causing an intense inflammatory reaction called _____.

6. Spilled contents from ruptured hollow organs may irritate the _____ _____ and cause the patient to report abdominal pain.

7. Closed abdominal injuries are also known as _____ _____.

8. Open abdominal injuries are also known as _____ _____.

9. The region below the rib cage and above the hip is called the _____.

10. An open wound that allows internal organs or fat to protrude through the wound is called _____.

Labeling

Label the following diagrams with the correct terms.

1. Hollow Organs

A. _____

B. _____

C. _____

D. _____

E. _____

F. _____

G. _____

H. _____

I. _____

J. _____

K. _____

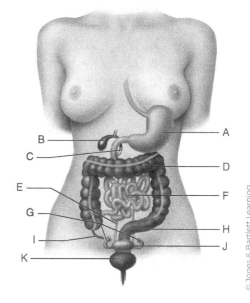

2. Solid Organs

A. _____

B. _____

C. _____

D. _____

E. _____

F. _____

G. _____

H. _____

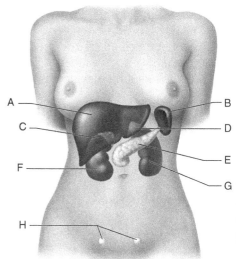

Critical Thinking

Short Answer

Complete this section with short written answers using the space provided.

1. List the hollow organs of the abdomen and urinary system.

_____

_____

_____

2. List the solid organs of the abdomen and urinary system.

_____

_____

_____

3. List the signs and symptoms of an abdominal injury.

_____

_____

_____

4. List the major history or physical findings associated with possible kidney damage.

_____

_____

_____

Ambulance Calls

The following case scenarios provide an opportunity to explore the concerns associated with patient management and to enhance critical-thinking skills. Read each scenario and answer each question to the best of your ability.

1. You are dispatched to a local bar where your patient, a 26-year-old man, was involved in an altercation. He has several superficial lacerations to his arms, and a knife is impaled in his right upper quadrant. He is lying supine on the floor. He is alert. The bar patrons tell you that he did not fall but that they helped him to the floor.

   How would you best manage this patient?

_____

_____

_____

2. You are dispatched to assist police with a mentally ill patient who has threatened harm to himself and others. Police officers found the man running around his home with a knife and blood all over his lower body. The man tells you that "the voices" told him to cut off his penis.

   How would you best manage this patient?

   _____

   _____

   _____

3. You are dispatched to a construction site where a man has fallen onto a piece of rebar. You arrive to find a man sitting on the ground with his legs drawn toward his chest. He tells you that he fell from a ladder onto a piece of rebar. He says, "Something's sticking out of me." As you visualize his abdomen, you can clearly see a portion of his bowel on the outside of his body.

   How would you best manage this patient?

   _____

   _____

   _____

Skills

Assessment Review

Answer the following questions pertaining to the assessment of the types of emergencies discussed in this chapter.

_____ 1. If you are treating a patient with an abdominal evisceration, you should use a(n):

   A. moist, sterile dressing

   B. dry, sterile dressing

   C. adhesive dressing

   D. triangular bandage

_____ 2. You have a male patient who has no immediate life threat but does have bleeding genitalia. You should bandage with a(n):

   A. dry dressing

   B. moist dressing

   C. occlusive dressing

   D. adhesive dressing

_____ 3. You have a patient with suspected kidney injury but no spinal injury. How should he be positioned?

   A. Supine

   B. Prone

   C. Lateral recumbent

   D. Position of comfort

_____ 4. Your patient has his penis caught in his zipper. What do you need to do to relieve the pressure?

   A. Pull the pants off the patient.

   B. Force the zipper open.

   C. Remove the foreskin.

   D. Cut the zipper out of the pants.

_____ 5. Whenever possible, you should always provide the sexual assault patient with:

   A. a police escort

   B. privacy to use the restroom

   C. an attendant of the same gender

   D. the name of the assailant

Orthopaedic Injuries

General Knowledge

Matching

Match each of the items in the left column to the appropriate definition in the right column.

_____	**1.** Skeletal muscle	**A.** A fracture causing deformity or distortion of the injured limb
_____	**2.** Fascia	**B.** Any fracture in which the skin has not been broken
_____	**3.** Smooth muscle	**C.** A thin layer of cartilage covering the articular surface of bones in synovial joints
_____	**4.** Joint	**D.** An involuntary form of muscle found in the gastrointestinal (GI) tract, blood vessels, and other tubular structures of the body.
_____	**5.** Ligaments	**E.** Any break in the bone in which the overlying skin has also been damaged
_____	**6.** Closed fracture	**F.** Bands of fibrous tissue that strengthen joint capsules
_____	**7.** Point tenderness	**G.** Also called striated or voluntary muscle because it is under direct voluntary control of the brain
_____	**8.** Displaced fracture	**H.** The act of pulling on a body structure in the direction of its normal alignment
_____	**9.** Articular cartilage	**I.** Where two bones come into contact
_____	**10.** Open fracture	**J.** Fibrous tissue that covers all skeletal muscle
_____	**11.** In-line traction	**K.** Pain elicited by palpation with a finger at the site of an injury

Multiple Choice

Read each item carefully and then select the one best response.

_____ **1.** Blood in the urine is known as:

  A. hematuria

  B. hemoptysis

  C. hematocrit

  D. hemoglobin

_____ **2.** Smooth muscle is found in the:

  A. back

  B. blood vessels

  C. heart

  D. leg

_____ **3.** The bones in the skeleton produce _____ in the bone marrow.

  A. blood cells

  B. minerals

  C. electrolytes

  D. hormones

_____ **4.** _____ are held together in a tough fibrous structure known as a capsule.
    A. Tendons
    B. Joints
    C. Ligaments
    D. Bones

_____ **5.** Joints are bathed and lubricated by _____ fluid.
    A. cartilaginous
    B. articular
    C. synovial
    D. cerebrospinal

_____ **6.** A _____ is a disruption of a joint in which the bone ends are no longer in contact.
    A. torn ligament
    B. dislocation
    C. fracture-dislocation
    D. sprain

_____ **7.** A _____ occurs when a joint is twisted or stretched beyond its normal range of motion.
    A. dislocation
    B. strain
    C. sprain
    D. torn ligament

_____ **8.** A _____ is a stretching or tearing of the muscle and/or tendon.
    A. strain
    B. sprain
    C. torn ligament
    D. split

_____ **9.** The zone of injury includes all of the following EXCEPT:
    A. adjacent nerves
    B. adjacent blood vessels
    C. surrounding soft tissue
    D. the incident scene

_____ **10.** A(n) _____ fractures the bone at the point of impact.
    A. direct blow
    B. indirect force
    C. twisting force
    D. high-energy injury

_____ **11.** A(n) _____ may cause a fracture or dislocation at a distant point.
    A. direct blow
    B. resultant force
    C. twisting force
    D. high-energy injury

_____ **12.** When caring for patients who have fallen, you must identify the _____ and the mechanism of injury so that you will not overlook associated injuries.
    A. site of injury
    B. height of fall
    C. point of contact
    D. twisting forces

_____ **13.** _____ produce severe damage to the skeleton, surrounding soft tissues, and vital internal organs.
  A. Direct blows
  B. Indirect forces
  C. Twisting forces
  D. High-energy injuries

_____ **14.** Regardless of the extent and severity of the damage to the skin, you should treat any injury that breaks the skin as a possible:
  A. closed fracture
  B. open fracture
  C. nondisplaced fracture
  D. displaced fracture

_____ **15.** A(n) _____ is also known as a hairline fracture.
  A. closed fracture
  B. open fracture
  C. nondisplaced fracture
  D. displaced fracture

_____ **16.** A(n) _____ produces actual deformity, or distortion, of the limb by shortening, rotating, or angulating it.
  A. closed fracture
  B. open fracture
  C. nondisplaced fracture
  D. displaced fracture

_____ **17.** You respond to a 19-year-old woman who was kicked in the leg by a horse. She is alert and oriented. Respirations are 20 breaths/min, regular and unlabored. Pulse is 110 beats/min and regular. Distal pulses are present. She has point tenderness at the site of the injury. You should compare the limb to:
  A. the opposite uninjured limb
  B. one of your limbs or one of your partner's limbs
  C. an injury chart
  D. other limb injuries you have seen

_____ **18.** _____ is the most reliable indicator of an underlying fracture.
  A. Crepitus
  B. Deformity
  C. Point tenderness
  D. Absence of distal pulse

_____ **19.** A(n) _____ fracture occurs in a growth section of a child's bone, which may prematurely stop growth if not properly treated.
  A. greenstick
  B. comminuted
  C. pathologic
  D. epiphyseal

_____ **20.** A(n) _____ fracture is an incomplete fracture that passes only partway through the shaft of a bone but may still cause severe angulation.
  A. greenstick
  B. comminuted
  C. pathologic
  D. epiphyseal

_____ **21.** You are called to the local assisted living facility where a 94-year-old man has fallen. He is alert and oriented and denies passing out. His respirations are 18 breaths/min and regular. Pulse is 106 beats/min, regular and strong. Distal pulses are present. He states that he was walking, heard a pop, and fell to the floor. You suspect a(n) _____ fracture.

    A. greenstick

    B. comminuted

    C. pathologic

    D. epiphyseal

_____ **22.** A(n) _____ fracture is a fracture in which the bone is broken into more than two fragments.

    A. greenstick

    B. comminuted

    C. pathologic

    D. epiphyseal

_____ **23.** Your 24-year-old patient fell off a balance beam and landed on his arm. He is complaining of pain in the upper arm, and there is obvious swelling. You know that swelling is a sign of:

    A. bleeding

    B. laceration

    C. a locked joint

    D. compartment syndrome

_____ **24.** Fractures are almost always associated with _____ of the surrounding soft tissue.

    A. laceration

    B. crepitus

    C. ecchymosis

    D. swelling

_____ **25.** Signs and symptoms of a dislocated joint include all of the following EXCEPT:

    A. marked deformity

    B. tenderness or palpation

    C. locked joint

    D. ecchymosis

_____ **26.** Signs and symptoms of sprains include all of the following EXCEPT:

    A. point tenderness

    B. pain preventing the patient from moving or using the limb normally

    C. marked deformity

    D. instability of the joint indicated by increased motion

_____ **27.** Which of the following is NOT considered one of the 6 Ps of the musculoskeletal assessment?

    A. Pain

    B. Pulselessness

    C. Pressure

    D. Peristalsis

_____ **28.** Which of the following statements about compartment syndrome is FALSE?

    A. It occurs 6 to 12 hours after an injury.

    B. It most commonly occurs with a fractured femur.

    C. It is usually a result of excessive bleeding, a severely crushed extremity, or the rapid return of blood to an ischemic limb.

    D. It is characterized by pain that is out of proportion to the injury.

_____ **29.** Checking neurovascular function is required at all of the following times EXCEPT:

    A. after any manipulation of the limb

    B. before applying a splint

    C. after applying a splint

    D. during history taking

_____ **30.** You respond to a 19-year-old woman who was involved in a motor vehicle collision. She is alert and oriented. Her airway is open, and respirations are 18 breaths/min and unlabored. Pulse is 94 beats/min and is strong and regular. Distal pulses are present. Her upper arm has obvious deformity. You splint the upper arm. You know that splinting will do all of the following EXCEPT:

    A. prevent the need for surgery

    B. make it easier to transfer the patient

    C. help prevent restriction of distal blood flow

    D. reduce pain

_____ **31.** In-line _____ is the act of exerting a pulling force on a body structure in the direction of its normal alignment.

    A. stabilization

    B. immobilization

    C. traction

    D. direction

_____ **32.** Which of the following is NOT a basic type of splint?

    A. Rigid

    B. Formable

    C. Pelvic binder

    D. Sling

_____ **33.** For which of the following should you use a traction splint?

    A. Injuries of the pelvis

    B. An isolated femur fracture

    C. Partial amputation or avulsions with bone separation

    D. Lower leg or ankle injury

_____ **34.** All of the following are hazards of improper splinting EXCEPT:

    A. an increase of distal circulation

    B. a delay in the transport of a patient with a life-threatening injury

    C. a reduction of distal circulation

    D. a compression of nerves, tissues, and blood vessels

_____ **35.** The _____ is one of the most commonly fractured bones in the body.

    A. scapula

    B. clavicle

    C. humerus

    D. radius

_____ **36.** What joint is frequently separated during football and hockey when a player falls and lands on the point of the shoulder?

    A. Glenohumeral joint

    B. Acromioclavicular joint

    C. Sternoclavicular joint

    D. Sacroiliac joint

_____ **37.** Signs and symptoms associated with hip dislocation include all of the following EXCEPT:

    A. severe pain in the hip

    B. lateral and posterior aspects of the hip region are tender on palpation

    C. being able to palpate the femoral head deep within the muscles of the buttock

    D. decreased resistance to any movement of the joint

_____ **38.** There is often a significant amount of blood loss, as much as _____ mL, after a fracture of the shaft of the femur.

    A. 100 to 250

    B. 250 to 500

    C. 500 to 1,000

    D. 1,000 to 1,500

_____ **39.** The knee is especially susceptible to _____ injuries, which occur when abnormal bending or twisting forces are applied to the joint.

   A. tendon

   B. ligament

   C. dislocation

   D. fracture-dislocation

_____ **40.** Signs and symptoms of knee ligament injury include all of the following EXCEPT:

   A. swelling

   B. point tenderness

   C. joint effusion

   D. the affected leg being externally rotated

_____ **41.** Although substantial ligament damage always occurs with a knee dislocation, the more urgent injury is to the _____ artery, which is often lacerated or compressed by the displaced tibia.

   A. tibial

   B. femoral

   C. popliteal

   D. dorsalis pedis

_____ **42.** Because of local tenderness and swelling, it is easy to confuse a nondisplaced or minimally displaced fracture at the knee with a:

   A. tendon injury

   B. ligament injury

   C. dislocation

   D. fracture-dislocation

_____ **43.** Fractures of the tibia and fibula are sometimes associated with _____ as a result of the distorted positions of the limb following injury.

   A. vascular injury

   B. muscular injury

   C. tendon injury

   D. ligament injury

_____ **44.** Dislocation of the _____ is usually associated with fractures of one or both malleoli.

   A. knee

   B. elbow

   C. ankle

   D. hip

True/False

If you believe the statement to be more true than false, write the letter "T" in the space provided. If you believe the statement to be more false than true, write the letter "F."

_____ **1.** All extremity injuries should be splinted before moving a patient unless the patient's life is in immediate danger.

_____ **2.** Splinting reduces pain and prevents the motion of bone fragments.

_____ **3.** It may be necessary to force bone fragments back into place when applying traction.

_____ **4.** When applying traction, the direction of pull is in the direction of the limb's normal alignment.

_____ **5.** Cover wounds with a dry, sterile dressing before applying a splint.

_____ **6.** When splinting a fracture, you should be careful to immobilize only the joint above the injury site.

_____ **7.** One of the steps of the neurologic examination is to palpate the pulse distal to the site of injury.

_____ **8.** White blood cells and platelets are produced in the marrow cavity.

_____ **9.** Compartment syndrome can develop in the forearm in children with a fracture of the humerus.

_____ **10.** Fractures of the distal radius are known as Colles fractures.

Fill-in-the-Blank

Read each item carefully and then complete the statement by filling in the missing words.

1. The _____ is the largest of the tarsal bones.

2. Bone marrow produces _____ _____.

3. The humerus connects with the radius and ulna to form the _____ elbow joint.

4. The _____ is a slender, S-shaped bone attached by ligaments to the sternum on one end and to the acromion process on the other.

5. A patient who has a significant _____ _____ _____ but whose condition appears otherwise stable should also be transported promptly to the closest appropriate hospital.

6. Any damage or open wound in the skin should alert you to the possibility of a(n) _____ _____.

7. The _____ _____ is the largest peripheral nerve in the body; it controls the activity of muscles in the thigh and below the knee.

8. _____ _____ are used to splint the bony pelvis to reduce hemorrhage from bone ends, venous disruption, and pain.

9. A grating or grinding sensation known as _____ can be felt and sometimes even heard when fractured bone ends rub together.

10. A dislocated joint sometimes will spontaneously _____, or return to its normal position.

11. If you suspect that a patient has compartment syndrome, splint the affected limb, keeping it at the level of the heart, and provide immediate transport, reassessing _____ _____ frequently during transport.

Labeling
Label the following diagrams with the correct terms.

1. Pectoral Girdle

A. _____

B. _____

C. _____

D. _____

E. _____

F. _____

G. _____

H. _____

I. _____

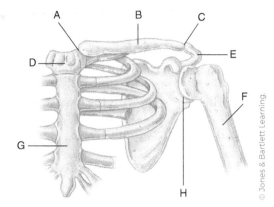

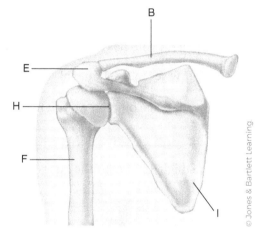

2. Anatomy of the Wrist and Hand

A. _____

B. _____

C. _____

D. _____

E. _____

F. _____

G. _____

H. _____

I. _____

J. _____

K. _____

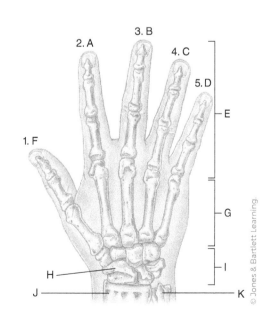

3. Bones of the Thigh, Leg, and Foot

A. _____

B. _____

C. _____

D. _____

E. _____

F. _____

G. _____

H. _____

I. _____

J. _____

K. _____

L. _____

M. _____

N. _____

© Jones & Bartlett Learning.

Critical Thinking

Short Answer

Complete this section with short written answers using the space provided.

1. List the four types of forces that may cause injury to a limb.

_____

_____

2. List at least five of the signs associated with a possible fracture.

_____

_____

_____

3. List the 6 Ps of musculoskeletal assessment.

_____

_____

_____

4. List the general principles of splinting.

_____

_____

_____

5. What are the three goals of in-line traction?

_____

_____

_____

Ambulance Calls

The following case scenarios provide an opportunity to explore the concerns associated with patient management and to enhance critical-thinking skills. Read each scenario and answer each question to the best of your ability.

1. You are dispatched to care for a 17-year-old boy who jumped from the top of a three-story home into a pool. He landed directly on his feet just short of the pool. He is now complaining of low back pain and numbness and tingling of his legs.

How would you best manage this patient?

_____

_____

_____

2. You are called to a local park where an 11-year-old girl fell off the parallel bars onto her right elbow. She is cradling the arm to her chest. She has obvious swelling and deformity in the area. She has good pulse, motor, and sensation at the wrist. ABCs are normal.

How would you best manage this patient?

_____

_____

_____

3. You are dispatched to a fall at a local personal care home. You arrive to find an 82-year-old female complaining of severe pain in her right hip, and the right leg is extended straight out and externally rotated.

How would you best manage this patient?

_____

_____

Skills

Skill Drills
Skill Drill 32-1: Caring for Musculoskeletal Injuries

Test your knowledge of this skill by filling in the correct words in the photo captions.

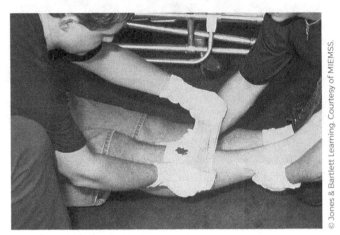

1. Cover open wounds with a(n) _____, _____ dressing and apply pressure to control _____. Assess distal pulse and motor and sensory function. If bleeding cannot be controlled, quickly apply a tourniquet.

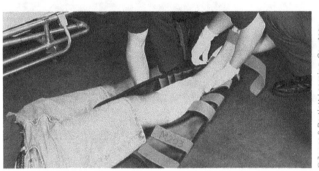

2. Apply a(n) _____, and elevate the extremity about 6 inches (15 cm) (slightly above the level of the heart). Assess distal pulse and motor and sensory function.

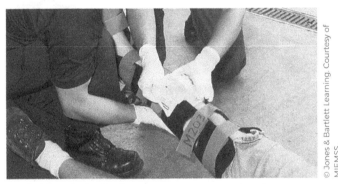

3. Apply cold packs if there is _____, but do not place them directly on the skin.

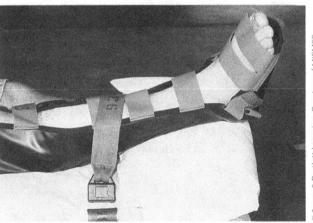

4. Position the patient for transport, and secure the _____ _____.

Skill Drill 32-2: Applying a Rigid Splint

Test your knowledge of this skill by filling in the correct words in the photo captions.

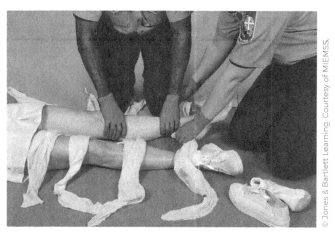

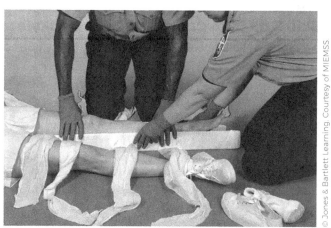

1. Provide gentle _____ and _____ _____ for the limb. Assess distal pulse and motor and sensory function.

2. Place the splint _____ or _____ the limb. _____ between the limb and the splint as needed to ensure even pressure and contact.

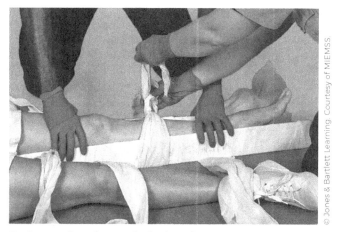

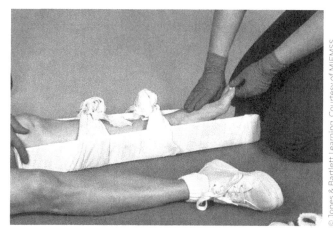

3. Secure the splint to the limb with _____.

4. Assess and record _____ _____ function.

Skill Drill 32-3: Applying a Vacuum Splint

Test your knowledge of this skill by filling in the correct words in the photo captions.

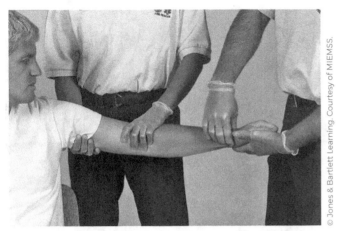

1. Assess distal pulse and motor and sensory function. Your partner _____ and _____ the injury.

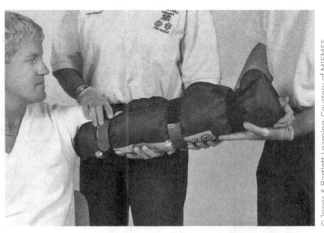

2. Place the splint, and _____ it around the limb.

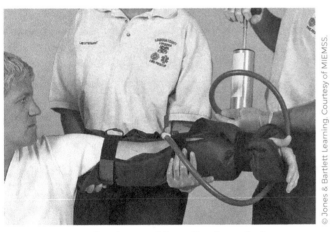

3. _____ the air out of the splint through the _____ _____, and then _____ the valve. Assess distal pulse and motor and sensory function.

Skill Drill 32-5: Applying a Hare Traction Splint

Test your knowledge of this skill by placing the following photos in the correct order. Number the first step with a "1," the second step with a "2," etc.

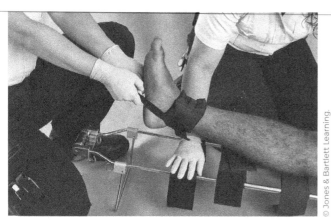

1. _____ Slide the splint into position under the injured limb.

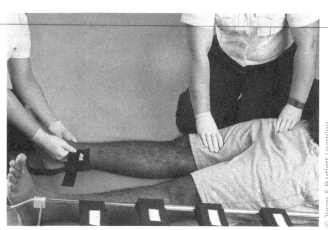

2. _____ Support the injured limb as your partner fastens the ankle hitch about the foot and ankle.

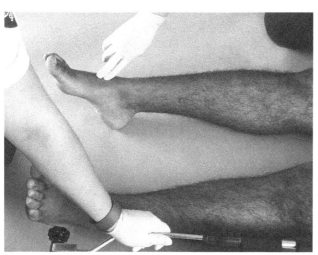

3. _____ Expose the injured limb and check pulse, motor, and sensory function. Place the splint beside the uninjured limb, adjust the splint to proper length, and prepare the straps.

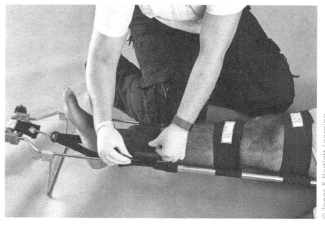

4. _____ Secure and check support straps. Assess pulse and motor and sensory functions.

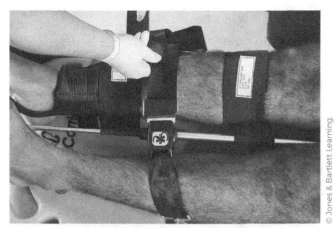

5. _____ Secure the patient and splint to the backboard in a way that will prevent movement of the splint during patient movement and transport. _____

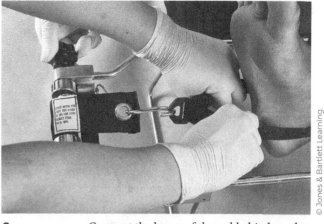

6. _____ Connect the loops of the ankle hitch to the end of the splint as your partner continues to maintain traction. Carefully tighten the ratchet to the point that the splint holds adequate traction.

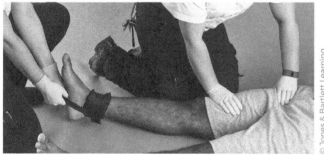

7. _____ Continue to support the limb as your partner applies gentle in-line traction to the ankle hitch and foot.

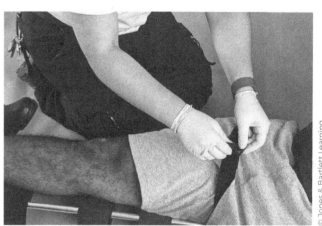

8. _____ Pad the groin and fasten the ischial strap.

Skill Drill 32-4: Splinting the Hand and Wrist

Test your knowledge of this skill by filling in the correct words in the photo captions.

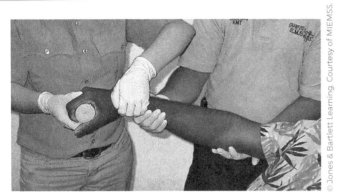

1. Support the injured limb and move the hand into the
_____ of _____. Place a soft _____
_____ in the palm.

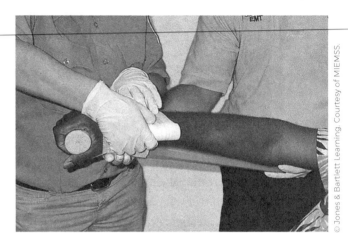

2. Apply a(n) _____ _____ splint on the
_____ side with fingers _____.

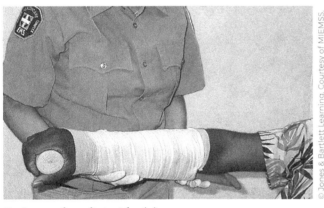

3. Secure the splint with a(n) _____ _____.

Skills

Assessment Review

Answer the following questions pertaining to the assessment of the types of emergencies discussed in this chapter.

_____   **1.** You respond to a motorcycle accident for a 41-year-old man who is unconscious. He has obvious
deformity to both lower legs and is bleeding moderately from an open fracture. His airway is open, and
he is making gurgling noises. Pulse is rapid and weak. Distal pulses are very weak. Your first priority
with this patient is to:

    A. control life-threatening bleeding

    B. apply splints

    C. maintain an airway

    D. apply a pneumatic antishock garment

_____ 2. You have loaded the patient from Question 1 and are en route to the hospital. You have secured the airway and immobilized the fractures. How often should you reassess his vital signs?

    A. Every 3 minutes

    B. Every 5 minutes

    C. Every 10 minutes

    D. Every 15 minutes

_____ 3. You are called to the local junior high school where a 12-year-old boy fell and hurt his wrist. There is obvious deformity. He is alert and oriented. Respirations and pulse are within normal limits. Distal pulse is present. It is important to remember to:

    A. use a zippered air splint

    B. splint in a position of function

    C. splint the wrist only

    D. completely cover the wrist and hand

_____ 4. When you have applied a traction splint and confirmed that pulse, motor, and sensory function are intact, the last thing that you do is:

    A. call in your patient report to the hospital

    B. release traction if the pulse disappears

    C. apply elasticized straps

    D. secure the patient to a backboard

CHAPTER

33 Environmental Emergencies

General Knowledge

Matching

Match each of the items in the left column to the appropriate definition in the right column.

_____ **1.** Conduction

_____ **2.** Air embolism

_____ **3.** Evaporation

_____ **4.** Hyperthermia

_____ **5.** Diving reflex

_____ **6.** Core temperature

_____ **7.** Convection

_____ **8.** Laryngospasm

_____ **9.** Turgor

_____ **10.** Radiation

_____ **11.** Hypothermia

_____ **12.** Ambient temperature

_____ **13.** Heat cramps

_____ **14.** Drowning

_____ **15.** Hymenoptera

A. The slowing of heart rate caused by submersion in cold water

B. The ability of the skin to resist deformation

C. A spasm of the larynx and vocal cords

D. Respiratory impairment from submersion or immersion in liquid

E. Heat transfer between the body and a radiant energy source; examples include standing close to a fire or inside of a cold room

F. Bees, wasps, ants, and yellow jackets

G. A core temperature less than 95°F (35°C)

H. Condition caused by air bubbles in the blood vessels

I. Heat transfer between the body and circulating air; examples include exposure to windy, wintry weather with inadequate thermal insulation

J. Heat transfer between the body and an object or substance that it is in direct contact with; examples include sitting in snow

K. Conversion of any liquid to a gas; examples include the body cooling itself through sweating

L. Painful muscle spasms that occur after vigorous exercise

M. The temperature of the surrounding environment

N. The temperature of the heart, lungs, and vital organs

O. A core temperature greater than 101°F (38.3°C)

Multiple Choice

Read each item carefully and then select the one best response.

_____ **1.** _____ causes body heat to be lost as warm air in the lungs is exhaled into the atmosphere and cooler air is inhaled.

    A. Convection

    B. Conduction

    C. Radiation

    D. Respiration

_____ **2.** Evaporation, the conversion of a liquid to a gas, is a process that requires:

    A. energy

    B. circulating air

    C. a warmer ambient temperature

    D. high humidity

_____ **3.** The rate and amount of heat loss by the body can be modified by all of the following EXCEPT:
   A. increasing heat production
   B. moving to an area where heat loss is decreased
   C. wearing insulated clothing
   D. increasing fluid intake

_____ **4.** The characteristic appearance of blue lips and/or fingertips seen in hypothermia is the result of:
   A. lack of oxygen in venous blood
   B. frostbite
   C. blood vessels constricting
   D. bruising

_____ **5.** Signs and symptoms of severe systemic hypothermia include all of the following EXCEPT:
   A. weak pulse
   B. coma
   C. shivering
   D. very slow respirations

_____ **6.** Hypothermia is more common among all of the following EXCEPT:
   A. older individuals
   B. long-distance athletes
   C. infants and children
   D. those who are already ill

_____ **7.** To assess a patient's core body temperature, pull back your glove and place the back of your hand on the patient's:
   A. abdomen, underneath the clothing
   B. forehead
   C. forearm, on the inside of the wrist
   D. neck, at the area where you check the carotid pulse

_____ **8.** Never assume that a(n) _____, pulseless patient is dead.
   A. apneic
   B. cyanotic
   C. cold
   D. hyperthermic

_____ **9.** Management of hypothermia in the field consists of all of the following EXCEPT:
   A. applying heat packs to the groin, axillary, and cervical regions
   B. removing wet clothing
   C. preventing further heat loss
   D. massaging the cold extremities

_____ **10.** All of the following conditions refer to when exposed parts of the body become very cold, but not frozen, EXCEPT:
   A. frostnip
   B. trench foot
   C. immersion foot
   D. frostbite

_____ **11.** When heat gain exceeds heat loss, _____ result(s).
   A. hyperthermia
   B. heat cramps
   C. heat exhaustion
   D. heatstroke

_____ **12.** Contributing factors to the development of heat illnesses include all of the following EXCEPT:
   A. high air temperature
   B. vigorous exercise
   C. high humidity
   D. increased fluid intake

_____ **13.** When obtaining a SAMPLE history for a patient with a diving emergency, pay special attention to all of the following dive parameters EXCEPT:
   A. depth
   B. length of time the patient was underwater
   C. the time of onset of symptoms
   D. time of day

_____ **14.** Which of the following statements about heat cramps is FALSE?
   A. They only occur when it is hot outdoors.
   B. They may be seen in well-conditioned athletes.
   C. The exact cause of heat cramps is not well understood.
   D. Dehydration may play a role in the development of heat cramps.

_____ **15.** Signs and symptoms of heat exhaustion and associated hypovolemia include all of the following EXCEPT:
   A. cold, clammy skin with ashen pallor
   B. dizziness, weakness, or faintness
   C. normal vital signs
   D. moist oral mucosa

_____ **16.** Most spinal injuries in diving incidents affect the:
   A. cervical spine
   B. thoracic spine
   C. lumbar spine
   D. sacrum/coccyx

_____ **17.** Often, the first sign of heatstroke is:
   A. a change in behavior
   B. an increase in pulse rate
   C. an increase in respirations
   D. hot, dry, flushed skin

_____ **18.** The least common but most serious illness caused by heat exposure, occurring when the body is subjected to more heat than it can handle and normal mechanisms for getting rid of the excess heat are overwhelmed, is:
   A. hyperthermia
   B. heat cramps
   C. heat exhaustion
   D. heatstroke

_____ **19.** _____ is the body's reaction to inhaling very small amounts of water.
   A. Bronchoconstriction
   B. Laryngospasm
   C. Esophageal spasms
   D. Swelling in the oropharynx

_____ **20.** Treatment of drowning and/or near drowning begins with:
   A. opening the airway
   B. ventilation with 100% oxygen via a bag-mask device.
   C. suctioning the lungs to remove the water
   D. rescue and removal from the water

_____ **21.** In a diving emergency, _____ occurs when bubbles of gas, especially nitrogen, obstruct the blood vessels.
- **A.** compression sickness
- **B.** decompression sickness
- **C.** pulmonary sickness
- **D.** nitrogen toxicity

_____ **22.** Young children can drown in as little as _____ of water if left unattended.
- **A.** 1 inch
- **B.** 2 inches
- **C.** 3 inches
- **D.** 4 inches

_____ **23.** You should never give up on resuscitating a cold-water drowning victim because:
- **A.** when the patient is submerged in water colder than body temperature, heat is maintained in the body
- **B.** the resulting hypothermia can protect vital organs from the lack of oxygen
- **C.** the resulting hypothermia raises the metabolic rate
- **D.** heat is conducted from the water to the body

_____ **24.** The three phases of a dive, in the order they occur, are:
- **A.** ascent, descent, and bottom
- **B.** descent, bottom, and ascent
- **C.** orientation, bottom, and ascent
- **D.** descent, orientation, and ascent

_____ **25.** Areas usually affected by descent problems include:
- **A.** the lungs
- **B.** the skin
- **C.** the joints
- **D.** vision

_____ **26.** Potential problems associated with rupture of the lungs include all of the following EXCEPT:
- **A.** air emboli
- **B.** pneumomediastinum
- **C.** pneumothorax
- **D.** hemopneumothorax

_____ **27.** The organs most severely affected by air embolism are the:
- **A.** brain and spinal cord
- **B.** brain and heart
- **C.** heart and lungs
- **D.** brain and lungs

_____ **28.** Black widow spiders may be found in all of the following EXCEPT:
- **A.** New Hampshire
- **B.** woodpiles
- **C.** Georgia
- **D.** Alaska

_____ **29.** Coral snake venom is a powerful toxin that causes _____ of the nervous system.
- **A.** paralysis
- **B.** hyperactivity
- **C.** hypoactivity
- **D.** hemiparesis

_____ **30.** Rocky Mountain spotted fever and Lyme disease are both spread through the tick's:
  A. saliva
  B. blood
  C. hormones
  D. excrement

_____ **31.** Signs of envenomation by a pit viper include all of the following EXCEPT:
  A. swelling
  B. chest pain
  C. ecchymosis
  D. severe burning pain at the site of the injury

_____ **32.** Removal of a tick should be accomplished by:
  A. suffocating it with gasoline
  B. burning it with a lighted match to cause it to release its grip
  C. using fine tweezers to pull it straight out of the skin
  D. suffocating it with Vaseline

_____ **33.** Which of the following statements regarding the brown recluse spider is FALSE?
  A. It is larger than the black widow spider.
  B. It lives mostly in the southern and central parts of the country.
  C. Venom is not neurotoxic.
  D. Bites rarely cause systemic signs and symptoms.

_____ **34.** Treatment of a snakebite from a pit viper includes all of the following EXCEPT:
  A. calming the patient
  B. not giving anything by mouth
  C. marking the skin with a pen over the swollen area to note whether swelling is spreading
  D. providing water to drink

Questions 35–38 are derived from the following scenario: At 1400 in July, the weather is 105°F (41°C) and very humid. You have been called for a "man down" at the park. As you arrive, you recognize him as an alcoholic who has been a "frequent flyer" with your service. As you begin to assess him, his speech is unintelligible, and he is clearly weak and confused.

_____ **35.** As you assess the patient, he has cold, clammy skin and a dry tongue. You suspect that:
  A. he is well hydrated
  B. he has suffered heat exhaustion
  C. he is hypothermic
  D. he has heatstroke

_____ **36.** The patient suddenly loses consciousness, and you note that his skin is flushed, hot, and dry in many areas. You also note that he is no longer actively perspiring. You begin to suspect that his condition has evolved into:
  A. hyperthermia
  B. hypothermia
  C. intoxication
  D. heatstroke

_____ **37.** The direct transfer of heat from the hot air surrounding him to his body is:
  A. conduction
  B. convection
  C. radiation
  D. evaporation

_____ **38.** Treat this patient by doing all of the following EXCEPT:
   A. promote conduction heat loss
   B. promote convection heat loss
   C. remove the patient from the environment
   D. handle him roughly

_____ **39.** Small infants have a poor ability to thermoregulate and are unable to shiver to control heat loss until about the age of:
   A. 4 to 6 months
   B. 6 to 12 months
   C. 12 to 18 months
   D. 18 to 24 months

_____ **40.** Most heatstroke cases occur when the temperature is above _____ and the humidity is 80%.
   A. 80°F (27°C)
   B. 90°F (32°C)
   C. 100°F (38°C)
   D. 110°F (43°C)

_____ **41.** Often, the first sign of heatstroke is a change in _____.
   A. behavior
   B. skin turgor
   C. blood pressure
   D. perspiration

True/False

If you believe the statement to be more true than false, write the letter "T" in the space provided. If you believe the statement to be more false than true, write the letter "F."

_____ **1.** Normal body temperature is 98°F (36.7°C).

_____ **2.** To assess the skin temperature in a patient experiencing a generalized cold emergency, you should feel the patient's skin.

_____ **3.** Mild hypothermia occurs when the core temperature drops to 85°F (29°C).

_____ **4.** The body's most efficient heat-regulating mechanisms are sweating and dilation of skin blood vessels.

_____ **5.** The people who are at greatest risk for heat illnesses are the elderly and children.

_____ **6.** The strongest stimulus for breathing is an elevation of oxygen in the blood.

_____ **7.** Immediate bradycardia after jumping in cold water is called the diving reflex.

_____ **8.** Ice should be promptly applied to any snakebite with swelling.

_____ **9.** The most common type of pit viper is the copperhead.

_____ **10.** Cottonmouths are known for aggressive behavior.

_____ **11.** Ticks should be removed by firmly grasping them with tweezers while rotating them counterclockwise.

_____ **12.** The pain of coelenterate stings may respond to flushing with cold water.

_____ **13.** If you are unsure as to whether a hypothermic patient has a pulse present, palpate the carotid artery for 15 to 20 seconds.

_____ **14.** The goal with the patient with moderate to severe hypothermia is to prevent further heat loss.

_____ **15.** After a lightning strike, you should practice reverse triage.

_____ **16.** Extremes in temperature and humidity are needed to produce hot or cold injuries.

_____ **17.** When approaching a water rescue scene, it is better to drive through moving water than through stagnant water.

_____ **18.** Potential safety hazards in the environment can include wet grass, mud, or icy streets.

_____ **19.** Long-sleeved shirts and long pants are considered dangerous for EMS responders in extreme heat and are not necessary because they provide only minimal protection from exposure.

Fill-in-the-Blank

Read each item carefully and then complete the statement by filling in the missing words.

1. Active rewarming of patients who have _____ to _____ is best accomplished in the emergency department.

2. Most serious diving injuries occur during _____.

3. When treating a patient with frostbite, never attempt _____ if there is any chance that the part may freeze again before the patient reaches the hospital.

4. A patient at an altitude above 8,000 feet (3,048 m) with shortness of breath and cough with pink sputum is likely to be suffering from _____ _____ _____.

5. _____, a common effect of hypothermia, is the body's attempt to increase its heat production.

6. Whenever a person dives or jumps into very cold water, the _____ _____ may cause immediate bradycardia.

7. _____ is the transfer of heat by radiant energy.

8. Mild hypothermia occurs when the core temperature is between _____ and _____.

9. The _____ and _____ systems are the most commonly injured during a lightning strike.

10. _____ is the fifth most common cause of death from isolated environmental phenomena.

11. _____ is a serum containing antibodies that counteracts venom.

12. _____ (bees, wasps, ants, and yellow jackets) stings are painful but are not medical emergencies unless the patient is allergic to the venom.

13. Most snakebites occur between _____ and _____, when the animals are active.

14. In the United States, the most common form of pit viper is the _____.

15. _____ are eight-legged arachnids with a venom gland and stinger at the end of their tails.

16. Tick bites occur most commonly during the _____ months.

17. The first symptoms of Lyme disease are generally fever and flulike symptoms, sometimes associated with a _____ rash.

18. To treat a sting from a jellyfish, pour _____ on the affected area.

19. Coelenterates are responsible for more _____ than any other marine animals.

20. Toxins from the spines of urchins and stingrays are _____ _____.

Critical Thinking

Short Answer

Complete this section with short written answers using the space provided.

1. What are three ways to modify heat loss? Give an example of each.

_____

_____

_____

2. What are the steps in treating heatstroke?

_____

_____

_____

3. What is an air embolism, and how does it occur?

_____

_____

_____

4. For what diving emergencies are hyperbaric chambers used?

_____

_____

_____

5. How should a frostbitten foot be treated?

_____

_____

_____

6. What are four "Do Nots" in relation to local cold injuries?

_____

_____

_____

7. What treatments for a snakebite assist with slowing and monitoring the spread of venom?

_____

_____

_____

8. What are the two most common poisonous spiders in the United States, and how do their bites differ?

_____

_____

_____

Ambulance Calls

The following case scenarios provide an opportunity to explore the concerns associated with patient management and to enhance critical-thinking skills. Read each scenario and answer each question to the best of your ability.

1. You are called to the local airport for a 52-year-old man who is the pilot of his own aircraft. He tells you that he is having severe abdominal pain and joint pain. History reveals that the patient is returning from a dive trip off the coast. He says he has had "the bends" before, and this feels similar.

   How would you best manage this patient?

   _____

   _____

   _____

2. You are dispatched to a long-term care facility for an Alzheimer's patient with an "unknown problem." You arrive to find a staff member who greets you at the front door and escorts you to a resident's room. He explains that the patient wandered out the back exit door of the Alzheimer's unit when the nurse was on her other rounds. They aren't sure how this happened because each patient wears a necklace that triggers an alarm if the patient leaves this specialized wing of the facility. They found the man outside in the snow, and he was possibly outdoors for 45 minutes.

   How would you best manage this patient?

   _____

   _____

   _____

3. You are dispatched to the local high school for a "person down." On arrival, you are directed to the football field, where the team is practicing for an upcoming game. You find a 16-year-old boy sitting on the bench, confused and lethargic. The coach tells you that they have been practicing for a couple of hours, and the temperature is 97°F (36°C). He says that he has encouraged the guys to drink continuously and that he thought they were all well hydrated. During your assessment of the patient, you notice that his skin is cool and clammy, with a rapid, weak pulse. His temperature is 102.9°F (39.4°C) orally. He says he is thirsty but also feels nauseated, so he stopped drinking a while ago.

   How would you best manage this patient?

   _____

   _____

   _____

Skills

Skill Drills

Skill Drill 33-1: Treating for Heat Exhaustion

Test your knowledge of this skill by filling in the correct words in the photo captions.

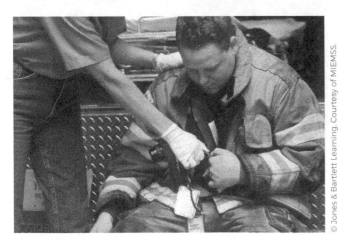

© Jones & Bartlett Learning. Courtesy of MIEMSS.

1. Move the patient to a(n) _____ _____.
Remove extra _____.

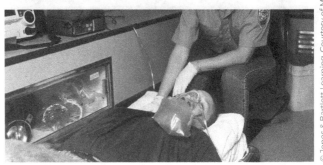

© Jones & Bartlett Learning. Courtesy of MIEMSS.

2. Give _____ if indicated. Check the patient's blood glucose level if indicated. Perform cold-water immersion or other cooling measures as available. Place the patient in a(n) _____ position and fan the patient.

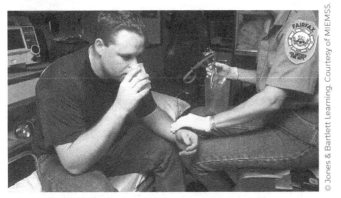

© Jones & Bartlett Learning. Courtesy of MIEMSS.

3. If the patient is fully alert, give _____ by mouth.

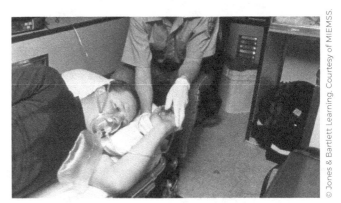

© Jones & Bartlett Learning. Courtesy of MIEMSS.

4. If _____ develops, secure and transport the patient on his or her left side.

Skill Drill 33-2: Stabilizing a Suspected Spinal Injury in the Water

Test your knowledge of this skill by placing the following photos in the correct order. Number the first step with a "1," the second step with a "2," etc.

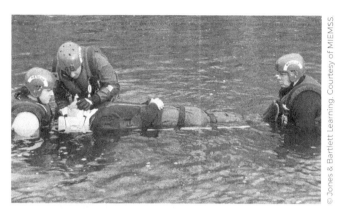

1. _____ Secure the patient to the backboard.

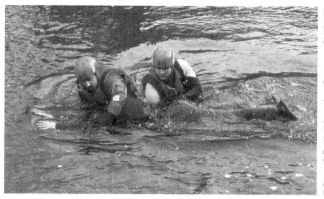

2. _____ Turn the patient to a supine position by rotating the entire upper half of the body as a single unit.

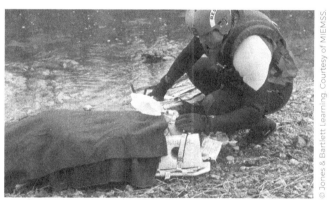

3. _____ Maintain the body's normal temperature and apply oxygen if the patient is breathing. Begin CPR if breathing and pulse are absent.

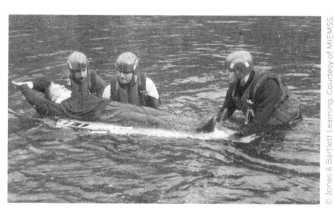

4. _____ Float a buoyant backboard under the patient.

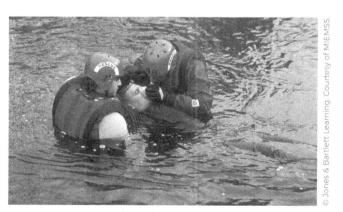

5. _____ As soon as the patient is turned, begin artificial ventilation using the mouth-to-mouth method or a pocket mask.

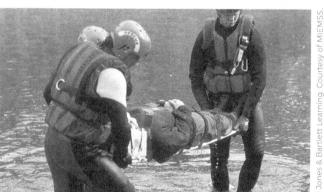

6. _____ Remove the patient from the water.

Assessment Review

Answer the following questions pertaining to the assessment of the types of emergencies discussed in this chapter.

_____ **1.** Most frostbitten parts are:

   A. soft and moist

   B. hard and waxy

   C. soft and waxy

   D. hard and moist

_____ **2.** If a patient has a cold skin temperature, he or she is likely:

   A. hypothermic

   B. hyperthermic

   C. hypovolemic

   D. hypoglycemic

_____ **3.** If a patient has a hot skin temperature, he or she is likely:

   A. hypothermic

   B. hyperthermic

   C. hypoglycemic

   D. hypervolemic

_____ **4.** When treating multiple victims of lightning strikes, whom should you concentrate your efforts on first?

   A. Conscious patients

   B. Unconscious patients in respiratory or cardiac arrest

   C. All unconscious patients

   D. Conscious patients with burn wounds.

_____ **5.** What is the best method of inactivating a jellyfish sting?

   A. Urinating on it

   B. Flushing the site with cold water

   C. Applying vinegar

   D. Applying an ice pack

CHAPTER

Obstetrics and Neonatal Care

34

General Knowledge

Matching

Match each of the items in the left column to the appropriate definition in the right column.

_____	**1.** Cervix	**A.** An umbilical cord that is wrapped around the infant's neck
_____	**2.** Crowning	**B.** A fluid-filled, baglike membrane inside the uterus in which the fetus develops
_____	**3.** Placenta	**C.** The appearance of the infant's head at the vaginal opening during labor
_____	**4.** Amniotic sac	**D.** The lower third of the uterus
_____	**5.** Fetus	**E.** Connects mother and infant through the placenta
_____	**6.** Embryo	**F.** The sensation felt by a pregnant patient when the fetus descends in the pelvis and positions itself for delivery
_____	**7.** Primigravida	**G.** The body part of the infant that is delivered first
_____	**8.** Umbilical cord	**H.** The stage from 0 to 10 weeks after fertilization
_____	**9.** Lightening	**I.** A woman who has had previous pregnancies
_____	**10.** Breech presentation	**J.** Spontaneous abortion prior to 20 weeks of gestation without any medical or surgical intervention
_____	**11.** Limb presentation	**K.** Delivery in which the presenting part is a single arm, leg, or foot
_____	**12.** Multigravida	**L.** A disk-shaped structure attached to the uterine wall that provides nourishment to the fetus
_____	**13.** Nuchal cord	**M.** First pregnancy
_____	**14.** Presentation	**N.** The stage from 10 weeks until delivery
_____	**15.** Miscarriage	**O.** Delivery in which the buttocks are delivered first

Multiple Choice

Read each item carefully and then select the one best response.

_____ **1.** Which of the following is NOT true regarding delivery with a nuchal cord?

   A. Gently slip the cord over the infant's head or shoulder.

   B. Encourage the woman to push harder and more often after cutting the cord.

   C. Clamp the cord, then suction the airway before cutting the cord.

   D. Clamp the cord and cut it, then gently unwind it from around the neck if wrapped around more than once.

_____ **2.** Which of the following refers to green or foul-smelling amniotic fluid?

   A. Nuchal rigidity

   B. Meconium

   C. Placenta previa

   D. Bloody show

_____ **3.** Approximately _____ of deliveries are complicated by the presence of meconium in the amniotic fluid.

    A. 7%

    B. 17%

    C. 57%

    D. 97%

_____ **4.** You may help control bleeding by massaging the _____ after delivery of the placenta.

    A. perineum

    B. fundus

    C. lower back

    D. inner thighs

_____ **5.** The Apgar score should be calculated at _____ minutes after birth.

    A. 1 and 5

    B. 3 and 7

    C. 2 and 10

    D. 4 and 8

_____ **6.** Once the infant is delivered, feel for a brachial pulse or the pulsations in the umbilical cord. If the pulse rate is below _____ beats/min, begin assisted ventilations.

    A. 60

    B. 80

    C. 100

    D. 120

_____ **7.** In situations where assisted ventilation is required, you should use a newborn bag-mask device and ventilate with high-flow oxygen at a rate of _____ breaths/min.

    A. 20 to 30

    B. 30 to 50

    C. 35 to 45

    D. 40 to 60

_____ **8.** When performing CPR on a newborn, a compression to ventilation ratio of 3:1 should be used; this will yield a total of _____ "actions" per minute.

    A. 90

    B. 100

    C. 110

    D. 120

_____ **9.** You cannot successfully deliver a _____ presentation in the field.

    A. limb

    B. breech

    C. vertex

    D. cephalic

_____ **10.** Which of the following is NOT performed when caring for a mother with a prolapsed cord?

    A. Clamp and cut the cord.

    B. Provide high-flow oxygen and rapid transport.

    C. Use your fingers to physically hold the infant's head off the cord.

    D. Position the mother to keep the weight of the infant off the cord.

_____ **11.** When handling a delivery involving a drug- or alcohol-addicted mother, your first concern should be for:

    A. the mother's airway

    B. your personal safety

    C. the infant's airway

    D. the need for CPR for the infant

12. Which of the following is NOT a stage of labor?
    A. Rupture of amniotic fluid
    B. Delivery of the fetus
    C. Delivery of the placenta
    D. Dilation of the cervix

13. The first stage of labor begins with the onset of contractions and ends when:
    A. the infant is born
    B. the cervix is fully dilated
    C. the water breaks
    D. the placenta is delivered

14. Which of the following is NOT a sign of the *beginning* of labor?
    A. Bloody show
    B. Contractions of the uterus
    C. Crowning
    D. Rupture of the amniotic sac

15. The second stage of labor begins when the cervix is fully dilated and ends when:
    A. the infant is born
    B. the water breaks
    C. the placenta delivers
    D. the uterus stops contracting

16. The third stage of labor begins with the birth of the newborn and ends with the:
    A. release of milk from the breasts
    B. cessation of uterine contractions
    C. delivery of the placenta
    D. cutting of the umbilical cord

17. The difference between preeclampsia and eclampsia is the onset of:
    A. seeing spots
    B. seizures
    C. swelling in the hands and feet
    D. headaches

18. You should consider the possibility of a(n) _____ in women who have missed a menstrual cycle and complain of a sudden stabbing and usually unilateral pain in the lower abdomen.
    A. pelvic inflammatory disease (PID)
    B. ectopic pregnancy
    C. miscarriage
    D. abruptio placentae

19. Which of the following is NOT a reason for delivery of the fetus at the scene?
    A. Delivery can be expected within a few minutes.
    B. There is a natural disaster.
    C. There is severe inclement weather.
    D. The amniotic sac has ruptured.

20. Which of the following statements regarding pregnancy is TRUE?
    A. A patient in the third trimester is at a decreased risk for aspiration.
    B. As the pregnancy continues, the patient will experience slower and deeper breathing.
    C. By the 20th week of pregnancy, the uterus is at or above the belly button.
    D. Maternal blood volume increases up to 10% by the end of pregnancy.

_____ 21. Low blood pressure resulting from compression of the inferior vena cava by the weight of the fetus when the mother is supine is called:
   A. pregnancy-induced hypertension
   B. placenta previa
   C. abruptio placentae
   D. supine hypotensive syndrome

_____ 22. _____ is a situation in which the umbilical cord comes out of the vagina before the infant.
   A. Eclampsia
   B. Placenta previa
   C. Abruptio placentae
   D. Prolapsed cord

_____ 23. Premature separation of the placenta from the wall of the uterus is known as:
   A. eclampsia
   B. placenta previa
   C. abruptio placentae
   D. prolapsed cord

_____ 24. _____ is a condition in which the placenta develops over and covers the cervix.
   A. Eclampsia
   B. Placenta previa
   C. Abruptio placentae
   D. Prolapsed cord

_____ 25. _____ is heralded by the onset of convulsions, or seizures, resulting from severe hypertension in the pregnant woman.
   A. Eclampsia
   B. Placenta previa
   C. Abruptio placentae
   D. Supine hypotensive syndrome

_____ 26. Which of the following is NOT considered a possible effect to the fetus when the mother is a known substance abuser?
   A. Low birth weight
   B. Spina bifida
   C. Prematurity
   D. Severe respiratory depression

Questions 27–31 are derived from the following scenario: You have been dispatched to the side of a highway where a woman is reported to be delivering a baby. As you approach the vehicle, you see her lying down in the back seat.

_____ 27. Which of the following signs tells you that the birth is imminent?
   A. Her water has not broken.
   B. Her contractions are 3 to 6 minutes apart.
   C. She is a primigravida.
   D. The infant is crowning.

_____ 28. If the baby is crowning and the amniotic sac has not yet ruptured, you should:
   A. leave it in place and wait for ALS
   B. puncture the sac only after ordered to do so by medical control
   C. puncture the sac, allow the fluid to drain, and leave the sac in place
   D. puncture the sac away from the head and then push the sac away from the infant's face

_____ 29. As you perform a visual exam, you note crowning. This means that:
   A. the baby is making a crowing-type of sound
   B. the baby cannot be visualized
   C. the top of the head is visible
   D. the father is excited and needs care

_____ **30.** Bleeding that exceeds approximately _____ mL is considered a high risk for maternal mortality and morbidity.
- **A.** 100
- **B.** 250
- **C.** 500
- **D.** 1,000

_____ **31.** Concerning the delivery of the placenta, which of the following is NOT an emergency situation?
- **A.** More than 30 minutes have elapsed and the placenta has not delivered.
- **B.** There is more than 500 mL of bleeding before delivery of the placenta.
- **C.** There is significant bleeding after delivery of the placenta.
- **D.** Delivery of the placenta occurs 10 minutes after the birth.

_____ **32.** Ovulation occurs approximately _____ before menstruation.
- **A.** 1 week
- **B.** 2 weeks
- **C.** 3 weeks
- **D.** 4 weeks

_____ **33.** Fertilization usually occurs when the egg is inside the:
- **A.** ovary
- **B.** uterus
- **C.** fallopian tube
- **D.** endometrium

_____ **34.** Which of the following statements is FALSE?
- **A.** Gestational diabetes will clear up in most women after delivery.
- **B.** The leading cause of abruptio placentae is an ectopic pregnancy.
- **C.** As pregnancy progresses, the uterus enlarges and rises out of the pelvis.
- **D.** Some cultures may not permit male EMTs to examine a female patient.

_____ **35.** The "P" in Apgar stands for:
- **A.** perfusion
- **B.** pulse
- **C.** pupils
- **D.** position

_____ **36.** Which of the following statements regarding multiple gestations is FALSE?
- **A.** You should consider the possibility of twins when the first infant is small and the mother's abdomen remains fairly large after the birth.
- **B.** You should record the time of birth on each twin separately.
- **C.** There are always two placentas with the birth of twins.
- **D.** The second baby will usually be born within 45 minutes of the first.

_____ **37.** An infant delivered before _____ weeks is considered premature.
- **A.** 36
- **B.** 37
- **C.** 38
- **D.** 39

_____ **38.** All of the following are correct regarding postterm pregnancy EXCEPT:
- **A.** infants can be larger, sometimes weighing 10 pounds (4.5 kg) or more
- **B.** there is an increased risk of meconium aspiration
- **C.** postterm is considered past 42 weeks' gestation
- **D.** the likelihood of cesarean section delivery is decreased

_____ **39.** A patient presents with a sudden onset of shortness of breath 3 days following a delivery. What is the likely underlying cause of this condition?

    A. Pulmonary hypertension

    B. Pulmonary inflammation

    C. Pulmonary cmbolism

    D. Pulmonary fibrosis

_____ **40.** After delivery, if the infant does not begin breathing after _____ seconds, you should begin resuscitation efforts.

    A. 10

    B. 20

    C. 30

    D. 60

True/False

If you believe the statement to be more true than false, write the letter "T" in the space provided. If you believe the statement to be more false than true, write the letter "F."

_____ **1.** The small mucous plug from the cervix that is discharged from the vagina, often at the beginning of labor, is called a bloody show.

_____ **2.** Crowning occurs when the baby's head obstructs the birth canal, preventing normal delivery.

_____ **3.** Labor begins with the rupture of the amniotic sac and ends with the delivery of the baby's head.

_____ **4.** A woman who is having her first baby is called a multigravida.

_____ **5.** Once labor has begun, it can be slowed by holding the patient's legs together.

_____ **6.** Delivery of the buttocks before the baby's head is called a breech delivery.

_____ **7.** Massaging the abdomen after delivery helps to control bleeding.

_____ **8.** The placenta and cord should be properly disposed of in a biohazard container after delivery.

_____ **9.** The umbilical cord may be gently pulled to aid in delivery of the placenta.

_____ **10.** A limb presentation occurs when the baby's arm, leg, or foot is emerging from the vagina first.

_____ **11.** Multiple births may have more than one placenta.

_____ **12.** Pregnant teenagers may not know that they are pregnant.

_____ **13.** The secondary assessment of a pregnant patient should include a complete set of vital signs and pulse oximetry.

_____ **14.** Abuse during pregnancy increases the chance of miscarriage, premature delivery, and low birth weight.

_____ **15.** If called to deliver an infant who may have died in the uterus, you could notice skin blisters and dark discoloration to the infant.

_____ **16.** Most premature infants have vernix on their skin when delivered.

_____ **17.** Excessive bleeding after birth is usually caused by the muscles of the uterus not fully contracting.

Fill-in-the-Blank

Read each item carefully and then complete the statement by filling in the missing words.

1. After delivery, the _____, or afterbirth, separates from the uterus and is delivered.

2. The umbilical cord contains two _____ and one _____.

3. The amniotic sac contains about _____ to _____ mL of amniotic fluid, which helps to insulate and protect the floating fetus as it develops.

4. A pregnancy is considered full term once it reaches _____ weeks but has not gone beyond _____ weeks, _____ days.

5. By the end of pregnancy, the pregnant patient's heart rate increases up to 20%, or about _____ beats more per minute.

6. Blood volume may increase by as much as _____ by the end of the pregnancy.

7. The sudden onset of severe abdominal pain and vaginal bleeding in the first trimester of pregnancy should be considered a(n) _____ _____ until proven otherwise.

8. With a breech presentation, if the woman does not deliver within _____ minutes of the buttocks' presentation, provide prompt transport.

9. During the delivery, be careful that you do not poke your fingers into the infant's eyes or into the two soft spots, called _____, on the head.

10. _____ _____ is a developmental defect in which a portion of the spinal cord protrudes outside the vertebrae.

11. Passage of the fetus and placenta before 20 weeks without medical or surgical intervention is called _____ _____.

12. False labor is commonly referred to as _____ contractions.

13. The _____ _____ carries oxygenated blood from the woman to the heart of the fetus.

14. The _____ is the area of skin between the vagina and the anus.

15. Due to hormonal changes that cause joints in the musculoskeletal system to "loosen," a pregnant patient has a greater risk of _____.

Fill-in-the-Table

Fill in the missing parts of the table.

Apgar Scoring System			
Area of Activity	**Score**		
	2	**1**	**0**
Appearance			
Pulse			
Grimace or irritability			
Activity or muscle tone			
Respiration			

Labeling

Label the following diagram with the correct terms.

1. Anatomic Structures of the Pregnant Woman

A. _____

B. _____

C. _____

D. _____

E. _____

F. _____

G. _____

H. _____

I. _____

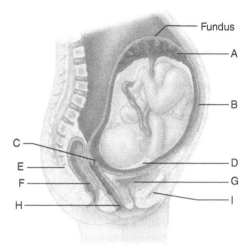

Critical Thinking

Multiple Choice

Read each item carefully and then select the one best response. Determine the Apgar score for each of the following scenarios.

_____ 1. You assess an infant newborn after delivery and note that the child has a loud cry and withdraws to pain. The heart rate is 94 beats/min, the extremities are cyanotic but the trunk is pink, respirations are rapid, and the newborn strongly resists your attempts to straighten the knees.

    A. 2

    B. 10

    C. 8

    D. 4

_____ 2. You arrive at the scene of a home delivery. On entering the scene, the father appears upset and hands you a limp baby. The child has a weak cry with slow respirations, is completely cyanotic, and has a pulse of 70 beats/min.

    A. 3

    B. 9

    C. 2

    D. 7

_____ 3. You arrive on scene to assist another crew with a delivery. On arrival, the crew on scene informs you that the delivery has already taken place and that you are going to be responsible for the care of the newborn. As you approach, you hear a very loud cry. The newborn appears completely pink and moves his foot away when you flick the sole of his foot. The pulse is 120 beats/min, and respirations are rapid. The newborn has excellent muscle tone and resists your attempt to straighten the hips.

    A. 6

    B. 10

    C. 1

    D. 8

Short Answer

Complete this section with short written answers using the space provided.

1. What are some possible causes of vaginal hemorrhage in early and late pregnancy?

_____

_____

_____

2. In what position should pregnant patients who are not delivering be transported, and why?

_____

_____

_____

3. List three signs that indicate the beginning of labor.

_____

_____

_____

4. When determining whether delivery is imminent and whether there are complications, what questions should you ask the patient?

_____

_____

_____

5. Once the baby's head emerges, what actions should be taken to prevent a too rapid delivery?

_____

_____

_____

6. Why is it important to avoid pushing on the fontanelles?

_____

_____

_____

7. How can you help decrease perineal tearing?

_____

_____

_____

8. What are the two situations in which an EMT may insert his or her fingers into a patient's vagina?

_____

_____

_____

9. What are three fetal effects of maternal drug or alcohol addiction?

_____

_____

_____

10. List five signs/symptoms associated with preeclampsia.

_____

_____

_____

Ambulance Calls

The following case scenarios provide an opportunity to explore the concerns associated with patient management and to enhance critical-thinking skills. Read each scenario and answer each question to the best of your ability.

1. You are dispatched to a grocery store for an "unknown medical problem." You arrive to find a 20-year-old woman who is in her 32nd week of pregnancy. She tells you that this is her first pregnancy, and she had made an appointment to see her obstetrician later that day because she was not feeling well. She's been experiencing a headache, swelling in her hands and feet, and transient problems with her vision. She states that she suddenly felt lightheaded and had to sit down. She appears unhurt.

How would you best manage this patient?

_____

_____

_____

2. You are on the scene with a 32-year-old woman who is 38 weeks pregnant. Delivery is imminent. As the infant starts to crown, you notice that the amniotic sac is still intact.

How would you best manage this patient?

_____

_____

_____

Skills

Skill Drills

Test your knowledge of this skill by placing the following photos in the correct order. Number the first step with a "1," the second step with a "2," etc.

Skill Drill 34-1: Delivering the Newborn

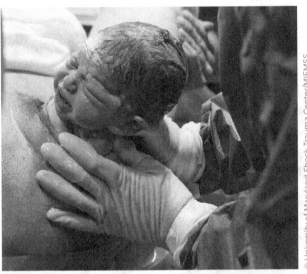

1. _____ Support the head and upper body as the lower shoulder delivers; guide the head up if needed.

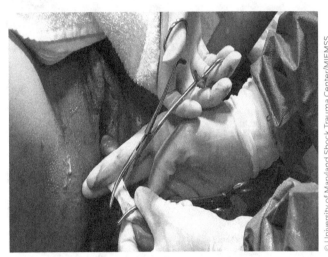

2. _____ Wait for the umbilical cord to stop pulsing. Place a clamp on the cord. Milk the blood from a small section of the cord on the placental side of the clamp. Place a second clamp 2 inches to 3 inches away from the first.

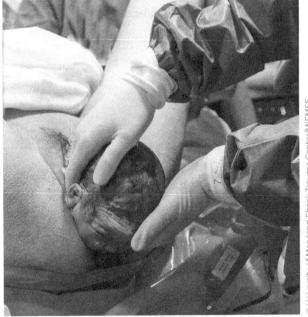

3. _____ Use your hands to support the bony parts of the head as it emerges. The child's body will naturally rotate to the right or left at this point in the delivery. Continue to support the head to allow it to turn in the same direction.

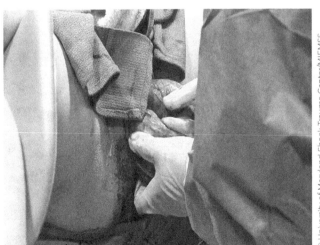

4. _____ Allow the placenta to deliver itself. Do not pull on the cord to speed delivery.

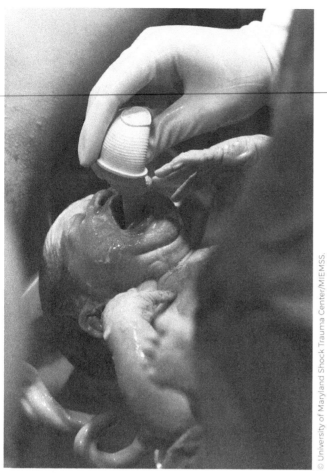

© University of Maryland Shock Trauma Center/MIEMSS.

5. _____ After delivery and prior to cutting the cord, if the child is gurgling or shows other signs of respiratory distress, suction the mouth and oropharynx to clear any amniotic fluid and ease the infant's initiation of air exchange.

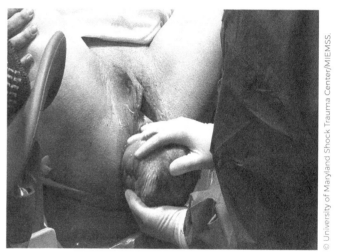

© University of Maryland Shock Trauma Center/MIEMSS.

6. _____ As the upper shoulder appears, guide the head down slightly by applying gentle downward traction to deliver the shoulder.

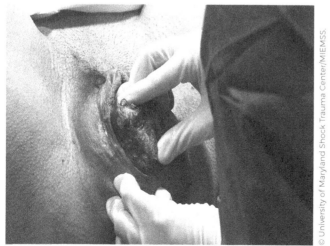

© University of Maryland Shock Trauma Center/MIEMSS.

7. _____ Crowning is the definitive sign that delivery is imminent and transport should be delayed until after the child has been born.

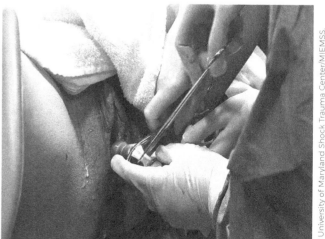

© University of Maryland Shock Trauma Center/MIEMSS.

8. _____ Cut between the clamps.

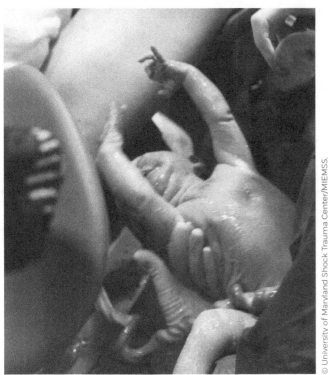

© University of Maryland Shock Trauma Center/MIEMSS.

9. _____ Handle the newborn firmly but gently, support the head, and keep the neck in a neutral position to maintain the airway. Consider placing the newborn on the mother's abdomen with the umbilical cord still intact, allow skin-to-skin contact to warm the newborn. Otherwise, keep the newborn approximately at the level of the vagina until the cord has been cut.

Assessment Review

Answer the following questions pertaining to the assessment of the types of emergencies discussed in this chapter.

_____ **1.** During delivery, after the head has been delivered and the shoulder appears:
   A. lower the head a little to deliver the upper shoulder
   B. apply a nasal cannula to the infant
   C. guide the head up slightly to deliver the shoulder
   D. pull gently

_____ **2.** If chest compressions are required for a newborn:
   A. use the hands-encircling technique for two-person resuscitation
   B. press the palm of your hand over the sternum, compressing 1 inch to 1.5 inches (2.5 cm to 3 cm) deep
   C. compress at a rate of 60 to 80 times a minute
   D. compress the sternum one-quarter the depth of the chest

_____ **3.** Which of the following would NOT be a typical question to ask when taking a history on a woman in labor?
   A. Are you having a boy or a girl?
   B. When is your due date?
   C. Did your physician mention the possibility of any complications?
   D. Is there a possibility of multiples?

_____ **4.** Once the infant is completely delivered, you should do all of the following EXCEPT:
   A. dry and wrap the infant in a blanket
   B. keep the infant at the level of the vagina until the umbilical cord is cut
   C. use sterile gauze and wipe out the infant's mouth
   D. gently pull on the umbilical cord to speed up delivery of the placenta

_____ **5.** When cutting the umbilical cord:
   A. place the clamps 7 inches to 10 inches (18 cm to 25 cm) apart
   B. place the clamps 2 inches to 4 inches (5 cm to 10 cm) apart
   C. place the clamps 1 inch to 2 inches (2 cm to 5 cm) apart
   D. place the clamps 4 inches to 7 inches (10 cm to 18 cm) apart

SPECIAL PATIENT POPULATIONS

CHAPTER

35

Pediatric Emergencies

General Knowledge

Matching

Match each of the items in the left column to the appropriate definition in the right column.

_____ **1.** Adolescents

_____ **2.** Croup

_____ **3.** Infancy

_____ **4.** Grunting

_____ **5.** Neglect

_____ **6.** Pediatrics

_____ **7.** Pertussis

_____ **8.** Preschool age

_____ **9.** Sniffing position

_____ **10.** Toddler

A. An "uh" sound heard during exhalation, reflecting an attempt to keep the lower airways open

B. The optimal neutral head position for uninjured airway management

C. 12 to 18 years of age

D. Failure to provide life necessities

E. Infant to 3 years of age

F. The first year of life

G. A medical practice devoted to care of the young

H. 3 to 6 years of age

I. An infection below the level of the vocal cords usually caused by a virus; usually associated with a seal-bark cough

J. Also known as "whooping cough"; caused by a bacterium that is spread through respiratory droplets; seldom seen due to increased vaccination

Multiple Choice

Read each item carefully and then select the one best response.

_____ **1.** Making eye contact, recognizing caregivers, and following a bright light with their eyes are initially noticed in what age group?

    A. 0 to 2 months

    B. 2 to 6 months

    C. 6 to 12 months

    D. 12 to 18 months

_____ **2.** Saying their first word, sitting without support, and teething are initially noticed in what age group?

    A. 0 to 2 months

    B. 2 to 6 months

    C. 6 to 12 months

    D. 12 to 18 months

_____ **3.** Which of the following is NOT initially seen in children 12 to 18 months old?

    A. Speak four to six words

    B. Know the major body parts

    C. Can open doors

    D. Understand cause and effect

_____ **4.** Toilet training is typically mastered at what age level?
  A. 6 to 12 months
  B. 12 to 18 months
  C. Preschool age
  D. School age

_____ **5.** Which of the following is FALSE regarding the pediatric airway?
  A. The trachea is larger in diameter and shorter in length.
  B. The glottis opening is higher and positioned more anterior.
  C. The neck appears to be nonexistent.
  D. The lungs are smaller.

_____ **6.** Breath sounds in the pediatric population are more easily heard because:
  A. their chest walls are thinner
  B. the size of their lungs amplifies the sounds
  C. the chest cavity is small in proportion to the rest of the body
  D. children typically have upper airway problems

_____ **7.** An infant's heart can beat as many as _____ times or more per minute if the body needs to compensate for injury or illness.
  A. 110
  B. 120
  C. 140
  D. 160

_____ **8.** Which of the following is NOT a common cause of altered mental status in pediatric patients?
  A. Drug and alcohol ingestion
  B. Hypertension
  C. Seizure
  D. Hypoglycemia

_____ **9.** A fracture of the femur is rare and is a major source of _____ in the pediatric population.
  A. infection
  B. growth abnormalities
  C. blood loss
  D. nerve damage

_____ **10.** When you assess a pediatric patient, it is best to place _____ on the patient's chest to feel the rise and fall of the chest wall.
  A. the left hand
  B. the right hand
  C. both hands
  D. the stethoscope

_____ **11.** Tachycardia in pediatric patients may be an indication of all of the following EXCEPT:
  A. hypothermia
  B. hypoxia
  C. fever
  D. pain

_____ **12.** When assessing capillary refill in pediatric patients, the color should return after:
  A. 1 second
  B. 2 seconds
  C. 3 seconds
  D. 4 seconds

_____ 13. Pupillary response in pediatric patients may be abnormal in the presence of all of the following EXCEPT:
  A. anxiety
  B. hypoxia
  C. brain injury
  D. drugs

_____ 14. When obtaining information from the family regarding the pediatric patient's history, which of the following is NOT an appropriate inquiry?
  A. Does the child have any rashes?
  B. What has been the child's recent activity level?
  C. Has there been any vomiting or diarrhea?
  D. Is the child in public or private school?

_____ 15. When examining the head of a pediatric patient, which of the following statements is FALSE?
  A. You should look for bruising, swelling, and hematomas.
  B. Significant blood loss can come from the scalp.
  C. A bulging fontanelle suggests dehydration.
  D. The head is larger in proportion to the rest of the body.

_____ 16. _____ may increase the effort or work of breathing.
  A. Anxiety
  B. Agitation
  C. Crying
  D. All of the above

_____ 17. Which of the following is NOT a sign of increased work of breathing in pediatric patients?
  A. Nasal flaring
  B. Grunting
  C. Equal chest expansion
  D. Retractions

_____ 18. Which of the following is NOT an infection that can cause respiratory distress in pediatric patients?
  A. Pneumonia
  B. Asthma
  C. Croup
  D. Epiglottitis

_____ 19. Signs and symptoms of a lower airway obstruction in pediatric patients include:
  A. stridor
  B. friction rub
  C. drooling
  D. wheezing

_____ 20. Exposure to cold air, infection, and emotional stress are all triggers of:
  A. pneumonia
  B. asthma
  C. bronchiolitis
  D. epiglottitis

_____ 21. Which of the following statements regarding pediatric asthma is FALSE?
  A. Use strong, forceful breaths when ventilating to get air past the obstruction.
  B. The wheezing may be so loud that you can hear it without a stethoscope.
  C. The patient may be in the tripod position.
  D. A bronchodilator via a metered-dose inhaler may be helpful.

_____ **22.** All of the following are signs associated with pneumonia in pediatric patients EXCEPT:
   A. bradycardia
   B. grunting
   C. nasal flaring
   D. hypothermia

_____ **23.** Bronchiolitis usually occurs during the first _____ of life.
   A. 2 years
   B. 3 years
   C. 4 years
   D. 6 years

_____ **24.** Which of the following is NOT a common cause of shock in pediatric patients?
   A. Diseases of the heart
   B. Severe infection
   C. Dehydration
   D. Renal failure

_____ **25.** Signs of shock in children include all of the following EXCEPT:
   A. altered mental status
   B. poor capillary refill
   C. hypertension
   D. tachycardia

_____ **26.** A pediatric patient with hives, wheezing, increased work of breathing, and hypoperfusion is likely suffering from:
   A. pneumonia
   B. bronchiolitis
   C. asthma
   D. anaphylaxis

_____ **27.** Which of the following is NOT appropriate when treating pediatric patients with seizures?
   A. Clear the mouth with suction.
   B. Provide 100% oxygen.
   C. Consider placing the patient in the recovery position.
   D. Restrain the patient.

_____ **28.** Which of the following populations is at the greatest risk for contracting meningitis?
   A. Females
   B. Children who have had head trauma
   C. Children with preexisting heart conditions
   D. Children of parents with a history of meningitis

_____ **29.** A pediatric patient with a fever, pain on palpation of the right lower quadrant, and rebound tenderness is likely to be suffering from:
   A. cholecystitis
   B. gastroenteritis
   C. appendicitis
   D. constipation

_____ **30.** Which of the following is NOT a question you would ask if you suspected a poisoning emergency?
   A. Did the substance have an odor?
   B. Are there any changes in behavior or level of consciousness?
   C. What is the substance involved?
   D. Was there any choking or coughing after the exposure?

_____ **31.** Activated charcoal is indicated for pediatric patients who have ingested a(n):
- **A.** acid
- **B.** alkali
- **C.** petroleum product
- **D.** poison

_____ **32.** Which of the following is NOT a sign of severe dehydration in pediatric patients?
- **A.** Bulging fontanelles
- **B.** Very dry lips and gums
- **C.** Sunken eyes
- **D.** Sleepiness

_____ **33.** Young children can compensate for fluid losses by:
- **A.** decreasing blood flow to the brain and heart
- **B.** decreasing blood flow to the extremities
- **C.** increasing blood flow to the extremities
- **D.** increasing blood flow to the gastrointestinal tract

_____ **34.** All of the following are common causes of a fever in pediatric patients EXCEPT:
- **A.** infection
- **B.** status epilepticus
- **C.** drug ingestion
- **D.** cholecystitis

_____ **35.** A pediatric patient involved in a drowning emergency may present with:
- **A.** cerebral edema
- **B.** hypoglycemia
- **C.** abdominal distention
- **D.** chest pain

_____ **36.** Head and neck injuries are common after high-speed collisions in all of the following contact sports EXCEPT:
- **A.** wrestling
- **B.** football
- **C.** lacrosse
- **D.** basketball

_____ **37.** All children with abdominal injuries should be monitored for signs and symptoms of:
- **A.** pain
- **B.** shock
- **C.** hypothermia
- **D.** nausea

_____ **38.** Which of the following is NOT a common exposure when dealing with pediatric burns?
- **A.** Scalding water in a bathtub
- **B.** Electrocution from poor wiring
- **C.** Hot items on a stove
- **D.** Cleaning solvents

_____ **39.** How many triage categories are there in the JumpSTART system?
- **A.** Three
- **B.** Four
- **C.** Five
- **D.** Six

_____ **40.** Which of the following is NOT a known risk factor for sudden infant death syndrome (SIDS)?
   A. Mother younger than 20 years old
   B. Mother smoked during pregnancy
   C. Gestational diabetes
   D. Low birth weight

_____ **41.** Which of the following is considered to have a protective effect against SIDS?
   A. Use of extra padding in the crib
   B. Bumpers along the crib rails
   C. Formula feeding
   D. The use of a pacifier

_____ **42.** Incidents involving the death of a child pose extra stress for EMS workers. Which of the following is NOT a sign of posttraumatic stress?
   A. Cold intolerance
   B. Restlessness
   C. Difficulty sleeping
   D. Loss of appetite

True/False

If you believe the statement to be more true than false, write the letter "T" in the space provided. If you believe the statement to be more false than true, write the letter "F."

_____ **1.** You should avoid letting the parent or caregiver hold an infant during your assessment.

_____ **2.** Toddlers have a hard time describing or localizing pain because they do not have the verbal ability to be precise.

_____ **3.** It is considered acceptable to lie to a preschool-age child because he or she will not be able to understand the true medical condition.

_____ **4.** Adolescence is a time for experimentation and risk-taking behaviors.

_____ **5.** Adolescents often feel invincible or indestructible.

_____ **6.** Congenital cardiovascular problems are the leading cause of cardiopulmonary arrest in the pediatric population.

_____ **7.** Sprains are uncommon in the pediatric population.

_____ **8.** Infants and young children should be kept warm during a transport or when the patient is exposed to assess or reassess an injury.

_____ **9.** Bradypnea usually indicates that the pediatric patient's condition is improving.

_____ **10.** Pediatric patients weighing less than 18 kg (40 lb) should be transported by car seat.

_____ **11.** Blood pressure is usually not assessed in pediatric patients younger than 4 years.

_____ **12.** A prolonged asthma attack that is unrelieved may progress to a condition known as status asthmaticus.

_____ **13.** An oropharyngeal airway should be used for pediatric patients who are unconscious and in possible respiratory failure.

_____ **14.** Blow-by oxygen is as effective as a face mask or nasal cannula for delivering oxygen to a pediatric patient.

_____ **15.** A rectal temperature is the most accurate for infants to toddlers.

_____ **16.** At around 8 to 10 years of age, children no longer require padding underneath the torso to create a neutral position.

_____ **17.** Extremity injuries in the pediatric population are managed much differently than extremity injuries in adults.

18. EMTs in all states must report all cases of suspected abuse, even if the emergency department fails to do so.

19. Do not examine the genitalia of a young child unless there is evidence of bleeding or there is an injury that must be treated.

20. You should use a euphemism such as "passed away" when informing the family of a pediatric death to lessen their emotional pain.

Fill-in-the-Blank

Read each item carefully and then complete the statement by filling in the missing words.

1. Children not only have a higher metabolic rate but also a higher _____ _____, which is twice that of an adult.

2. Breathing requires the use of the _____ muscles and diaphragm.

3. Young children experience muscle fatigue much more quickly than older children, which can lead to _____ _____.

4. Located on the front (anterior) and back (posterior) portions of the head are soft spots, the _____.

5. The _____ _____ _____ is a structured assessment tool that allows you to rapidly form a general impression of the pediatric patient's condition without touching him or her.

6. Always position the airway in a neutral _____ _____.

7. Car seats are designed to be either _____ or _____; they cannot be mounted sideways on a bench seat.

8. A child in respiratory distress or possible respiratory failure needs supplemental _____.

9. _____ is an infection of the soft tissue in the area above the vocal cords.

10. _____ _____ are recommended to relieve a severe airway obstruction in an unconscious pediatric patient.

11. A prolonged asthma attack that is unrelieved may progress into _____ _____.

12. Inserting a(n) _____ _____ in a responsive patient may cause a spasm of the larynx and result in vomiting.

13. _____ is a congenital condition in which the patient lacks one or more of the normal clotting factors of blood.

14. _____ is common in pediatric patients and if left untreated can lead to peritonitis or shock.

15. _____ is the second most common cause of unintentional death among children in the United States.

16. In pediatric patients, chest injuries are usually the result of _____ _____, rather than penetrating trauma.

17. One common problem following burn injuries in children is _____ .

18. _____ is refusal or failure on the part of the caregiver to provide life necessities.

Critical Thinking

Short Answer

Complete this section with short written answers using the space provided.

1. What does each letter in the mnemonic TICLS mean?

_____

_____

_____

2. What are the signs of increased work of breathing in a pediatric patient, and what do they mean?

_____

_____

_____

3. List the indications for immediate transport of a pediatric patient.

_____

_____

_____

4. What tool is used to determine the appropriate blood pressure for a pediatric patient between 1 and 10 years of age?

_____

_____

_____

5. When assessing for circulation, what are the specific areas to focus on, and what questions should you ask yourself?

_____

_____

_____

Ambulance Calls

The following case scenarios provide an opportunity to explore the concerns associated with patient management and to enhance critical-thinking skills. Read each scenario and answer each question to the best of your ability.

1. You are dispatched to the residence of a toddler who has a history of fever and who is now unresponsive. You arrive to find a 13-year-old babysitter who tells you that she is not sure what is wrong with the 2-year-old boy. She tells you that he started "shaking all over," and she didn't know what to do. He is currently responsive to painful stimuli and warm to the touch.

   How would you best manage this patient?

   _____

   _____

   _____

2. You are dispatched to the residence of a 3-year-old child with a history of lung problems. The child, a very small boy, is cyanotic and lethargic. He is pain responsive. He has copious mucous secretions in his airway. The grandmother, who was sitting with the child, is hysterical.

   How would you best manage this patient?

   _____

   _____

   _____

3. You are called to a residence for a 2-year-old child with difficulty breathing. The little girl has stridor and expiratory wheezes, as well as intercostal retractions. She is very upset by your arrival and clings to her mother. Her breathing worsens with agitation. Her mother tells you that she is currently taking medication for an upper respiratory infection and has spent much of her life in and out of hospitals with respiratory problems.

   How would you best manage this patient?

   _____

   _____

   _____

4. It's 0530, and you are dispatched to the home of a 6-month-old girl who is not breathing. You arrive to find a crying, young mother holding a lifeless baby. The infant is not breathing, is cold to the touch, and appears to have dependent lividity.

   How would you best manage this patient?

   _____

   _____

   _____

Skills

Skill Drills

Test your knowledge of this skill by filling in the correct words in the photo captions.

Skill Drill 35-1: Positioning the Airway in a Pediatric Patient

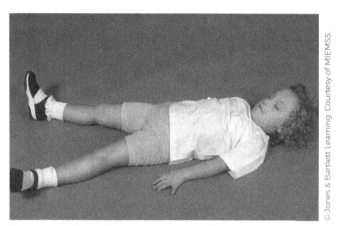

1. Position the pediatric patient on a(n) _____ surface.

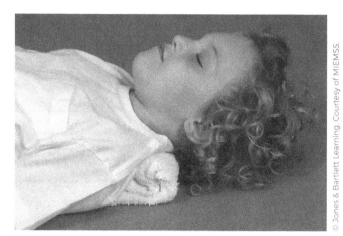

2. Place a(n) _____ towel about 1-inch (2.5-cm) thick under the _____ and _____.

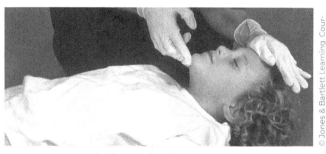

3. _____ the forehead to limit _____, and use the head tilt–chin lift maneuver to open the airway.

Test your knowledge of this skill by filling in the correct words in the photo captions.

Skill Drill 35-2: Inserting an Oropharyngeal Airway in a Pediatric Patient

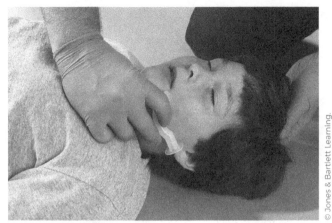

1. Determine the appropriately _____ airway. Confirm the correct size _____ by placing it next to the pediatric patient's _____.

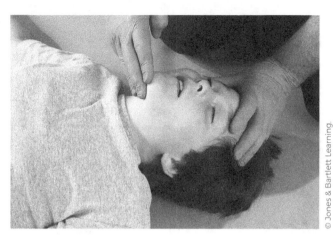

2. Position the pediatric patient's _____ with the appropriate method.

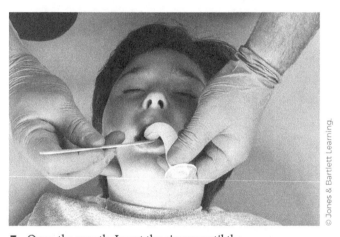

3. Open the mouth. Insert the airway until the _____ rests against the _____. _____ the airway.

Test your knowledge of this skill by filling in the correct words in the photo captions.

Skill Drill 35-3: Inserting a Nasopharyngeal Airway in a Pediatric Patient

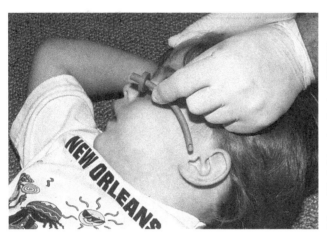

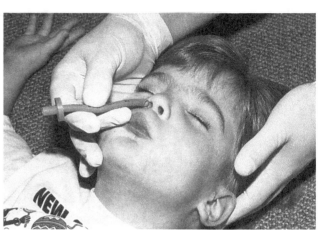

1. Determine the correct airway size by comparing its _____ to the opening of the _____ (nare). Place the airway next to the pediatric patient's _____ to confirm correct _____. _____ the airway.

2. _____ the airway. Insert the _____ into the right naris with the bevel pointing toward the _____.

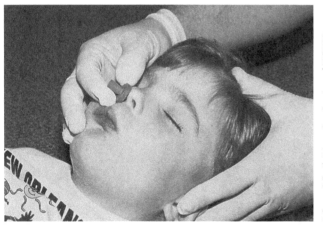

3. Carefully move the tip forward until the _____ rests against the _____ of the nostril. Reassess the _____.

Skill Drill 35-4: One-Person Bag-Mask Ventilation on a Pediatric Patient

Test your knowledge of this skill by placing the following photos in the correct order. Number the first step with a "1," the second step with a "2," etc.

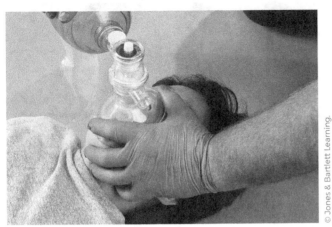

1. _____ Hold the mask on the patient's face with a one-handed head tilt–chin lift technique (EC clamp method). Ensure a good mask–face seal while maintaining the airway.

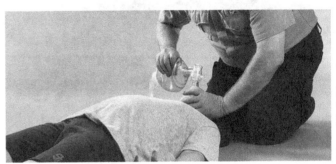

2. _____ Assess effectiveness of ventilation by watching bilateral rise and fall of the chest.

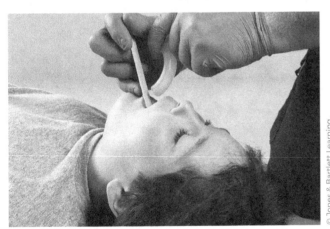

3. _____ Open the airway and insert the appropriate airway adjunct.

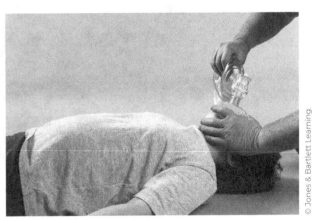

4. _____ Squeeze the bag using the correct ventilation rate of 1 breath every 3 to 5 seconds, or 12 to 20 breaths/min. Allow adequate time for exhalation.

Test your knowledge of this skill by filling in the correct words in the photo captions.

Skill Drill 35-6: Immobilizing a Patient in a Car Seat

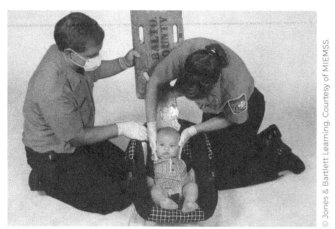

1. _____ the head in a(n) _____ position.

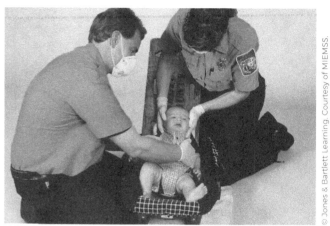

2. Place a(n) _____ _____ or pediatric _____ _____ between the patient and the surface he or she is resting on.

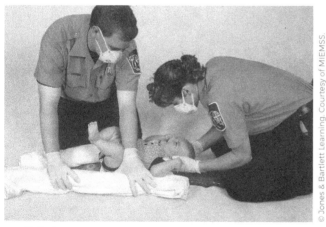

3. Slide the patient onto the _____ _____ or pediatric immobilization device.

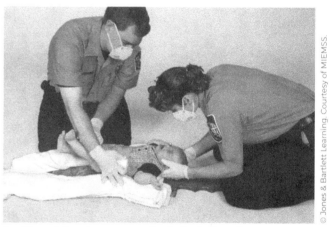

4. Place a(n) _____ under the back, from the _____ to the _____, to ensure _____ head position.

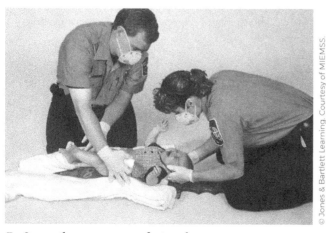

5. Secure the _____ first; pad any _____.

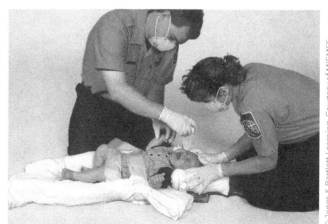

6. Secure the head to the short backboard or pediatric _____ _____.

SPECIAL PATIENT POPULATIONS

CHAPTER

Geriatric Emergencies

36

General Knowledge

Matching

Match each of the items in the left column to the appropriate definition in the right column.

_____	1. Aneurysm	**A.**	Forward curling of the back
_____	2. Cataract	**B.**	Fluid in the abdomen
_____	3. Delirium	**C.**	Clouding of the lens of the eye
_____	4. Dementia	**D.**	Reduced bone mass leading to fractures after minimal trauma
_____	5. Syncope	**E.**	Abnormal blood-filled dilation of a blood vessel
_____	6. Dyspnea	**F.**	Difficulty breathing
_____	7. Osteoporosis	**G.**	An inability to focus, think logically, or maintain attention
_____	8. Polypharmacy	**H.**	Use of multiple medications
_____	9. Kyphosis	**I.**	Slow onset of progressive disorientation
_____	10. Ascites	**J.**	Fainting due to interruption of blood flow to the brain

Multiple Choice

Read each item carefully and then select the one best response.

_____ 1. Which of the following is NOT one of the leading causes of death in the older population?
  A. Heart disease
  B. Diabetes
  C. AIDS
  D. Cancer

_____ 2. Geriatric patients present as a special problem for caregivers because:
  A. the classic presentation of disease is often altered
  B. geriatric patients tend not to understand their underlying conditions
  C. their medications are rather difficult to learn
  D. the typical diseases of the geriatric population are uncommon

_____ 3. Stereotyping of older adults that often leads to discrimination is called:
  A. geritism
  B. geriographics
  C. oldism
  D. ageism

_____ 4. Which of the following is NOT a common stereotype regarding geriatrics?
  A. Most older adults have dementia.
  B. Older adults are hard of hearing.
  C. Geriatric patients are likely to die on an EMS call.
  D. Older adults are immobile.

_____ 5. Which of the following is generally NOT acceptable when interviewing an older patient?
   A. Do not initiate eye contact because many geriatric patients might find this disrespectful.
   B. Speak slowly and distinctly.
   C. Give the patient time to respond unless the condition appears urgent.
   D. Explain what you are doing before you do it.

_____ 6. Which of the following is NOT considered a common condition of older adults?
   A. Hypertension
   B. Asthma
   C. Gastroenteritis
   D. Arthritis

_____ 7. Geriatric patients are commonly found living in all of the following locations EXCEPT:
   A. their homes
   B. nursing homes
   C. skilled nursing facilities
   D. churches

_____ 8. You are responding to the dementia unit at a nursing home for respiratory distress. When you arrive, you notice that the patient is experiencing mild dyspnea and has an altered mental status. What can you do to help determine if the patient's altered mental status is appropriate for her underlying dementia?
   A. As long as the patient is alert and able to answer most questions, there is no need to determine if this is normal behavior.
   B. Ask the patient's roommate if this is normal behavior for the patient.
   C. Find a staff member who can explain the patient's underlying mental status to you.
   D. Because the patient already has dementia, there is no need to investigate this further.

_____ 9. Anatomic changes that occur as a person ages predispose geriatric patients to:
   A. respiratory illness
   B. fungal infections
   C. communicable diseases
   D. mental status changes

_____ 10. Which of the following statements regarding geriatrics is FALSE?
   A. Chronic mental status impairment is a normal process of aging.
   B. Multiple disease processes and complaints can make assessment complicated.
   C. Communication may be more complicated with an older adult.
   D. You should find and account for all patient medications.

_____ 11. The last meal is particularly important in a patient with:
   A. hypertension
   B. myocardial infarction
   C. chronic obstructive pulmonary disease (COPD)
   D. diabetes

_____ 12. The heart rate should be in the normal adult range for a geriatric patient but can be altered by medications such as:
   A. insulin
   B. beta-blockers
   C. alpha-blockers
   D. aspirin

_____ 13. Which of the following is NOT a factor that predisposes an older patient to a serious head injury?
   A. Long-term abuse of alcohol
   B. Recurrent falls
   C. Family history
   D. Anticoagulant medication

_____ 14. The "E" of the GEMS diamond stands for:
   A. environmental assessment
   B. events leading to the incident
   C. extrication of the patient
   D. emergency assessment

_____ 15. The alveoli in an older patient's lung tissue can become enlarged and less elastic, making it:
   A. easier to inhale air
   B. harder to inhale air
   C. easier to exhale air
   D. harder to exhale air

_____ 16. _____ is the leading cause of death from infection in Americans older than 65 years.
   A. Chronic bronchitis
   B. Pneumonia
   C. Endocarditis
   D. Influenza

_____ 17. A patient with leg pain who complains of sudden shortness of breath, tachycardia, fever, chest pain, and a feeling of impending doom is likely experiencing a(n):
   A. pulmonary embolism
   B. pneumonia
   C. myocardial infarction
   D. aortic aneurysm

_____ 18. Geriatric patients are at risk for _____, an accumulation of fatty material in the arteries.
   A. vasculitis
   B. arteriosclerosis
   C. atherosclerosis
   D. varicose veins

_____ 19. A drop in blood pressure with a change in position is referred to as:
   A. orthostatic hypotension
   B. metastatic hypotension
   C. malignant hypotension
   D. psychogenic hypotension

_____ 20. Which of the following is NOT considered a risk factor for geriatric patients to develop a pulmonary embolism?
   A. Paralyzed extremities
   B. Sedentary behavior
   C. History of heart failure
   D. Exercise

_____ 21. All of the following are true of delirium EXCEPT:
   A. it may have metabolic causes
   B. the patient may be hypoglycemic
   C. it develops slowly over a period of years
   D. the memory remains mostly intact

_____ 22. An 82-year-old woman has slurred speech, weakness on the left side of her body, visual disturbances, and a headache. This patient is likely to be suffering from a:
   A. myocardial infarction
   B. stroke
   C. diabetic emergency
   D. spinal cord injury

_____ **23.** The brain decreases in terms of _____ and volume as a person ages.
  A. length
  B. width
  C. size
  D. weight

_____ **24.** Older adults develop an inability to differentiate colors and have:
  A. increased sensitivity to light
  B. decreased eye movement
  C. decreased daytime vision
  D. decreased night vision

_____ **25.** _____ and long-term exposure to loud noises are the main factors that contribute to hearing loss.
  A. Heredity
  B. Injury
  C. Infection
  D. Medications

_____ **26.** Which of the following statements regarding dementia is FALSE?
  A. Patients may have anxiety about going to the hospital.
  B. Some patients are confused and angry.
  C. There may be a decreased ability to communicate.
  D. Due to memory loss, they are able to adapt easily to changes in their daily routine.

_____ **27.** Which of the following statements about changes to the gastrointestinal system is correct?
  A. Gastric secretions are reduced as a person ages.
  B. Dental loss is not a normal result of the aging process.
  C. Blood flow to the liver is increased as a person ages.
  D. Gastric motility increases and results in an increase in gastric emptying.

_____ **28.** All of the following are common specific gastrointestinal problems in older adults EXCEPT:
  A. ulcerative colitis
  B. diverticulitis
  C. peptic ulcer disease
  D. gallbladder disease

_____ **29.** A patient with an abdominal aortic aneurysm most commonly complains of abdominal pain that radiates to the:
  A. chest
  B. lower legs
  C. back
  D. shoulders

_____ **30.** Changes to the kidney and genitourinary tract in older patients can cause all of the following EXCEPT:
  A. urinary incontinence
  B. urinary retention
  C. an increased response to sodium deficiency
  D. enlargement of the prostate

_____ **31.** A patient experiencing weight gain, fatigue, cold intolerance, drier skin and hair, and a slower heart rate could be suffering from:
  A. hyperglycemia
  B. ketosis
  C. hyperthyroidism
  D. hypothyroidism

_____ **32.** Which of the following is NOT a factor that affects the development of osteoporosis?
  A. Hypertension
  B. Smoking
  C. Level of activity
  D. Alcohol consumption

_____ **33.** _____ is a progressive disease of the joints that destroys cartilage and leads to joint spurs and stiffness.
  A. Osteoporosis
  B. Osteosarcoma
  C. Osteoarthritis
  D. Osteoplegia

_____ **34.** All of the following are considered to be reasons for medication noncompliance EXCEPT:
  A. financial challenges
  B. patient disagrees with the diagnosis
  C. impaired cognitive ability
  D. inability to open pill bottles

_____ **35.** Which of the following statements regarding depression is TRUE?
  A. Treatment typically involves medication because counseling usually does not work.
  B. Older adults in skilled nursing facilities are less likely to develop depression.
  C. It generally does not interfere with the ability to function in older adults.
  D. It is diagnosed three times more commonly in women than in men.

_____ **36.** Older pedestrians struck by a vehicle commonly sustain injuries to the:
  A. chest
  B. abdomen
  C. extremities
  D. back

_____ **37.** All of the following are common predisposing events that can lead to suicide in older adults EXCEPT:
  A. death of a loved one
  B. hallucinations
  C. alcohol abuse
  D. physical illness

_____ **38.** Older adults are more likely to experience burns because of all of the following EXCEPT:
  A. altered mental status
  B. inattention
  C. compromised neurologic status
  D. osteoporosis

_____ **39.** Signs and symptoms of possible abuse include all of the following EXCEPT:
  A. chronic pain with no medical explanation
  B. no history of repeated visits to the emergency department or clinic
  C. depression or lack of energy
  D. self-destructive behavior

_____ **40.** Because the brain tissue shrinks with age, older patients are more likely to sustain:
  A. basilar skull fractures
  B. depressed skull fractures
  C. open head injuries
  D. closed head injuries

_____ **41.** The most important piece of information to establish immediately when responding to a skilled nursing facility is determining:
   A. when someone last saw the patient
   B. which nurse is overseeing patient care
   ~~**C.** what is wrong with the patient~~
   D. how often this patient is transported to the hospital

_____ **42.** Methicillin-resistant _Staphylococcus aureus_ (MRSA) is NOT commonly found on which of the following?
   A. Decubitus ulcers
   B. Feeding tubes
   C. Indwelling catheters
   D. Patient charts

_____ **43.** In the presence of a do not resuscitate (DNR) order, if the patient is still alive, you are obligated to provide all of the following supportive measures EXCEPT:
   A. oxygen delivery
   B. pain relief
   C. comfort
   D. resuscitation

_____ **44.** Burns in elder abuse typically do NOT result from which of the following?
   A. Cigarettes
   B. Matches
   C. Hot liquids
   D. Fireplaces

_____ **45.** Clues that might indicate elder abuse would include all of the following EXCEPT:
   A. bruises on the buttocks and lower back
   B. weight gain
   C. wounds in various stages of healing
   D. lack of hygiene

True/False

If you believe the statement to be more true than false, write the letter "T" in the space provided. If you believe the statement to be more false than true, write the letter "F."

_____ **1.** Some older adults may not take all of their medications to save money.

_____ **2.** Your first words to the patient and the attitude behind them can gain or lose a patient's trust.

_____ **3.** Hip fractures are less likely to occur when the patient has osteoporosis.

_____ **4.** The heart hypertrophies with age, likely in response to the chronically increased afterload imposed by stiffened blood vessels.

_____ **5.** A general complaint of weakness and dizziness can be an indication of something more serious, such as a heart problem or pneumonia.

_____ **6.** Multiple disease processes and multiple and/or vague complaints can make assessment complicated.

_____ **7.** The "S" in the GEMS diamond stands for social assessment.

_____ **8.** Loss of mechanisms to protect the upper airway include increased cough and gag reflexes.

_____ **9.** Changes in the cardiovascular performance of a geriatric patient are the direct consequence of aging.

_____ **10.** Respiratory rates in a geriatric patient with chest pain tend to be lower.

_____ **11.** The treatment goal of a stroke is to salvage as much brain tissue as possible.

_____ **12.** Glaucoma, macular degeneration, and retinal detachment can all cause vision problems in the geriatric patient.

_____ **13.** Taste can be diminished in an older patient due to a decrease in the number of taste buds.

_____ **14.** Neuropathy is a dysfunction of the central nervous system.

_____ **15.** Irritation of the lining of the stomach or ulcers can cause forceful vomiting that tears the esophagus.

_____ **16.** Inflammation of the gallbladder will present with left upper quadrant pain and fever.

_____ **17.** The blood glucose level will be greater than 600 mg/dL in diabetic ketoacidosis (DKA).

_____ **18.** Pneumonia and urinary tract infections are common in patients who are bedridden.

_____ **19.** Decreased liver function makes it easier for the liver to detoxify the blood.

_____ **20.** Most geriatric suicides occur in people who have recently been diagnosed with depression.

_____ **21.** There is a lower mortality from penetrating trauma in older adults.

_____ **22.** Trauma is always isolated to a single issue when you are assessing and caring for a geriatric patient.

_____ **23.** Broken bones are common in the geriatric population and should be splinted in a manner appropriate to the injury.

_____ **24.** Most indoor hypothermia deaths involve geriatric patients.

_____ **25.** A health care power of attorney is an advance directive that is exercised by a person who has been authorized by the patient to make medical decisions for the patient.

Fill-in-the-Blank

Read each item carefully and then complete the statement by filling in the missing words.

1. Using the patient's _____ shows respect and helps the patient to focus on your questions.

2. Hip fractures are more likely to occur when bones are weakened by _____ or infection.

3. _____ is a useful therapy for many geriatric problems, including vague complaints of weakness or dizziness.

4. _____ is an inflammation/infection of the lung from bacterial, viral, or fungal causes.

5. Increased _____ _____, pulmonary secretions, and the inflammatory effects of infection all interfere with the ability of the alveoli to oxygenate the blood.

6. _____ refers to stiffening of the blood vessel wall.

7. Severe blood loss can occur when a(n) _____ bursts.

8. With _____ heart failure, fluid backs up into the lungs.

9. _____ is the gradual hearing loss that occurs as we age.

10. An older person may have a decreased sense of _____ and _____ perception from the loss of end nerve fibers.

11. _____ is a condition in which small pouches protrude from the colon.

12. _____ _____ form when a patient is lying or sitting in the same position for a long time.

13. As you get older, the brain shrinks, leading to a higher risk of _____ _____ following a minimal mechanism of injury.

14. _____ _____ may help determine if a loss of consciousness occurred before an accident.

15. Dentures may cause a(n) _____ _____ in a patient with an altered level of consciousness.

16. When assessing the abdomen, remember that geriatric patients have a(n) _____ _____ _____ and may not show signs of rigidity in abdominal trauma.

17. Patients with _____ will require padding in order to keep the patient supine.

18. In addition to hip fractures, older adults with osteoporosis are at risk for _____ fractures.

19. _____ _____ are facilities that serve patients who need 24-hour care; they are sometimes a step down from a hospital.

20. _____ _____ are specific legal papers that direct relatives and caregivers about what kinds of medical treatment may be given to patients who cannot speak for themselves.

Fill-in-the-Table

Fill in the missing parts of the table.

Categories of Elder Abuse	
Physical	• _____ • _____ • _____ • _____ • _____ • _____
Psychological	• _____ • _____ • _____ • _____
Financial	• _____ • _____

Critical Thinking

Short Answer

Complete this section with short written answers using the space provided.

1. List the eight most common conditions found in the geriatric patient.

_____

_____

_____

2. What are the types of nerves affected in neuropathy, and what are the associated symptoms?

_____

_____

_____

3. What are the differences between hyperosmolar hyperglycemic nonketotic syndrome (HHNS) and DKA?

_____

_____

_____

4. List at least five informational items that may be important in assessing possible elder abuse.

_____

_____

_____

5. Briefly describe the three possible causes of syncope in the geriatric patient.

_____

_____

_____

Ambulance Calls

The following case scenarios provide an opportunity to explore the concerns associated with patient management and to enhance critical-thinking skills. Read each scenario and answer each question to the best of your ability.

1. It is 0300, and you are dispatched to a long-term care facility for a geriatric woman with an "unknown emergency." You arrive to find no staff around, but you hear someone crying for help. You follow the voice and find an older woman lying on the floor, holding her right hip. Her bed is made, and the side rails are up. When a staff member finally appears, you ask how long she's been lying there. The staff member responds, "We don't know. How are we supposed to know that? We don't have enough help around here."

    How would you best manage this patient?

    _____

    _____

    _____

2. You are dispatched to the home of a 65-year-old woman who is complaining of severe back pain. She tells you that she tried to pick up the lawnmower when she "heard a pop and felt a crack in her back." She is experiencing intense pain in her lower back and feels some numbness in her legs.

    How would you best manage this patient?

    _____

    _____

    _____

3. You are dispatched to a private residence for a woman who has fallen. She tells you that she tripped over her granddaughter's toys and fell onto the hardwood floor. She tried to get up several times but couldn't. She denies any head, neck, or back pain or loss of consciousness. Her only complaint is pain in her right hip.

    How would you best manage this patient?

    _____

    _____

    _____

4. It is early evening, and you are dispatched to the parking lot of a popular shopping mall. Over the past several hours, local weather conditions have consisted of a combination of freezing rain and snow, making for very icy road conditions. Your patient is an older woman who has fallen and now complains of back pain and shortness of breath. She has severe kyphosis and will not tolerate traditional methods of spinal immobilization.

    How would you best manage this patient?

    _____

    _____

    _____

Fill-in-the-Patient Care Report

Read the incident scenario and then complete the following patient care report (PCR).

You are dispatched at 0843 to an unknown medical emergency at 222 Orchard Lane. You note the incident number as 011727 and immediately mark your unit as responding with the dispatcher. The dispatcher informs you that the fire department was also dispatched to assist you.

You arrive 6 minutes later to find an older woman who greets you at the front door. She tells you that her 78-year-old husband is lying on the bathroom floor, and he's too heavy for her to lift. As you enter the small bathroom, you notice a large man on the floor with a laceration and hematoma on his forehead.

"I was on the toilet and must have fallen, but I don't remember exactly what happened," the patient tells you.

You immediately maintain cervical spine stabilization as the fire department personnel arrive on scene. Your partner grabs the necessary immobilization equipment as you interview the patient.

The patient continues to tell you that he does not remember what happened, but he states that his head hurts.

"I heard a loud 'thud' in the bathroom and came in to find him on the floor," the wife states. "He was awake when I came in, but I saw the blood and called 9-1-1."

You ask, "Are you having any other pain?"

"No, I feel OK other than my head," says the patient. The patient rates his pain as a 4 out of 10 and denies radiation. The patient also denies neck pain.

You inquire about dizziness, sweating, chest pain, shortness of breath, nausea, or vomiting, all of which the patient denies.

Your partner arrives, along with the fire personnel, with the immobilization equipment. While they immobilize the patient, you apply 15 L/min of oxygen via a nonrebreathing mask at 0851 and place a bandage on the patient's forehead to control the bleeding.

After the patient is immobilized, you complete a rapid full-body scan of the patient and find no other deformities/abnormalities other than a hematoma and a 3-cm (1.2-inch) laceration noted to the patient's right forehead, with minor bleeding, now controlled.

Your partner obtains vital signs 2 minutes after the patient is immobilized and finds the following: pulse, 86 beats/min; respirations, 20 breaths/min; blood pressure, 110/68 mm Hg; pulse oximetry, 98%.

The patient tells you that he is allergic to aspirin and that he takes metoprolol, Lisinopril, Actos, metformin, Zocor, Celebrex, allopurinol, Lasix, K-dur, Plavix, and a multivitamin. You're able to decipher much of the history from the medications, but you ask the patient to confirm. The patient tells you that he had a heart attack several years ago in which a stent was placed; he has congestive heart failure, hypertension, diabetes, arthritis, gout, and high cholesterol.

The fire personnel package the patient onto the litter and take the patient to the unit with your partner. The patient tells you that he wants to go to Mercy Hospital down the road. Because this is the closest trauma facility, you are happy to accommodate the patient's wishes.

You depart the scene at 0902 and reassess vital signs and physical exam. The vital signs are as follows: pulse, 84 beats/min; respirations, 18 breaths/min; blood pressure, 116/76 mm Hg; pulse oximetry, 100%. The patient's status remains stable through the transport, although he continues to complain about his head pain.

You arrive at Mercy Hospital 6 minutes later. The patient states that his head still hurts but that he otherwise feels fine. He states that his pain is still 4/10.

You bring the patient to room 4 and give your report to the nurse. You state that it appears the patient had a syncopal episode and bumped his head; however, he's been stable throughout your care.

You replace the supplies while your partner cleans the unit. The unit is back in service at 0915.

Fill-in-the-Patient Care Report

EMS Patient Care Report (PCR)					
Date:	Incident No.:	Nature of Call:		Location:	
Dispatched:	En Route:	At Scene:	Transport:	At Hospital:	In Service:

Patient Information	
Age: Sex: Weight (in kg [lb]):	Allergies: Medications: Past Medical History: Chief Complaint:

Vital Signs				
Time:	BP:	Pulse:	Respirations:	SpO$_2$:
Time:	BP:	Pulse:	Respirations:	SpO$_2$:
Time:	BP:	Pulse:	Respirations:	SpO$_2$:

EMS Treatment
(circle all that apply)

Oxygen @ ___ L/min via (circle one): NC NRM BVM	Assisted Ventilation	Airway Adjunct	CPR
Defibrillation	Bleeding Control	Bandaging	Splinting:	Other:

Narrative

CHAPTER

37

Patients With Special Challenges

General Knowledge

Matching

Match each of the items in the left column to the appropriate definition in the right column.

_____ **1.** Cerebral palsy

A. A surgical opening between the small intestine and the outside of the body

_____ **2.** Colostomy

B. A portion of the spinal cord that protrudes outside of the vertebrae

_____ **3.** Developmental disability

C. A group of disorders characterized by poorly controlled body movement

_____ **4.** Down syndrome

D. An excessive amount of body fat

_____ **5.** Ileostomy

E. A plastic tube placed in a stoma connecting the trachea to the outside skin

_____ **6.** Obesity

F. A group of conditions that may impair development in the areas of physical ability, learning, language development, or behavioral coping skills.

_____ **7.** Sensorineural deafness

G. Damage to the inner ear resulting in a permanent lack of hearing

_____ **8.** Shunts

H. A surgical opening between the colon and the outside of the body

_____ **9.** Spina bifida

I. Tubes that drain fluid from the ventricles of the brain

_____ **10.** Tracheostomy tube

J. Occurs when the two 21st chromosomes fail to separate; also called trisomy 21

Multiple Choice

Read each item carefully and then select the one best response.

_____ **1.** Which of the following is NOT considered a potential cause of a developmental disability?
   A. Genetic factors
   B. Complications at birth
   C. Poverty
   D. Malnutrition

_____ **2.** Which of the following statements is FALSE regarding patients with autism?
   A. They fail to use or understand nonverbal communication.
   B. If they cannot speak, they will not be able to understand when spoken to.
   C. They may have extreme difficulty with complex tasks that require many steps.
   D. They have difficulty making eye-to-eye contact.

_____ **3.** All of the following are associated with Down syndrome EXCEPT:
   A. a small face
   B. short, wide hands
   C. a protruding tongue
   D. narrow-set eyes

_____ 4. Down syndrome patients are at an increased risk for medical complications. Which of the following is NOT one of those potential complications?
   A. Olfactory complications
   B. Cardiovascular complications
   C. Gastrointestinal complications
   D. Endocrine complications

_____ 5. Which of the following is TRUE regarding airway management of patients with Down syndrome?
   A. Patients often have large tongues.
   B. Patients have large oral and nasal cavities.
   C. Mask ventilation is relatively easy to achieve.
   D. The head-tilt chin-lift maneuver is more effective than the jaw-thrust.

_____ 6. When caring for a patient with a previous brain injury, you should:
   A. speak in a loud, commanding tone
   B. expect the patient to be able to walk
   C. watch the patient for signs of anxiety
   D. never consider restraining the patient

_____ 7. Which of the following is NOT a possible cause of visual impairment?
   A. Disease
   B. Injury
   C. Congenital defect
   D. Upper respiratory infection

_____ 8. When caring for a patient with a visual impairment, which of the following is NOT appropriate?
   A. Identifying noises
   B. Avoid transporting the patient's service dog if possible
   C. Describing the situation and surroundings
   D. Telling the patient what is happening

_____ 9. Conductive hearing loss can be caused by:
   A. advanced age
   B. damage to the inner ear
   C. nerve damage
   D. a perforated eardrum

_____ 10. Which of the following is NOT considered a clue that your patient might be hearing impaired?
   A. Slurred speech
   B. Presence of hearing aids
   C. Poor pronunciation of words
   D. Failure to respond to your questions

_____ 11. All of the following are possible causes of cerebral palsy EXCEPT:
   A. meningitis during early childhood
   B. damage to the developing fetal brain in utero
   C. traumatic brain injury at birth
   D. postpartum infection

_____ 12. Cerebral palsy is associated with all of the following conditions EXCEPT:
   A. epilepsy
   B. cardiovascular complications
   C. difficulty communicating
   D. intellectual disabilities

_____ **13.** Which of the following statements is FALSE regarding the care of a patient with cerebral palsy?
    A. Do not assume these patients are mentally disabled.
    B. Limbs are often underdeveloped and are prone to injury.
    C. Walkers or wheelchairs should not be taken in the ambulance.
    D. Be prepared to care for a seizure if one occurs.

_____ **14.** Some patients with spina bifida have:
    A. partial or full paralysis of the lower extremities
    B. multiple cardiovascular problems
    C. daily episodes of neck pain
    D. a tendency to resist sitting

_____ **15.** When suctioning a tracheostomy tube, be sure not to suction for longer than:
    A. 5 seconds
    B. 10 seconds
    C. 15 seconds
    D. 20 seconds

_____ **16.** If a patient's home mechanical ventilator malfunctions, you should remove the patient from the ventilator and:
    A. place the patient on a nasal cannula
    B. place the patient on a nonrebreathing mask
    C. begin ventilations with a bag-mask device
    D. contact medical control

_____ **17.** An apnea monitor is indicated in all of the following situations EXCEPT:
    A. premature birth
    B. severe gastroesophageal reflux
    C. family history of sudden infant death syndrome (SIDS)
    D. asthma

_____ **18.** Which of the following is NOT a risk factor associated with the implantation of a left ventricular assist device?
    A. Excessive bleeding
    B. Acute heart failure
    C. Renal failure
    D. Stroke

_____ **19.** Central venous catheters are located in all of the following areas EXCEPT:
    A. the upper arm
    B. the lower leg
    C. the chest
    D. under the clavicle

_____ **20.** Patients with gastric tubes who have difficulty breathing should be transported sitting or lying on the:
    A. left side, with the head elevated 30°
    B. right side, with the head elevated 30°
    C. right side, with the head elevated 45°
    D. left side, with the head elevated 45°

_____ **21.** A ventricular atrium shunt drains excess fluid from the ventricles of the brain into the:
    A. right atrium of the heart
    B. left atrium of the heart
    C. right ventricle of the heart
    D. left ventricle of the heart

_____ **22.** Services offered by home care agencies include all of the following EXCEPT:

    A. providing personal hygiene

    B. wound care

    C. taking the patient to restaurants

    D. yard maintenance

_____ **23.** All of the following are diseases or conditions that are associated with patients receiving hospice EXCEPT:

    A. AIDS

    B. end-stage Alzheimer disease

    C. cancer

    D. pneumonia

_____ **24.** The term _obese_ is used when someone is _____ or more over his or her ideal body weight.

    A. 20%

    B. 30%

    C. 40%

    D. 50%

True/False

If you believe the statement to be more true than false, write the letter "T" in the space provided. If you believe the statement to be more false than true, write the letter "F."

_____ **1.** It is important to make sure you are at eye level when communicating with patients.

_____ **2.** Visually impaired patients can be guided, pulled, or pushed to help them move.

_____ **3.** Some patients with paralysis will have normal sensation.

_____ **4.** In severe or morbid obesity, the person is 11 kg to 34 kg (25 lb to 75 lb) over his or her ideal weight.

_____ **5.** Tracheostomy tubes are prone to obstruction from mucus plugs or foreign bodies.

_____ **6.** You can estimate the size of a suction catheter for a tracheostomy tube by doubling the inner diameter of the tracheostomy tube.

_____ **7.** Patients with tracheostomies breathe through their mouths and noses.

_____ **8.** You should never place defibrillator paddles or pacing patches directly over an implanted defibrillation device.

_____ **9.** Patients who have a gastric tube in place may still be at increased risk of aspiration.

_____ **10.** Interaction with the caregiver of a child or adult with special needs will be an important part of the patient assessment process.

Fill-in-the-Blank

Read each item carefully and then complete the statement by filling in the missing word.

1. _____ is an intellectual disability characterized by deficits in social communication and interactions, along with restricted, repetitive patterns of behavior, interests, and activities.

2. You may allow a patient with a visual impairment to rest his or her hand on your _____ because this may help with balance and security while moving.

3. _____ _____ can be either external or internal, depending on the type of hearing damage.

4. The two most common forms of hearing loss are _____ deafness and _____ hearing loss.

5. _____ _____ is a term for a group of disorders characterized by poorly controlled body movement.

6. To reduce the occurrence of spina bifida, pregnant women are advised to take _____ _____.

7. A(n) _____ _____ _____ is a special piece of medical equipment that takes over the function of either one or both heart ventricles.

8. _____ are tubes that drain excess cerebrospinal fluid from the ventricles of the brain to keep pressure from building up in the brain.

9. If you encounter a patient with a colostomy or ileostomy bag, assess for signs of _____ if the patient has been complaining of diarrhea or vomiting.

10. Comfort care, or _____ _____, improves the patient's quality of life before the patient dies.

Fill-in-the-Table
Complete the missing information to the right of the mnemonic.

DOPE Mnemonic	
D	
O	
P	
E	

Critical Thinking

Short Answer
Complete this section with short written answers using the space provided.

1. List at least four helpful hints for working with patients with hearing impairments.

_____

_____

_____

2. Describe the various troubleshooting methods for a hearing aid malfunction.

_____

_____

_____

3. List the four types of hearing aids.

_____

_____

_____

4. List at least eight helpful tips to use when moving a morbidly obese patient.

_____

_____

_____

5. List six questions you should ask when caring for a patient with an implanted pacemaker.

_____

_____

_____

Ambulance Calls

The following case scenarios provide an opportunity to explore the concerns associated with patient management and to enhance critical-thinking skills. Read each scenario and answer each question to the best of your ability.

1. You respond to a nursing home for a 75-year-old man whose internal defibrillator continues to fire. When you arrive on scene, you find the patient being assisted by the nursing staff. The patient is pale, with an altered mental status. You notice he "jumps" every few minutes.

How would you best manage this patient?

_____

_____

_____

2. You are dispatched to a residence for a 12-year-old girl having a seizure. When you arrive on scene, you are met at the door by the patient's mother. The mother tells you that her daughter has Down syndrome and is prone to seizures. She states that her daughter has had two "tonic-clonic seizures" today. When you walk into the room, you see the patient lying on the floor in what appears to be a postictal state. The patient is being attended by other family members.

How would you best manage this patient?

_____

_____

_____

Skills

Assessment Review

Answer the following questions pertaining to the assessment of the types of emergencies discussed in this chapter.

_____ **1.** When treating a patient with autism, remember that the patient:

    A. will be able to describe his or her underlying condition to you

    B. will speak in a clear, inflected voice

    C. is not likely to maintain eye contact with you

    D. will be able to follow most of your commands without difficulty

_____ **2.** What sign found at a scene might indicate that your patient is visually impaired?

    A. No carpet

    B. Animals

    C. No stairs

    D. A cane

_____ **3.** What can be done for a patient with a tracheostomy who needs oxygen when you do not have a proper tracheostomy collar?

    A. Immediately assist ventilations with a bag-mask device.

    B. Place a nasal cannula on the patient.

    C. Place a face mask over the patient's mouth.

    D. Place a face mask over the stoma.

_____ **4.** Which of the following is NOT a sign of infection at a colostomy site?

    A. Tenderness

    B. Intact skin

    C. Warm skin

    D. Redness

Transport Operations

General Knowledge

Matching

Match each of the items in the left column to the appropriate definition in the right column.

_____ **1.** Air ambulances

_____ **2.** Type II design

_____ **3.** Spotter

_____ **4.** Sterilization

_____ **5.** Ambulance

_____ **6.** Cleaning

_____ **7.** Disinfection

A. A standard van; forward-control integral cab-body ambulance

B. The killing of pathogenic agents by direct application of chemicals

C. The process of removing dirt, dust, blood, or other visible contaminants

D. Fixed- or rotary-wing aircraft used to rapidly transport patients to the appropriate facility

E. A person who assists a driver in backing up an ambulance

F. A specialized vehicle for treating and transporting sick and injured patients

G. Removes all microbial contamination

Multiple Choice

Read each item carefully and then select the one best response.

_____ **1.** Modern ambulances are designed according to strict government regulations based on _____ standards.

   A. FDA

   B. EPA

   C. NFPA

   D. USDA

_____ **2.** Features of the modern ambulance include all of the following EXCEPT:

   A. a self-contained breathing apparatus

   B. a patient compartment

   C. two-way radio communication

   D. a driver's compartment

_____ **3.** The first thing you do each day when you arrive at work is to make sure all equipment and supplies are functioning and in their assigned places. This is the _____ phase of transport operations.

   A. preparation

   B. dispatch

   C. arrival at scene

   D. transport

_____ **4.** The type _____ ambulance is a standard van with a forward-control integral cab body.

   A. I

   B. II

   C. III

   D. IV

_____ **5.** Suction units carried on ambulances must be powerful enough to generate a vacuum of _____ when the tube is clamped.

A. 100 mm Hg

B. 200 mm Hg

C. 300 mm Hg

D. 400 mm Hg

_____ **6.** Which of the following is FALSE regarding the use of oropharyngeal airways?

A. Oropharyngeal airways can be used on adults.

B. Oropharyngeal airways can be used on children.

C. Oropharyngeal airways can be used on infants.

D. Oropharyngeal airways cannot be used by EMTs.

_____ **7.** When attached to oxygen supply with the oxygen reservoir in place, a bag-mask device is able to supply almost _____ oxygen.

A. 100%

B. 95%

C. 90%

D. 85%

_____ **8.** Extrication equipment carried on an ambulance may include all of the following EXCEPT:

A. a rescue blanket

B. an adjustable wrench

C. duct tape

D. the jaws of life

_____ **9.** Basic wound care supplies include all of the following EXCEPT:

A. sterile sheets

B. an obstetrics (OB) kit

C. an assortment of adhesive bandages

D. aluminum foil

_____ **10.** Your supervisor asks you to make up jump kits for each ambulance. He has told you that he will leave it up to you as to what goes into the kit. You would want to include everything that you might need within the first _____ minutes of arrival at the patient's side.

A. 2

B. 3

C. 4

D. 5

_____ **11.** Deceleration straps over the shoulders prevent the patient from continuing to move _____ in case the ambulance suddenly slows or stops.

A. forward

B. backward

C. laterally

D. down

_____ **12.** The ambulance inspection should include checks of all of the following EXCEPT:

A. fuel level

B. brake fluid

C. wheels and tires

D. spark plugs

_____ 13. You are hired at the local EMS agency. During your orientation, you are given a tour of the station and the ambulances that you will be riding on. Your duties include station cleanup and checking the unit for mechanical problems. You should also check all medical equipment and supplies:

    A. after every call

    B. after every emergency transport

    C. every 12 hours

    D. every day

_____ 14. For every emergency request, the dispatcher should gather and record all of the following EXCEPT:

    A. the nature of the call

    B. the patient's location

    C. medications that the patient is currently taking

    D. the number of patients and possible severity of their condition

_____ 15. During the _____ phase, the team should review dispatch information and assign specific initial duties and scene management tasks to each team member.

    A. preparation

    B. dispatch

    C. en route

    D. transport

_____ 16. Basic requirements for the driver to operate an ambulance safely do NOT include:

    A. physical fitness

    B. emotional fitness

    C. proper attitude

    D. the driver taking cold medication

_____ 17. The _____ phase may be the most dangerous part of the call.

    A. preparation

    B. en route

    C. transport

    D. on scene

_____ 18. To operate an emergency vehicle safely, you must know how it responds to _____ under various conditions.

    A. steering

    B. braking

    C. acceleration

    D. steering, braking, and acceleration

_____ 19. You must always drive:

    A. offensively

    B. defensively

    C. under the speed limit

    D. recklessly

_____ 20. When driving with lights and siren, you are _____ drivers to yield the right-of-way.

    A. requesting

    B. demanding

    C. offering

    D. insisting

_____ 21. Vehicle size and _____ will greatly influence braking and stopping distances.

    A. length

    B. height

    C. weight

    D. width

_____ **22.** When on an emergency call, before proceeding past a stopped school bus with its lights flashing, you should stop before reaching the bus and wait for the driver to do all of the following EXCEPT:

    A. make sure the children are safe

    B. close the bus door

    C. turn off the warning lights

    D. An emergency vehicle does not need to stop for a school bus displaying its flashing lights.

_____ **23.** _____ must be secured when the vehicle is in motion.

    A. All equipment and cabinets

    B. The patient

    C. Any passengers accompanying the patient

    D. All equipment, cabinets, the patient, and any passengers

_____ **24.** The _____ is a specialized siren that emits low-frequency sound waves that may penetrate vehicles more effectively than traditional sirens.

    A. Shaker

    B. Saber

    C. Rumbler

    D. Rocker

_____ **25.** If you are involved in a motor vehicle collision while operating an emergency vehicle and are found to be at fault, you may be charged:

    A. civilly

    B. criminally

    C. both civilly and criminally

    D. neither civilly nor criminally

_____ **26.** _____ crashes are the most common and usually the most serious type of collision in which ambulances are involved.

    A. Roundabout

    B. Intersection

    C. Lateral

    D. Rollover

_____ **27.** You respond to a multiple-vehicle collision. You and your partner are reviewing dispatch information en route to the scene. You will be at a major intersection of two state highways. As you approach the scene, you review the guidelines for sizing up the scene. The guidelines include all of the following EXCEPT:

    A. looking for safety hazards

    B. evaluating the need for additional units or other assistance

    C. evaluating the need to stabilize the spine

    D. entering the scene even if there are hazards

_____ **28.** The main objectives in directing traffic include all of the following EXCEPT:

    A. warning other drivers

    B. preventing additional crashes

    C. keeping vehicles moving in an orderly fashion

    D. answering curious motorists' questions

_____ **29.** Transferring the patient to a receiving staff member occurs during the _____ phase.

    A. arrival

    B. transport

    C. delivery

    D. postrun

_____ **30.** The decision to activate the emergency lights and siren depends on all of the following factors EXCEPT:
   A. local protocols
   B. patient condition
   C. the anticipated clinical outcome of the patient
   D. wanting to go faster

_____ **31.** You have called for an air ambulance. While your partner is monitoring the patient, he tells you to go set up a landing zone for the helicopter. When establishing a landing site for an approaching helicopter, ensure all of the following EXCEPT:
   A. that loose debris is cleared away
   B. that the area is free of electric or telephone wires
   C. that the area is free of telephone poles
   D. that the area is on a hill

True/False

If you believe the statement to be more true than false, write the letter "T" in the space provided. If you believe the statement to be more false than true, write the letter "F."

_____ **1.** Equipment and supplies should be placed in the unit according to how urgently and how often they are needed.

_____ **2.** A CPR board is a pocket-sized reminder that the EMT carries to help recall CPR procedures.

_____ **3.** Specially trained medical flight crews accompany all air ambulance flights.

_____ **4.** The en route or response phase of the emergency call is the least dangerous for the EMT.

_____ **5.** The use of a police escort is a standard practice.

_____ **6.** Use the "4-second rule" in all conditions, to help you maintain a safe following distance.

_____ **7.** Always approach a helicopter from the front.

_____ **8.** Fixed-wing air ambulances are generally used for short-haul patient transfers.

_____ **9.** A clear landing zone of 50 feet by 50 feet (15 m by 15 m) is recommended for EMS helicopters.

Fill-in-the-Blank

Read each item carefully and then complete the statement by filling in the missing words.

1. A(n) _____ _____ is a portable kit containing items that are used in the initial 5 minutes of caring for the patient.

2. The six-pointed star that identifies vehicles that meet federal specifications as licensed or certified ambulances is known as the _____ _____ _____.

3. For many decades after the first motorized ambulance was used in the 1800s, a(n) _____ was the vehicle that was most often used as an ambulance.

4. _____-_____ _____ respond initially to the scene with personnel and equipment to treat the sick and injured until an ambulance can arrive.

5. An ambulance call has _____ phases.

6. Some states allow you to proceed through a controlled intersection "_____ _____ _____,"

using flashing lights and siren.

7. Suction tubing must reach the patient's _____, regardless of the patient's position.

8. A(n) _____ _____ provides a firm surface under the patient's torso so that you can give effective chest

compressions.

Labeling
Label the following diagrams with the correct terms.

1. Helicopter Hand Signals

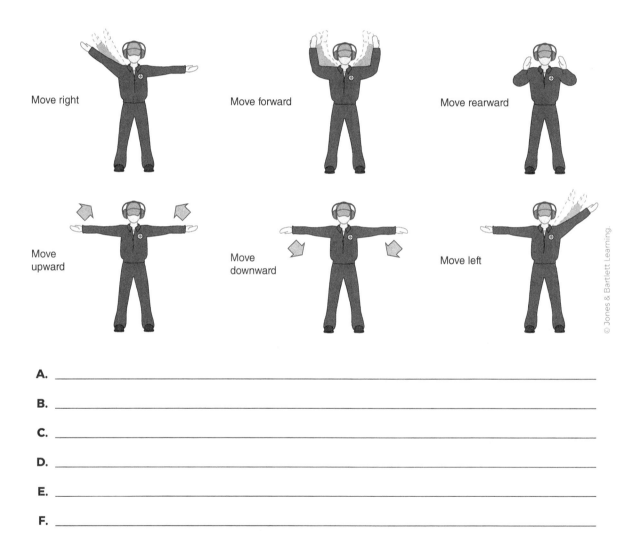

A. _____

B. _____

C. _____

D. _____

E. _____

F. _____

Critical Thinking

Multiple Choice

Read each critical-thinking item carefully and then select the one best response.

Questions 1–5 are derived from the following scenario: You are requested out to County Road 93 for a motor vehicle collision at a rural area known for serious crashes. After driving with lights and siren for nearly 20 minutes to reach the scene, you arrive at the intersection at the east end of the county. As you pull up, you see two pickup trucks crushed into a mass of twisted, smoking metal. A sheriff's deputy is shouting and waving you over to the passenger-side door of one of the demolished trucks. You quickly look down all four roads leading to the scene and note that they are deserted as far as you can see.

_____ 1. Specifically regarding the transport of patients from this scene, you should immediately consider _____ before stepping out of the ambulance.
   A. scene safety
   B. parking 100 feet (30 m) past the scene
   C. requesting a medical helicopter
   D. the risks versus benefits of using the siren

_____ 2. Which phase of an ambulance call does this scenario demonstrate?
   A. en route
   B. arrival at scene
   C. preparation
   D. postrun

_____ 3. Which of the following would you most likely NOT need for this incident?
   A. Jump kit
   B. Airway kit
   C. Extrication kit
   D. OB kit

_____ 4. How would you ensure the proper control of traffic around this scene?
   A. Lower or switch off warning lights so as not to blind oncoming motorists.
   B. Because the roads were deserted when you arrived, it is not a priority.
   C. Ask the law enforcement officer to control any traffic.
   D. Pull completely off the roadway and leave your hazard lights flashing.

_____ 5. You end up transporting an unstable trauma patient from this scene. Assuming that the patient is breathing adequately, what should you be doing about every 5 minutes during the transport phase?
   A. Reassessing vital signs
   B. Providing an update to the receiving facility
   C. Checking your ETA with the navigational equipment
   D. Attempting to rendezvous with an ALS crew

Short Answer

Complete this section with short written answers using the space provided.

1. Describe the three basic ambulance designs.

_____

_____

_____

2. List the phases of an ambulance call.

_____

_____

_____

3. Define the term _siren syndrome_.

_____

_____

_____

4. Describe the three basic principles that govern the use of warning lights and siren.

_____

_____

_____

5. List four guidelines for safe ambulance driving.

_____

_____

_____

6. List the general considerations used for selecting a helicopter landing site.

_____

_____

_____

Ambulance Calls

The following case scenarios provide an opportunity to explore the concerns associated with patient management and to enhance critical-thinking skills. Read each scenario and answer each question to the best of your ability.

1. You are cross-trained as a firefighter, and your station has been dispatched to a working structure fire. As you near the scene, another call is dispatched for "an unknown medical emergency." You are the closest unit to the medical emergency.

How would you best manage this situation?

_____

_____

_____

2. Your department's coverage area is quite large, including ALS coverage for the entire county, as well as surrounding areas out of state. You are dispatched to an unfamiliar address for "CPR in progress" and are working with a newly hired partner who is not familiar with your coverage area.

   How would you best manage this situation?

   _____

   _____

   _____

3. You are called to the scene of a motor vehicle collision. The car is situated in a curve, and traffic is heavy. Police are not on the scene. Your patient is alert and looking around but is stuck in the vehicle due to traffic. You see blood smeared across her face, but it appears to be minimal.

   How would you best manage this situation?

   _____

   _____

   _____

Fill-in-the-Patient Care Report

Read the incident scenario and then complete the following patient care report (PCR).

It is just before dawn (0512 by the clock on the dashboard), and the darkness is broken only by the occasional burst of lightning in the clouds above, which briefly illuminates the heavy rainfall that has been coming down all night long. You are just about to tell your partner, Alejandro, that you are surprised by the absence of vehicle collisions tonight with the weather the way it is when the dispatch tones burst from the speakers.

"4-0-9, Central Dispatch, emergency call to Highway 12 and Nest Creek Road for a motor vehicle collision."

"4-0-9 copies," Alejandro responds as you start the truck. "En route to Highway 12 and Nest Creek."

"Station time, 0513."

You drive carefully through the torrential rain, the flashing strobes mounted above the cab reflecting off the raindrops and reducing your visibility, turning what would normally be a 6-minute drive into 10. Thankfully, the heavy rain eases as you arrive on the scene, dissipating to a gentle shower. You park safely off the roadway, which has been shut down by highway patrol, and approach the scene while Alejandro pulls the equipment from the back.

"We've got two drivers and two cars involved," a highway patrol officer wearing a plastic-covered, wide-brimmed hat says as you approach. "One's not injured, but the other is bleeding pretty good from her nose. I think she hit the steering wheel."

You walk over to the small white car where the injured woman is still in the driver's seat and see that the highway patrol has chocked the wheels and disconnected the battery. You approach from the front, so the 41-year-old woman can see you directly out of the windshield, and Alejandro moves to the rear door.

"Ma'am," you say loudly through the windshield. "Keep looking straight ahead at me, and do not move your head. My partner is going to get in the back of your car right now and hold your head steady."

As soon as Alejandro is holding the woman's head in a neutral, in-line position, you set about applying a cervical collar, and finding no injuries other than a swollen (no longer bleeding) nose, you apply the vest-type extrication device and initiate high-flow oxygen therapy. Eight minutes after arriving on scene, and with the rain starting to fall harder again, you have the 90-kg (198-lb) patient secured to a long backboard and loaded into the back of the ambulance.

One minute after closing the back doors, you have obtained a baseline set of vital signs, and Alejandro has pulled out onto the roadway and has started driving to the nearest emergency department, 14 minutes south. The patient's vital signs are: blood pressure, 142/100 mm Hg; pulse, 100 beats/min; respirations, 16 breaths/min and unlabored (but she cannot breathe through her nose); and SpO$_2$ of 98%.

"What is your blood pressure normally?" you ask while filling out the PCR.

"It's high," she says. "I'm supposed to take Lisinopril, but I always forget. I had something like a stroke when I was 36. They called it a TIA or something."

"Do you have any other medical issues or allergies?"

"No. But my nose and cheeks are killing me."

"Okay," you say, patting her arm. "I'm sorry about that. We'll be at the hospital in a few minutes, and they will be able to help with that."

You then pick up the radio and contact the hospital to provide a patient report and your ETA.

Three minutes before arriving at the emergency department, you get a second set of vital signs and find that they are the same as the first, except that the patient's breathing has slowed by two breaths per minute as she relaxed. You and Alejandro unload the gurney from the ambulance and deliver the patient to the waiting staff of County Medical Center, where you provide a verbal report to the accepting nurse and properly turn over care.

A total of 45 minutes after the initial dispatch, you notify the dispatch center that you are available and ready for more calls.

Fill-in-the-Patient Care Report

EMS Patient Care Report (PCR)			
Date:	Incident No.:	Nature of Call:	Location:
Dispatched:	En Route:	At Scene:	Transport:	At Hospital:	In Service:

Patient Information	
Age: Sex: Weight (in kg [lb]):	Allergies: Medications: Past Medical History: Chief Complaint:

Vital Signs				
Time:	BP:	Pulse:	Respirations:	SpO$_2$:
Time:	BP:	Pulse:	Respirations:	SpO$_2$:

EMS Treatment (circle all that apply)				
Oxygen @ _____ L/min via (circle one): NC NRM BVM	Assisted Ventilation	Airway Adjunct	CPR
Defibrillation	Bleeding Control	Bandaging	Splinting	Other:

Narrative

CHAPTER

39 Vehicle Extrication and Special Rescue

General Knowledge

Matching

Match each of the items in the left column to the appropriate definition in the right column.

_____	1. Extrication	**A.**	Access requiring no special tools or force
_____	2. Simple access	**B.**	An individual who has overall command of the scene in the field
_____	3. Hazardous material	**C.**	An area where individuals can be exposed to sharp objects and hazardous materials
_____	4. Access	**D.**	Access requiring special tools and training
_____	5. Incident commander	**E.**	Removal from entrapment or a dangerous situation or position
_____	6. SWAT	**F.**	The ability to reach patients
_____	7. Complex access	**G.**	A fire in a house, apartment building, or other building
_____	8. Command post	**H.**	The location of the incident commander
_____	9. Technical rescue group	**I.**	Individuals trained to respond to special rescue situations
_____	10. Structure fire	**J.**	Special weapons and tactics team
_____	11. SCBA	**K.**	Self-contained breathing apparatus
_____	12. Danger zone	**L.**	Toxic, poisonous, radioactive, flammable, or explosive

Multiple Choice

Read each item carefully and then select the one best response.

_____ 1. During all phases of rescue, your primary concern is:
  A. extrication
  B. safety
  C. patient care
  D. rapid transport

_____ 2. When you arrive at the scene where there is a potential for hazardous materials exposure:
  A. turn off your warning light
  B. do not waste time waiting for the scene to be marked and protected
  C. park your unit downhill of the scene
  D. park your unit uphill of the scene

_____ 3. _____ is the ability to recognize any possible issues once you arrive on the scene and to act proactively to avoid a negative impact.
  A. Situational awareness
  B. Situational consciousness
  C. Situational alertness
  D. Situational disregard

_____ **4.** Controlling traffic at a scene is typically the responsibility of:
  A. a firefighter
  B. law enforcement
  C. the rescue group
  D. EMS personnel

_____ **5.** During a 360° walk around at an accident scene, you should look for all of the following EXCEPT:
  A. the mechanism of injury
  B. leaking fuels or fluids
  C. trapped or ejected patients
  D. the amount of air left in the tires

_____ **6.** You should communicate with members of _____ throughout the extrication process.
  A. law enforcement
  B. the media
  C. the rescue team
  D. the insurance company

_____ **7.** If there are downed power lines near a vehicle involved in a crash, you should:
  A. attempt to move the power lines yourself
  B. touch the power lines with an object to see if there is active electricity
  C. have the patient slowly exit the vehicle
  D. have the patient remain in the vehicle

_____ **8.** _____ is responsible for properly securing and stabilizing the vehicle and providing a safe entrance and access to the patient.
  A. Law enforcement
  B. The rescue team
  C. The EMS agency
  D. The HazMat unit

_____ **9.** Prior to attempting to gain access into a vehicle, the parking brake should be on, and the _____ should be disconnected.
  A. radio
  B. battery
  C. hydraulics
  D. brake lines

_____ **10.** Lighting at a scene, establishing a tool and equipment area, and marking for a helicopter landing all fall under:
  A. logistic operations
  B. EMS operations
  C. support operations
  D. law enforcement

_____ **11.** When removing an injured patient from a vehicle due to an environmental threat or the need to perform CPR, it is best to use the _____ technique.
  A. rapid extrication
  B. Kendrick Extrication Device (KED) board
  C. upright chest compression
  D. intermediate extrication

_____ **12.** When attempting simple access into a vehicle, you should:
  A. use complex tools
  B. try opening the doors using the door handles first
  C. break the windows initially
  D. make sure that all the windows are rolled up

_____ **13.** Which of the following is NOT considered a specialized rescue situation?
  A. Cave rescue
  B. Dive rescue
  C. Truck rescue
  D. Mine rescue

_____ **14.** When arriving at the scene of a cave-in or trench collapse, response vehicles should be parked at least _____ away from the scene.
  A. 50 feet (15 m)
  B. 150 feet (46 m)
  C. 250 feet (76 m)
  D. 500 feet (152 m)

_____ **15.** Which of the following statements regarding tactical emergency medical support is FALSE?
  A. Some incidents pose an increased risk to EMS.
  B. Once you have checked in at the command post, you are free to roam the area, looking for ways to help.
  C. Lights and siren should be turned off when nearing the scene.
  D. Planning measures and working with the incident commander will reduce the potential for chaos.

True/False

If you believe the statement to be more true than false, write the letter "T" in the space provided. If you believe the statement to be more false than true, write the letter "F."

_____ **1.** At a fire scene, you must ensure that your ambulance will not block or hinder other arriving equipment.

_____ **2.** Ambulances are not typically summoned to search and rescue scenes.

_____ **3.** When you arrive at the site of a technical rescue, you should identify the staging area where the technical rescue team will bring the patient.

_____ **4.** Following the termination of a rescue incident, all equipment used at the scene must be checked before being reloaded onto the apparatus.

_____ **5.** White-water rescue, structural collapse, and mountain-climbing rescue require specialized rescue teams.

_____ **6.** You should put on proper protective gear before exiting your vehicle at an emergency scene.

_____ **7.** Securing an injured arm to the body is generally considered to be acceptable until the patient is fully extricated.

_____ **8.** When determining a rescue plan, your input will be essential so that the patient's injuries will be considered during the rescue process.

_____ **9.** A short in a vehicle's electric system or a damaged battery may also cause a postcrash fire.

_____ **10.** Hybrid batteries have a higher voltage than traditional automotive batteries, and it may take up to 10 minutes for a high-voltage system to de-energize after the main battery is turned off.

_____ **11.** It is generally uncommon for EMTs to be in the vehicle with a patient during the disentanglement process.

_____ **12.** Providing medical care to a patient who is trapped in a vehicle is principally the same as for any other patient.

_____ **13.** Simple access typically involves breaking glass.

_____ **14.** When there are multiple patients, you should locate and rapidly triage each patient to determine who needs urgent care.

_____ **15.** A vehicle on its side is typically not a danger to you as long as the vehicle is not swaying.

_____ **16.** Airbags can be located in the steering wheel, doors, or seats.

_____ **17.** There are five phases to the extrication process.

Fill-in-the-Blank

Read each item carefully and then complete the statement by filling in the missing words.

1. In addition to posing a threat to you and others at the scene, _____ _____ may pose a threat to a much larger area and population.

2. A team of experienced EMTs should be able to perform _____ _____ in 1 minute or less.

3. _____ is the term used when a person is caught within a closed area with no way out or who has a limb or other body part trapped.

4. Once the patient has been freed or access has been gained, you should perform a(n) _____ _____ and provide care before further extrication begins.

5. _____ is the ongoing process of information gathering and scene evaluation to determine measures for managing an emergency.

6. Extrication is often extremely noisy, and appropriate _____ _____ should be worn by you and the patient.

7. _____ _____ are responsible for providing immediate assessment and treatment of injured people at rescue scenes.

8. Extinguishing fires, preventing additional ignition, and removing any spilled fuel is primarily the responsibility of _____.

9. The rescue team will set up a(n) _____ _____ that is off-limits to bystanders to protect their safety.

10. No matter what the fuel source of a crashed vehicle is, one common practice remains the same—the need to disconnect the _____.

11. You should not attempt to gain access into a vehicle until you are sure that it has been _____.

12. All EMS personnel should wear proper _____ _____ while in the working area.

13. The _____ _____ should provide you with the entrance you need to gain access to the patient.

14. _____ among team members and clear leadership are essential to safe, efficient provision of proper emergency care.

15. A lack of identifiable _____ at the scene hinders the rescue effort and patient care.

16. During disentanglement, cover the patient with a heavy, _____ _____ or place a(n) _____ between the windshield and the patient to protect him or her from breaking glass or other hazards.

17. Cave rescue, confined space rescue, and search and rescue are all considered to be _____ _____ situations.

18. You should consider using _____ _____ if the patient will need to be transported an extensive distance.

19. Unless otherwise instructed, only the _____ _____ should communicate any news or progress of a search and rescue to a victim's family.

20. _____ is a primary cause of secondary collapse in a trench collapse.

21. At no time should medical personnel enter a trench deeper than _____ _____ without proper shoring in place.

22. In most areas, an ambulance is dispatched with the fire department to any _____ _____.

Critical Thinking

Short Answer

Complete this section with short written answers using the space provided.

1. Explain the individual responsibilities of EMS, firefighters, law enforcement, and rescue teams at a rescue scene.

   _____

   _____

   _____

2. List the questions you and your team should consider whenever you need to determine the exact location and position of a patient.

   _____

   _____

   _____

3. List the steps for assessing and caring for a patient who is entrapped once access has been gained.

   _____

   _____

   _____

4. List the 10 phases of extrication.

_____

_____

_____

5. The reasons for rescue failure can be summarized by the mnemonic FAILURE. What does FAILURE stand for?

_____

_____

_____

Ambulance Calls

The following case scenarios provide an opportunity to explore the concerns associated with patient management and to enhance critical-thinking skills. Read each scenario and answer each question to the best of your ability.

1. You and your partner arrive on scene to find an extrication in progress. Your patient is a middle-aged female driver entrapped in a vehicle. One of the rescue team is yelling something about "bleeding" and waving you forward. The driver's side window is down, and the woman is screaming in pain. You note bright red blood spurting from her left upper arm. There are no immediate scene hazards to prevent you from approaching.

How would you best manage this situation?

_____

_____

_____

2. It is spring, and the water runoff from melting snow has caused the local viaduct to swell with cold, fast-moving waters. You are off duty when you hear a tone out for "small boy swept away by floodwaters." You arrive on the scene before your department's on-duty responders. You see a boy of approximately 13 years of age who is clinging to life in the middle of the channel, holding on to a trapped log. His mother is hysterical and screaming for you to "jump in and get him." You have no safety equipment available.

How would you best manage this patient?

_____

_____

_____

3. You are dispatched to a chemical spill where a train car derailed. The patient is the engineer; he was injured when he went to the back of the train to survey the damage. He is lying beside the tracks. From your vantage point at the staging area, he appears to be breathing. HazMat team members are suiting up to go in and retrieve the patient. They will decontaminate him before bringing him to the staging area.

How would you best manage this patient?

_____

_____

_____

CHAPTER

40 Incident Management

General Knowledge

Matching

Match each of the items in the left column to the appropriate definition in the right column.

_____ 1. Carboys
A. Shipping and storage vessels that may or may not be pressurized, holding between 4,000 and 6,000 gallons

_____ 2. Cold zone
B. Areas designated as hot, warm, and cold

_____ 3. Control zone
C. Initial triage done in the field

_____ 4. Freelancing
D. Patient sorting used in the treatment sector; involves retriage of patients

_____ 5. Decontamination
E. Removing or neutralizing hazardous materials from patients and equipment

_____ 6. Demobilization
F. Controlling spills when the main containment vessel fails

_____ 7. Disaster
G. Required on all four sides of vehicles transporting hazardous materials

_____ 8. Hot zone
H. Glass, plastic, or steel containers ranging in volume from 5 to 15 gallons

_____ 9. Intermodal tanks
I. The area surrounding a hazardous materials spill/incident that is the most contaminated area

_____ 10. Placards
J. Individual units or different organizations make independent and often inefficient decisions about the next appropriate action.

_____ 11. Primary triage
K. The area located between a hot zone and a cold zone

_____ 12. Secondary containment
L. A widespread event that disrupts community resources and function

_____ 13. Secondary triage
M. The supervisor-to-worker ratio

_____ 14. Span of control
N. A safe area where protective equipment is generally not required

_____ 15. Warm zone
O. Responders return to their facilities when work at a disaster is completed.

Multiple Choice

Read each item carefully and then select the one best response.

_____ 1. Major incidents require the involvement and coordination of all of the following EXCEPT:
   A. multiple jurisdictions
   B. local and national media
   C. multiple agencies
   D. emergency response disciplines

_____ **2.** Which of the following is NOT part of National Incident Management System (NIMS) standardization?
  A. Personnel training
  B. Resource classification
  C. Terminology
  D. Funding

_____ **3.** In the incident command system (ICS), organizational divisions may include sections, branches, divisions, and:
  A. groups
  B. teams
  C. platoons
  D. squads

_____ **4.** Which of the following is NOT considered a function of the finance section in the ICS?
  A. Time unit
  B. Procurement unit
  C. Cost unit
  D. Logistics unit

_____ **5.** Which of the following statements regarding the function of the public information officer is TRUE?
  A. Positions headquarters away from the incident
  B. Is not responsible for the safety of the media
  C. Monitors the scene for conditions that may be unsafe
  D. Relays information and concerns among the command and general staff

_____ **6.** What is one of the three main questions used during the scene size-up at a potential mass-casualty incident (MCI)?
  A. Is my ambulance stocked for an MCI?
  B. Where am I?
  C. What resources do I need?
  D. How long will it take to get help here?

_____ **7.** Which of the following is considered a priority when determining "what needs to be done" during the scene size-up?
  A. Rescue operations
  B. Incident stabilization
  C. Notifying hospitals
  D. Establishing operations

_____ **8.** Once you have performed a good scene size-up, _____ should be established by the most senior official.
  A. operations
  B. communications
  C. command
  D. rescue

_____ **9.** The primary duty of the triage supervisor is to:
  A. begin basic treatment
  B. establish zones for categorized patients
  C. communicate with the treatment division
  D. ensure that every patient is counted and prioritized

_____ **10.** Documenting and tracking of transporting vehicles, transported patients, and facility destinations is the responsibility of the:
  A. operations supervisor
  B. transportation supervisor
  C. logistics supervisor
  D. triage supervisor

_____ **11.** Which of the following is NOT a sign of stress that a rehabilitation supervisor is responsible for recognizing?
  A. Fatigue
  B. Headache
  C. Complete collapse
  D. Altered thinking patterns

_____ **12.** Which of the following definitions of MCI is correct?
  A. Any call that involves three or more patients
  B. Any situation that meets the demand of equipment or personnel
  C. Any incident that does not require a mutual-aid response
  D. Any call that has at least one motor vehicle involved

_____ **13.** Triaged patients are primarily divided into how many categories?
  A. Two
  B. Four
  C. Six
  D. Eight

_____ **14.** Delayed patients would be identified by using the color:
  A. black
  B. red
  C. yellow
  D. green

_____ **15.** Immediate patients would be identified by using the color:
  A. black
  B. red
  C. yellow
  D. green

_____ **16.** Minimal patients are the third priority and are identified using the color:
  A. black
  B. red
  C. yellow
  D. green

_____ **17.** Patients who are dead or whose injuries are so severe that they have, at best, a minimal chance of survival are categorized using what color?
  A. Black
  B. Gray
  C. White
  D. Brown

_____ **18.** Facilities, food, lighting, and medical equipment are the responsibility of the:
  A. operations section
  B. planning section
  C. logistics section
  D. finance section

_____ **19.** When using the START triage system, a patient who is breathing faster than 30 breaths/min is triaged as:
  A. immediate
  B. delayed
  C. minimal
  D. expectant

_____ **20.** "If you can hear my voice and are able to walk . . ." is said to immediately identify patients categorized as:

   A. immediate

   B. delayed

   C. minimal

   D. expectant

_____ **21.** A pediatric patient who is breathing 12 breaths/min would be categorized as:

   A. immediate

   B. delayed

   C. minimal

   D. expectant

_____ **22.** You are at the scene on a hazardous materials incident when your partner slips and falls, injuring his leg. He is alert and responds appropriately to your questions. His respirations are 20 breaths/min, and he has a radial pulse. What triage category does your partner fall into?

   A. Immediate

   B. Delayed

   C. Minimal

   D. Expectant

_____ **23.** Clues that you may be dealing with a hazardous material include all of the following EXCEPT:

   A. dead grass

   B. animals near the scene

   C. discolored pavement

   D. visible vapors or puddles

_____ **24.** Rail tank cars, intermodal tanks, and highway cargo tanks are all considered:

   A. oversize storage containers

   B. gross storage containers

   C. mass storage containers

   D. bulk storage containers

_____ **25.** Soap flakes, sodium hydroxide pellets, and food-grade materials are sometimes found in:

   A. bags

   B. carboys

   C. drums

   D. cylinders

_____ **26.** The US Department of Transportation (DOT) uses all of the following for hazardous identification EXCEPT:

   A. placards

   B. labels

   C. signals

   D. markings

_____ **27.** Some materials are so hazardous that shipping any amount of them requires a placard. Which of the following is NOT considered to be one of those hazards?

   A. Poison gases

   B. Low-level radioactive substances

   C. Water-reactive solids

   D. Explosives

_____ **28.** Which of the following statements regarding safety data sheets (SDSs) is FALSE?

   A. Facilities are no longer required by law to have an SDS on file for each chemical used.

   B. They provide basic information about the chemical makeup of a substance.

   C. They list the potential hazards associated with a substance.

   D. They list appropriate first aid in the event of an exposure.

_____ **29.** Control zones at HazMat incidents are labeled as all of the following EXCEPT:
    A. hot
    B. warm
    C. cold
    D. lukewarm

_____ **30.** Nonencapsulated protective clothing, eye protection, and a breathing device that contains an air supply fall into what level of personal protective equipment?
    A. Level A
    B. Level B
    C. Level C
    D. Level D

True/False

If you believe the statement to be more true than false, write the letter "T" in the space provided. If you believe the statement to be more false than true, write the letter "F."

_____ **1.** Some of the most challenging situations you can be called to are disasters and MCIs.

_____ **2.** The individuals who will participate in the many tasks in an MCI or a disaster should use the ICS.

_____ **3.** The purpose of the ICS is to designate the support agencies in several kinds of MCIs.

_____ **4.** Safety priorities include your life, then your patient's, and then your partner's.

_____ **5.** A key role of the transportation supervisor is to communicate with the area hospitals to determine where to transport patients.

_____ **6.** The staging supervisor should be established near the scene.

_____ **7.** The morgue should be out of view of the living patients and other responders.

_____ **8.** A way of tracking and accounting for patients is to issue only 20 to 25 triage tags at a time with a scorecard.

_____ **9.** Infants and children not developed enough to walk or follow commands should be taken as soon as possible to the treatment area for immediate secondary triage.

_____ **10.** When you approach a hazardous scene, you should stay downhill and upwind.

_____ **11.** The farther you are from the incident when you notice a problem, the safer you will be.

_____ **12.** The nature of the chemical dictates the construction of the storage drum.

_____ **13.** The DOT system requires that all chemical shipments be marked with placards and labels.

_____ **14.** Some substances are not hazardous but can become highly toxic when mixed with another substance.

_____ **15.** If you are treating a patient who was partially decontaminated, you will not need to wear additional protective clothing.

Fill-in-the-Blank

Read each item carefully and then complete the statement by filling in the missing words.

1. Two important underlying principles of the NIMS are _____ and _____.

2. One of the organizing principles of the ICS is limiting the _____ _____ _____ of any one individual.

3. A(n) _____ command system is one in which one person is in charge, even if multiple agencies respond.

4. The _____ section solves problems as they arise during the MCI.

5. _____ involves the decisions made and basic planning done before an incident occurs.

6. The _____ _____ is ultimately in charge of counting and prioritizing patients.

7. _____ _____ ensure that secondary triage of patients is performed.

8. The main information needed on a triage tag is a unique _____ and a triage _____.

9. The _____ and type of _____ are two good indicators of the possible presence of a hazardous material.

10. Containers of material are divided into two categories: _____ and _____ storage containers.

11. _____ _____ may be constructed of plastic, paper, or plastic-lined paper.

12. _____ _____ are established at a HazMat incident based on the chemical and physical properties of the released material and the environmental factors.

13. The _____ _____ is where personnel and equipment transition into and out of the hot zone.

14. Anyone who leaves a hot zone must pass through the _____ area.

15. A(n) _____ _____ is shipped to a facility, where it is stored and used, and then returned to the shipper for refilling.

Fill-in-the-Table

Fill in the missing parts of the table.

Triage Priorities	
Triage Category	**Typical Injuries**
Red tag: first priority (immediate) Patients who need immediate care and transport Treat these patients first and transport as soon as possible	• _____ • _____ • _____ • _____ • _____ • _____
Yellow tag: second priority (delayed) Patients whose treatment and transport can be temporarily delayed	• _____ • _____ • _____
Green tag: third priority, minimal (walking wounded) Patients who require minimal or no treatment and whose transport can be delayed until last	• _____ • _____
Black tag: fourth priority (expectant) Patients who are already dead or have little chance for survival; treat salvageable patients before treating these patients	• _____ • _____ • _____ • _____

Critical Thinking

Short Answer

Complete this section with short written answers using the space provided.

1. List the major components of the NIMS.

   _____

   _____

   _____

2. List the five factors that are included in mobilization and deployment.

   _____

   _____

   _____

3. What information should be communicated from the triage supervisor to the branch medical director?

_____

_____

_____

4. Based on the HAZWOPER regulation, what are the competencies that a first responder should be able to demonstrate at the awareness level?

_____

_____

_____

5. What information is typically included on an SDS?

_____

_____

_____

Ambulance Calls

The following case scenarios provide an opportunity to explore the concerns associated with patient management and to enhance critical-thinking skills. Read each scenario and answer each question to the best of your ability.

1. You are dispatched to a multiple-vehicle collision where you encounter three patients: a 4-year-old boy with bilateral femur fractures and absent radial pulse, a 27-year-old woman with a laceration to the head and a humerus fracture, and a 42-year-old man who is apneic and pulseless with an open skull fracture.

   How should you triage these patients?

   _____

   _____

   _____

2. Your response area contains a large portion of farming and other agricultural lands, including many orchards and vineyards. Right at shift change, there is a tone out for a "crop-duster accident" in a remote area of your jurisdiction. It appears that 15 to 30 agricultural workers were accidentally sprayed with pesticides and other chemicals from a crop-dusting plane. They are now experiencing a variety of signs and symptoms, including nausea, vomiting, and eye and upper airway irritation.

   How would you best manage this situation?

   _____

   _____

   _____

3. You and your partner are enjoying an unusually uneventful evening at work when you receive a dispatch for "overturned semitruck." As you approach the scene, you see a semi-tractor trailer that has left the roadway and rolled down a steep embankment. You see the driver attempting to climb up to the roadway, where many passersby have stopped to see what has happened. He is vigorously coughing, and you can see a liquid dripping from the truck's tank.

How would you best manage this situation?

_____

_____

_____

Skills

Assessment Review

Answer the following questions pertaining to the assessment of the types of emergencies discussed in this chapter.

_____ 1. You are at the scene of a multiple-vehicle collision involving eight people. Your partner has established command and is requesting additional resources as you begin to triage patients. You see patients in various areas as you visually inspect the scene. "If any of you are able to walk to me, please do so," you state to the patients. Three of the eight people are able to walk to you. What category of triage do these patients initially fall into?

    A. Immediate

    B. Delayed

    C. Minimal

    D. Expectant

_____ 2. As you continue moving through the scene, you come across two people in a vehicle. The first person has obvious bleeding from her forehead and is emotionally upset. She is slow to respond to your questions and cannot tell you what today's date is. When you ask her to show you "two fingers," she is able to but with some delay. Her radial pulse is 106 beats/min, and her respirations are 22 breaths/min and nonlabored. What category of triage does this patient initially fall into?

    A. Immediate

    B. Delayed

    C. Minimal

    D. Expectant

_____ 3. The next patient in the vehicle has an obvious open femur fracture. The patient is breathing at a rate of 32 breaths/min but is completely alert, oriented, and able to follow commands without hesitation. The patient's radial pulse is 102 beats/min and weak. What category of triage does this patient initially fall into?

    A. Immediate

    B. Delayed

    C. Minimal

    D. Expectant

_____ 4. Additional EMS have arrived on the scene, and you are being assisted by two other EMTs in the triage process. The last patient you encounter is a 7-year-old boy with neck and back pain. He is quite upset and keeps asking for his parents. His respirations are 38 breaths/min, and his radial pulse is 110 beats/min. What category of triage does this patient initially fall into?

    A. Immediate

    B. Delayed

    C. Minimal

    D. Expectant

CHAPTER

41

Terrorism Response and Disaster Management

General Knowledge

Matching

Match each of the items in the left column to the appropriate definition in the right column.

_____ **1.** Mutagen	**A.** A substance that emits radiation
_____ **2.** Vesicants	**B.** Describes how long a chemical agent will stay on a surface before it evaporates
_____ **3.** Disease vector	**C.** The period of time from exposure to onset of symptoms
_____ **4.** Phosgene	**D.** An agent that enters the body through the respiratory tract
_____ **5.** Neurotoxins	**E.** An animal that, once infected, spreads the disease to another animal
_____ **6.** Bacteria	**F.** An agent that affects the body's ability to use oxygen
_____ **7.** Volatility	**G.** Germs that require a living host to multiply and survive
_____ **8.** Cyanide	**H.** The means by which a terrorist will spread a disease
_____ **9.** Vapor hazard	**I.** A neurotoxin derived from mash that is left from the castor bean
_____ **10.** Lymph nodes	**J.** Biologic agents that are the most deadly substances known to humans
_____ **11.** Incubation	**K.** Microorganisms that reproduce by binary fission
_____ **12.** Ricin	**L.** A substance that mutates and damages the structures of DNA in the body's cells
_____ **13.** Dissemination	**M.** An area of the lymphatic system where infection-fighting cells are housed
_____ **14.** Radioactive material	**N.** A pulmonary agent that is a product of combustion
_____ **15.** Viruses	**O.** Blister agents

Multiple Choice

Read each item carefully and then select the one best response.

_____ **1.** All of the following are examples of terrorist groups EXCEPT:
  A. doomsday cults
  B. extremist political groups
  C. single-issue groups
  D. most organized religions

_____ **2.** An example of a single-issue group is:
  A. antiabortion groups
  B. separatist groups
  C. Aum Shinrikyo
  D. the KKK

_____ **3.** When were chemical agents first introduced?
   A. Spanish–American War
   B. World War I
   C. World War II
   D. Korean War

_____ **4.** During _____, Hiroshima and Nagasaki were devastated when they were targeted with nuclear bombs.
   A. World War I
   B. World War II
   C. the Vietnam War
   D. the Korean War

_____ **5.** You are called to the scene of an unexplained explosion at the local shopping mall. The reports are that there are multiple injuries. You are the first unit to arrive on the scene. Your first responsibility is to:
   A. ensure scene safety
   B. set up the incident command system
   C. start triage
   D. request additional resources

_____ **6.** In the previous scenario, you have been informed that there are numerous agencies responding with many different types of apparatus. They are approaching the scene from all directions and will be arriving shortly. You need to:
   A. set up a staging area
   B. separate the different types of apparatus
   C. let them continue as they are
   D. have them come in from downwind

_____ **7.** _____ agents can remain on a surface for long periods, usually longer than 24 hours.
   A. Volatile
   B. Persistent
   C. Secondary
   D. Vapor

_____ **8.** _____ is a brownish/yellowish oily substance that is generally considered very persistent.
   A. Lewisite
   B. Phosgene oxime
   C. Sulfur mustard
   D. Vesicant

_____ **9.** An example of a pulmonary agent is:
   A. chlorine
   B. phosgene oxime
   C. a G agent
   D. lewisite

_____ **10.** The most lethal of all the nerve agents is:
   A. V agent
   B. sarin
   C. soman
   D. tabun

_____ **11.** What two medications do DuoDote Auto-Injector antidote kits contain?
   A. Atropine and 2-PAM chloride
   B. Atropine and epinephrine
   C. Epinephrine and 2-PAM chloride
   D. Lidocaine and atropine

_____ **12.** You are dispatched to a local farm where an unconscious 41-year-old man has been discovered. The patient's airway is open, but he has been vomiting. Respirations are within normal limits, and distal pulses are present. The patient has muscle twitches and has urinated on himself. There is a funny odor that seems to be coming from the patient's clothing. You would suspect:

    A. alcohol poisoning

    B. organophosphate poisoning

    C. drug overdose

    D. respiratory agent

_____ **13.** You are dispatched to a patient who is having respiratory problems. He is awake but is working so hard to breathe that he can't answer questions. His distal pulses are present and strong. There is an odor of almonds in the air. You would suspect:

    A. cyanide

    B. sarin

    C. soman

    D. tabun

_____ **14.** The period of time between the person becoming exposed to an agent and when symptoms begin is called:

    A. contagious

    B. incubation

    C. communicability

    D. remission

_____ **15.** Which of the following is NOT an example of a viral hemorrhagic fever?

    A. Ebola

    B. Rift Valley

    C. Yellow fever

    D. Smallpox

_____ **16.** Which of the following statements regarding anthrax is FALSE?

    A. It enters the body through inhalation, cutaneous, and gastrointestinal routes.

    B. It is caused by a deadly bacterium that lies dormant in a spore.

    C. A vaccine is available to prevent anthrax infections.

    D. Pulmonary anthrax is associated with the lowest risk of death if left untreated.

_____ **17.** Bubonic plague infects the:

    A. respiratory system

    B. circulatory system

    C. lymphatic system

    D. digestive system

_____ **18.** The deadliest substances known to humans are:

    A. nerve agents

    B. hemotoxins

    C. plagues

    D. bacteria

_____ **19.** The least toxic route for ricin is:

    A. oral

    B. inhalation

    C. injection

    D. absorption

_____ **20.** The role of the EMS in helping to determine a biologic event is to:
    A. administer medications
    B. be aware of an unusual number of calls for unexplainable symptom clusters
    C. quarantine infected individuals
    D. set up field hospitals

_____ **21.** The most powerful of all radiation is:
    A. alpha
    B. neutron
    C. beta
    D. gamma

_____ **22.** To protect yourself from radiation exposure, you should do all of the following EXCEPT:
    A. limit the time of exposure
    B. increase the distance between yourself and the source
    C. use shielding
    D. wear a mask to prevent respiratory exposure

_____ **23.** Which organ is most susceptible to pressure changes during an explosion?
    A. Liver
    B. Lung
    C. Heart
    D. Kidney

True/False

If you believe the statement to be more true than false, write the letter "T" in the space provided. If you believe the statement to be more false than true, write the letter "F."

_____ **1.** The 2013 Boston Marathon bombing is an example of international terrorism.

_____ **2.** Weapons of mass destruction (WMDs) are easy to obtain or create.

_____ **3.** Most acts of terrorism occur after a warning is given to the general public.

_____ **4.** Understanding and being aware of the current threat are only the beginning of responding safely.

_____ **5.** Failure to park your ambulance in a safe location can place you and your partner in danger.

_____ **6.** You should have all units responding to an explosion converge on the main entrance to the building.

_____ **7.** Vapor hazards enter the body through the pores in the skin.

_____ **8.** The primary route of exposure of vesicants is through inhalation.

_____ **9.** Phosgene and phosgene oxime are two different classes of agents.

_____ **10.** Tabun looks like baby oil.

_____ **11.** Seizures are the most common symptom of nerve agent exposure.

_____ **12.** Organophosphate is the basic ingredient in nerve agents.

_____ **13.** Cyanide binds with the body's cells, preventing oxygen from being used.

_____ **14.** When dealing with smallpox, gloves are all the standard precautions you need.

_____ **15.** Outbreaks of the viral hemorrhagic fevers are extremely rare worldwide.

_____ **16.** Pulmonary anthrax infections are associated with a 90% death rate if untreated.

_____ **17.** Pneumonic plague is deadlier than bubonic plague.

_____ **18.** Ricin is deadlier than botulinum.

_____ **19.** Ingestion of ricin causes necrosis of the lungs.

_____ **20.** The dirty bomb is an ineffective WMD.

_____ **21.** Being exposed to a radiation source does not make a patient contaminated or radioactive.

_____ **22.** Neurologic injuries and head trauma are common causes of death from blast injuries.

Fill-in-the Blank

Read each item carefully and then complete the statement by filling in the missing words.

1. The bombing of the Alfred P. Murrah Federal Building in Oklahoma City is an example of _____ _____.

2. Any agent designed to bring about mass death, casualties, and/or massive damage to property and infrastructure is a(n) _____ _____ _____.

3. _____ _____ is when a nation has close ties with terrorist groups.

4. Like other burns, the primary complication associated with vesicant blisters is _____ _____.

5. _____ occurs when you come into contact with a contaminated person who has not been decontaminated.

6. _____ _____ _____ is a term used to describe how the agent most effectively enters the body.

7. An agent that gives off very little or no vapor and enters the body through the skin is called a(n) _____ _____.

8. _____ _____ are among the most deadly chemicals developed.

9. _____ means that vapors are continuously released over a period of time.

10. _____ is the means by which a terrorist will spread the agent.

11. _____ is a simple organism that requires a living host to multiply and survive.

12. The group of viruses that cause the blood in the body to seep out from the tissues and blood vessels is called _____ _____ _____.

13. _____ is a deadly bacterium that lies dormant in a spore.

14. Buboes are formed when the _____ _____ become infected and grow.

15. The most potent neurotoxin is _____.

16. _____ _____ _____ are existing facilities that are established in a time of need for the mass distribution of antibiotics, antidotes, vaccinations, and other medical supplies.

17. Any device that is designed to disperse a radioactive device is called a(n) _____ _____ _____.

18. A(n) _____ _____ _____ results from being struck by flying debris, such as projectiles or secondary missiles, that have been set in motion by the explosion.

Critical Thinking

Short Answer

Complete this section with short written answers using the space provided.

1. What are the key questions you should ask yourself when dealing with WMDs?

_____

_____

_____

2. List the four classes of chemical agents.

_____

_____

_____

3. What things should you observe on every call to determine the potential for a terrorist attack?

_____

_____

_____

4. List the signs of vesicant exposure to the skin.

_____

_____

_____

5. What are some of the later signs and symptoms of chlorine inhalation?

_____

_____

_____

6. What does the mnemonic SLUDGEM stand for?

_____

_____

_____

7. What are the signs and symptoms of high doses of cyanide?

_____

_____

_____

8. List the signs and symptoms of ricin ingestion.

_____

_____

_____

9. List three places that radioactive waste may be found.

_____

_____

_____

10. What should you use to best protect yourself from the effects of radiation?

_____

_____

_____

Ambulance Calls

The following case scenarios provide an opportunity to explore the concerns associated with patient management and to enhance critical-thinking skills. Read each scenario and answer each question to the best of your ability.

1. You are dispatched to an explosion at a nearby shopping mall. No other information is available regarding the nature of the explosion, only that there are possibly upward of 5 fatally wounded and 50 severely injured.

How would you best manage this situation?

_____

_____

_____

2. Your emergency system is suddenly inundated with numerous calls for people experiencing fever, chills, headache, muscle aches, nausea/vomiting, diarrhea, severe abdominal cramping, and gastrointestinal bleeding. All of the patients attended a local indoor sporting event 6 hours earlier.

How would you best manage this situation?

_____

_____

_____

3. You are dispatched to treat numerous patients with known exposure to cyanide. This occurred in a neighboring jurisdiction, and they have requested your assistance. The local fire department has set up a decontamination area, and you are asked to transport patients to the nearest appropriate medical facility.

What are important considerations to note about cyanide exposure?

_____

_____

_____

Skills

Assessment Review

Answer the following questions pertaining to the assessment of the types of emergencies discussed in this chapter.

_____ 1. A patient complains of a high fever for the past few days and now has blisters on the face and extremities. This is most consistent with:

    A. viral hemorrhagic fever

    B. bubonic plague

    C. smallpox

    D. anthrax

_____ 2. A patient complains of a fever, headache, muscle pain, shortness of breath, and extreme lymph node pain and enlargement. This is most consistent with:

    A. viral hemorrhagic fever

    B. bubonic plague

    C. smallpox

    D. anthrax

_____ 3. A patient was exposed to a package containing an unknown powder. The patient now complains of 3 to 5 days of flulike symptoms, difficulty breathing, and fever. The patient is also showing signs of shock, pulmonary edema, and respiratory failure. This is most consistent with:

    A. viral hemorrhagic fever

    B. bubonic plague

    C. smallpox

    D. anthrax

_____ 4. A patient complains of a sudden onset of fever, weakness, muscle pain, headache, and sore throat. Signs of external and internal hemorrhaging are noted, along with vomiting. This is most consistent with:

    A. viral hemorrhagic fever

    B. bubonic plague

    C. smallpox

    D. anthrax

PREPARATORY

EMS Systems

General Knowledge

Matching

1. H	(page 3; Introduction)	
2. N	(page 10; Public Basic Life Support and Immediate Aid)	
3. M	(page 11; Emergency Medical Technician)	
4. G	(page 11; Advanced Emergency Medical Technician)	
5. A	(page 11; Paramedic)	
6. K	(page 14; Medical Direction)	
7. B	(page 16; Continuous Quality Improvement)	

8. O	(page 3; Introduction)	
9. L	(page 15; Mobile Integrated Health Care and Community Paramedicine)	
10. C	(page 12; Public Access)	
11. I	(page 14; Legislation and Regulation)	
12. D	(page 14; Medical Direction)	
13. J	(page 7; Licensure Requirements)	
14. E	(page 16; Evaluation)	
15. F	(pages 22–23; Professional Attributes)	

Multiple-Choice

1. A	(pages 7–8; History of EMS)	
2. B	(page 14; Medical Direction)	
3. D	(page 15; Mobile Integrated Health Care and Community Paramedicine)	
4. C	(page 16; Continuous Quality Improvement)	
5. A	(pages 22–23; Professional Attributes)	

6. C	(page 14; Medical Direction)	
7. C	(page 14; Medical Direction)	
8. D	(page 9; Table 1-2)	
9. A	(page 3; Introduction)	
10. B	(page 10; Public Basic Life Support and Immediate Aid)	

True/False

1. F	(pages 9–10; Levels of Training)	
2. T	(pages 9–10; Levels of Training)	
3. T	(pages 10–11; Emergency Medical Responder)	
4. T	(pages 22–23; Professional Attributes)	
5. T	(pages 20–21; EMS Research)	
6. F	(pages 22–23; Professional Attributes)	

7. T	(pages 7–8; History of EMS)	
8. F	(page 14; Medical Direction)	
9. F	(page 11; Advanced Emergency Medical Technician)	
10. T	(pages 7–8; History of EMS)	

Fill-in-the-Blank

1. Continuous quality improvement (page 16; Continuous Quality Improvement)
2. medical director (page 14; Medical Direction)
3. automated external (page 10; Public Basic Life Support and Immediate Aid)
4. service (page 14; Legislation and Regulation)
5. access point (page 12; Public Access)

Critical Thinking

Short-Answer

1. The EMT is one of the four levels of prehospital care. The EMT provides basic life support, including automated external defibrillation, use of airway adjuncts, and assisting patients with certain medications. (pages 9–10; Levels of Training)

2. The Department of Transportation has developed a series of guidelines, curricula, funding sources, and assessment tools that are designed to develop and improve EMS in the United States. (pages 7–9; History of EMS)

3. • Keep vehicles and equipment ready for an emergency.

   • Ensure the safety of yourself, your partner, the patient, and bystanders.

   • Initiate the emergency vehicle operation.

   • Be an on-scene leader.

   • Perform an evaluation of the scene.

   • Call for additional resources as needed.

   • Gain patient access.

   • Perform a patient assessment.

   • Give emergency medical care to the patient while awaiting the arrival of additional medical resources.

   • Move patients only when absolutely necessary to preserve life.

   • Give emotional support to the patient, the patient's family, and other responders.

   • Maintain continuity of care by working with other medical professionals.

   • Resolve emergency incidents.

   • Uphold medical and legal standards.

   • Ensure and protect patient privacy.

   • Provide administrative support.

   • Constantly continue your professional development.

   • Cultivate and sustain community relations.

   • Give back to the profession.
   (pages 21–22; Roles and Responsibilities of the EMT)

4. Online medical direction is provided through radio or telephone connections between the EMT and the medical control facility. Off-line medical direction is provided through written protocols, training, and standing orders. (page 14; Medical Direction)

Ambulance Calls

1. You would decline the assistance of an ALS ambulance crew. ALS, or advanced life support, means that the crew would have a higher level of training and could perform more advanced patient care procedures than you or your partner could. Because there were no injuries resulting from this motor vehicle collision, there was no reason to summon advanced care. (page 9; Levels of Training)

2. Because none of the EMT-level airway skills were successful, it would be critical to request or rendezvous with a provider capable of using advanced airway techniques. You would contact dispatch and arrange to have an ALS crew either meet you at the patient's location or load the patient and meet up with an ALS crew while en route to the hospital. (page 9; Levels of Training)

Workforce Safety and Wellness

General Knowledge

Matching

1. D (page 38; Infectious and Communicable Diseases)
2. A (page 38; Donning and Doffing Full Personal Protective Equipment, page 41; Table 2-4)
3. C (page 41; Standard Precautions)
4. F (page 71; Posttraumatic Stress Disorder)
5. B (page 69; Stress Management on the Job)
6. E (page 38; Infectious and Communicable Diseases)
7. M (pages 38–40; Routes of Transmission)
8. G (page 53; General Postexposure Management)
9. L (pages 55–57; Hazardous Materials)
10. O (pages 38–39; Routes of Transmission)
11. J (page 38; Infectious and Communicable Diseases)
12. N (page 41; Standard Precautions)
13. H (pages 76–77; Sexual Harassment)
14. K (page 38; Infectious and Communicable Diseases)
15. I (pages 60–61; Mass Violence)

Multiple-Choice

1. C (pages 54–55; Scene Safety)
2. C (page 68; The Grieving Process)
3. A (page 68; The Grieving Process)
4. D (page 64; Eye Protection)
5. B (pages 35–36; Sleep)
6. A (pages 68–69; What Can the EMT Do?)
7. B (page 53; General Postexposure Management)
8. C (page 72; Compassion Fatigue)
9. B (page 32; Table 2-1)
10. D (pages 45–46; Masks, Respirators, and Barrier Devices)
11. B (page 37; Alcohol Abuse, pages 37–38; Drug Use)
12. A (pages 54–55; Scene Safety)
13. B (page 67; Helping the Family)
14. C (pages 38–40; Routes of Transmission)
15. B (page 41; Donning and Doffing Full Personal Protective Equipment)
16. D (pages 58–59; Fire)
17. B (pages 69–70; Stress Management on the Job)
18. A (pages 69–70; Stress Management on the Job)
19. A (pages 33–35; Nutrition)
20. B (pages 33–35; Nutrition)
21. A (page 71; Posttraumatic Stress Disorder)
22. A (pages 52; 51–53; Immunizations)
23. C (pages 55–57; Hazardous Materials)
24. B (pages 75–76; Cultural Diversity on the Job)

True/False

1. F (page 42; Table 2-4)
2. T (page 42; Table 2-4)
3. T (page 68; The Grieving Process)
4. F (page 41; Standard Precautions)
5. F (page 31; Introduction)
6. T (pages 32–36; Wellness and Stress Management)
7. F (page 53; General Postexposure Management)
8. T (page 63; Helmets)
9. T (page 76; Your Effectiveness as an EMT)
10. F (pages 75–76; Cultural Diversity on the Job)

Fill-in-the-Blank

1. Distress (page 32; Wellness and Stress Management)
2. Foodborne transmission (page 40; Routes of Transmission)
3. infectious disease (page 38; Infectious and Communicable Diseases)
4. hazardous (pages 55–57; Hazardous Materials)
5. handwashing (pages 41–43; Proper Hand Hygiene)
6. Cover (page 61; Mass Violence)
7. death, difficult (page 68; The Grieving Process)
8. stress management (pages 32–33; Strategies for Wellness and Resilience)
9. sleep (pages 35–36; Sleep)
10. Eye protection (page 45; Eye Protection and Face Shields)

Critical Thinking

Multiple Choice

1. C   (pages 65–66; Techniques for Communicating with the Critical Patient)
2. D   (pages 32–36; Strategies for Wellness and Resilience)
3. B   (pages 71–72; Posttraumatic Stress Disorder)
4. D   (page 72; Table 2-8)
5. A   (pages 54–55; Scene Safety)

Short-Answer

1. Standard precautions are protective measures based on the assumption that every person is potentially infected or can spread an organism that could be transmitted in the health care setting. Therefore, you must apply infection-control procedures to reduce infection in patients and health care personnel. (page 41; Standard Precautions)

2. 1. Denial
   2. Anger/hostility
   3. Bargaining
   4. Depression
   5. Acceptance (page 68; The Grieving Process)

3. • Irritability toward coworkers, family, and friends
   • Inability to concentrate
   • Difficulty sleeping, increased sleeping, or nightmares
   • Feelings of sadness, anxiety, or guilt
   • Loss of appetite (gastrointestinal disturbances)
   • Loss of interest in sexual activities
   • Isolation
   • Loss of interest in work
   • Increased use of alcohol
   • Recreational drug use
   • Physical symptoms such as chronic pain (e.g., headache, backache)
   • Feelings of hopelessness (page 72; Table 2-8)

4. • Minimize or eliminate stressors.
   • Change partners to avoid a negative or hostile personality.
   • Change work hours.

- Change the work environment.

- Cut back on overtime.

- Change your attitude about the stressor.

- Talk about your feelings with people you trust.

- Seek professional counseling if needed.

- Do not obsess over frustrating situations; focus on delivering high-quality care.

- Try to adopt a more relaxed, philosophical outlook.

- Expand your social support system outside of your coworkers.

- Sustain friends and interests outside emergency services.

- Minimize the physical response to stress by employing various techniques. (page 33; Table 2-2)

5. 1. Hepatitis B

  2. Influenza (yearly)

  3. Measles, mumps, and rubella (MMR)

  4. Varicella (chickenpox) vaccine, or having had chickenpox

  5. Tetanus, diphtheria, pertussis (Tdap) (every 10 years) (page 52; Table 2-6; Immunizations)

6. 1. Thin inner layer

  2. Thermal middle layer

  3. Outer layer (page 62; Cold Weather Clothing)

7. 1. Increased respiration and heart rate

  2. Increased blood pressure

  3. Constricted blood vessels near the skin surface (cool, clammy skin)

  4. Dilated pupils

  5. Tensed muscles

  6. Increased blood glucose levels

  7. Perspiration

  8. Decreased blood flow to the gastrointestinal tract (page 69; Stress Management on the Job)

8. • Smoke

  - Oxygen deficiency

  - High ambient temperature

  - Toxic gases

  - Building collapse

  - Equipment

  - Explosions (page 58; Fire)

Ambulance Calls

1. Continue to treat the patient appropriately and transport. Allow the cut to bleed, so long as the bleeding is minimal. This will help to wash/clean it out. Clean the wound with an alcohol gel, if available. Once patient care has been transferred to the receiving facility, immediately wash thoroughly with soap and water and report to your supervisor. Follow up with prompt medical attention.

2. As always, you should wear exam gloves and consider using eye protection. Because this call is for a respiratory issue and the possibility of tuberculosis is high, you should also don a particulate air respirator and place a surgical mask on the patient. Because the patient is complaining of respiratory distress, a nonrebreathing mask attached to oxygen will suffice as well. It is also very important that you pass the information about potential infection to the receiving facility staff in your patient report while en route and again when you hand off care to the emergency department.

Fill-in-the-Patient Care Report

EMS Patient Care Report (PCR)							
Date: Today's date	**Incident No.:** 2011-1234		**Nature of Call:** Overdose		**Location:** 7979 Fisher Blvd.		
Dispatched: 0912	**En Route:** 0912	**At Scene:** 0929		**Transport:** 0947	**At Hospital:** 0952		**In Service:** 1005
Patient Information							
Age: 16 years **Sex:** Female **Weight (in kg [lb]):** 48 kg (106 lb)				**Allergies:** None			
				Medications: None			
				Past Medical History: Attempted suicide 2 years ago—aspirin overdose			
				Chief Complaint: Unresponsive/overdose			
Vital Signs							
Time: 0934	**BP:** 116/76		**Pulse:** 56	**Respirations:** 8 GTV		**SpO$_2$:** 96%	
Time: 0947	**BP:** 114/74		**Pulse:** 48	**Respirations:** 8 GTV		**SpO$_2$:** 95%	
EMS Treatment (circle all that apply)							
Oxygen @ _15_ L/min via (circle one): NC (NRB) BVM			Assisted Ventilation		Airway Adjunct		CPR
Defibrillation	Bleeding Control		Bandaging		Splinting		Other:
Narrative							
Dispatched for an overdose. Arrived on scene to find a 16-year-old female, unresponsive on the bathroom floor, with a hypodermic needle next to her. The patient's airway was patent, and breathing was adequate. She was moved from the bathroom to the living room using an extremity lift in order to allow better assessment and treatment. History provided by the patient's mother indicated that the patient attempted suicide 2 years ago via aspirin ingestion. She has recently been struggling with heroin addiction, according to the mother. According to law enforcement on scene, the patient had apparently been arguing with her mother prior to today's events. Vital signs indicated that she was initially stable, but I chose to start her on high-flow oxygen therapy due to the potential for respiratory compromise. The patient was moved to the gurney and placed in the ambulance. I immediately obtained a second set of vitals, which showed a slight decrease in heart rate and oxygen saturation. I continued to monitor her en route to the receiving hospital without incident. While en route, I called the report in to the hospital, and upon turning care of the patient over to the emergency department, I gave a verbal report to the charge nurse.**End of Report**							

Skills

Skill Drills

Skill Drill 2-1: Proper Glove Removal Technique (page 44; Skill Drill 2-1)

1. Partially remove the first glove by pinching at the **wrist**. Be careful to touch only the outside of the glove.

2. Remove the **second** glove by pinching the **exterior** with your partially gloved hand.

3. Pull the second glove inside out toward the **fingertips**.

4. Grasp both gloves with your **free** hand, touching only the clean **interior** surfaces.

CHAPTER

3 Medical, Legal, and Ethical Issues

General Knowledge

Matching

1. H   (page 102; Assault and Battery and Kidnapping)
2. I   (page 101; Abandonment)
3. G   (pages 93–95; Advance Directives)
4. E   (page 102; Assault and Battery and Kidnapping)
5. L   (page 27; Vital Vocabulary, page 100; Certification and Licensure)
6. A   (page 93; Advance Directives)
7. D   (page 86; Consent)
8. F   (page 100; Duty to Act)
9. O   (page 106; Ethical Responsibilities)
10. B   (page 87; Expressed Consent)
11. C   (pages 89–90; Forcible Restraint)
12. M   (page 88; Implied Consent)
13. N   (page 115; Vital Vocabulary)
14. J   (page 101; Negligence)
15. K   (page 98; Standards of Care)

Multiple Choice

1. C   (page 98; Scope of Practice)
2. A   (page 98; Standards of Care)
3. D   (page 27; Vital Vocabulary, page 100; Certification and Licensure)
4. D   (page 101; Negligence)
5. C   (pages 86–89; Consent, pages 101–102; Abandonment, pages 90–91; The Right to Refuse Treatment)
6. B   (page 103; Good Samaritan Laws and Immunity)
7. D   (page 91; Confidentiality)
8. D   (page 104; Records and Reports)
9. B   (page 100; Duty to Act)
10. C   (page 95; Presumptive Signs of Death Table 3-1)
11. A   (pages 95–96; Definitive Signs of Death)
12. D   (page 96; Medical Examiner Cases)
13. B   (pages 91–92; HIPAA)

True/False

1. T   (page 101; Negligence)
2. F   (page 87; Expressed Consent)
3. T   (page 88; Implied Consent)
4. T   (pages 89–90; Forcible Restraint)
5. F   (pages 93–95; Advance Directives)
6. T   (page 93; Advance Directives)
7. T   (page 100; Standards Imposed by Textbooks)
8. F   (page 104; Special Mandatory Reporting Requirements)
9. T   (page 105; Scene of a Crime)
10. F   (pages 108–109; The EMT in Court)

Fill-in-the-Blank

1. scope of practice (page 98; Scope of Practice)
2. standard of care (page 98; Standards of Care)
3. duty to act (page 100; Duty to Act)
4. negligence (page 101; Negligence)
5. termination (page 101; Abandonment)
6. Expressed, implied (pages 87–88; Consent)
7. assault, battery (page 102; Assault and Battery and Kidnapping)

8. advance directive, DNR order (pages 93–95; Advance Directives)

9. refuse treatment (pages 90–91; The Right to Refuse Treatment)

10. special reporting (pages 104–105; Special Mandatory Reporting Requirements)

Critical Thinking

Multiple Choice

1. B   (page 88; Implied Consent)
2. A   (page 88; Implied Consent)
3. A   (page 88; Implied Consent)
4. C   (page 88; Implied Consent)
5. B   (pages 90–91; The Right to Refuse Treatment)
6. D   (page 101; Negligence)

Short Answer

1. Member of the armed services, married, a parent, or pregnant (pages 88–89; Minors and Consent)

2. You must continue to care for the patient until the patient is transferred to another medical professional of equal or higher skill level or another medical facility. (page 101; Abandonment)

3. 1. Obtain the refusing party's signature on an official medical release form that acknowledges refusal.

   2. Obtain a signature from a witness of the refusal.

   3. Keep the refusal form with the incident report.

   4. Note the refusal on the incident report.

   5. Keep a department copy of the records for future reference. (pages 90–91; The Right to Refuse Treatment)

4. 1. If an action or procedure is not documented, it did not happen.

   2. Incomplete or untidy records are evidence of incomplete or inexpert medical care. (page 104; Records and Reports)

5. 1. Duty

   2. Breach of duty

   3. Damages

   4. Causation (page 101; Negligence)

Ambulance Calls

1. This patient needs to be evaluated at the hospital. Her parents will likely feel a right to be informed of their child's medical conditions and medical care. Laws regarding the reproductive rights of minors vary from state to state. Some states allow minors to make decisions regarding birth control, prenatal care, or pregnancy termination without consenting parents, whereas others do not. You must know your local laws. You will have to provide information regarding the pregnancy to other health care providers directly involved in her care, and you should explain that fact and the necessity of such to the patient. Be tactful. Don't unnecessarily break your patient's trust by immediately sharing this knowledge with her parents. Document carefully and consult medical control.

2. The duty to act in this situation may vary from state to state; however, from an ethical perspective, you did the right thing by stopping to help the child. Once you have initiated care, you must ensure that the child's parent(s) or legal guardian is notified. Although the grandfather is home, you now have another dilemma. The condition of the house/capability of the grandfather to care for the child while the mother is away is such that the question of neglect arises. You should speak with the grandfather and attempt to contact the mother of the child. If you believe that neglect or abuse of a child is occurring, then you are most likely legally required to intervene (most states require this by law). You should notify law enforcement and/or child protective serves in accordance with your local statutes.

3. Assess the patient's mental status. If he is intoxicated or has an altered mental status, he is treated under implied consent. If he is alert and oriented, you may attempt to talk him into being treated by explaining what you feel is necessary and what may happen if he does not receive care. If he has an altered mental status, orders from medical control may be obtained to restrain the patient with the help of law enforcement and to transport him to the hospital.

Fill-in-the-Patient Care Report

EMS Patient Care Report (PCR)					
Date: Today's date	**Incident No.:** 2010-555		**Nature of Call:** MCA		**Location:** Grand and Hopper
Dispatched: 2115	**En Route:** 2116	**At Scene:** 2122	**Transport:** 2132	**At Hospital:** 2138	**In Service:** 2152

Patient Information	
Age: 24 years **Sex:** Female **Weight (in kg [lb]):** 52 kg (114 lb)	**Allergies:** N/A **Medications:** N/A **Past Medical History:** N/A **Chief Complaint:** N/A

Vital Signs				
Time: 2127	**BP:** 90/54	**Pulse:** 100 weak/irregular	**Respirations:** 12	**SpO$_2$:** 94%
Time: N/A	**BP:** N/A	**Pulse:** N/A	**Respirations:** N/A	**SpO$_2$:** N/A
Time: N/A	**BP:** N/A	**Pulse:** N/A	**Respirations:** N/A	**SpO$_2$:** N/A

EMS Treatment (circle all that apply)				
Oxygen @ 15 L/min via (circle one): NC (NRM) BVM	(Assisted Ventilation)	(Airway Adjunct)		CPR
Defibrillation	(Bleeding Control)	(Bandaging)	(Splinting)	Other:

Narrative
9-1-1 dispatch for a motorcycle versus automobile. On arrival, found the driver of the automobile unhurt and the motorcycle operator unresponsive in the street. She was bleeding heavily from a forehead laceration and did not have a patent airway—snoring respirations observed. Appropriate c-spine precautions taken, OPA inserted, and provided assisted ventilations using BVM with 15 L/min oxygen. Fire crew arrived on scene and assisted in bleeding control, obtaining vitals, and immobilizing patient to long backboard. Once adequately immobilized, patient was moved to the stretcher and loaded into the ambulance for transport to the university trauma center. Reassessment not completed while en route because of continuation of assisted ventilations. Delivered patient to trauma center and provided verbal report and copy of this written report to the charge nurse. **End of Report**

CHAPTER

4

Communications and Documentation

General Knowledge

Matching

1. M (pages 146–147; Base Station Radios)
2. G (page 147; Mobile and Portable Radios)
3. J (page 147; Mobile and Portable Radios)
4. K (pages 147–148; Repeater-Based Systems)
5. H (page 148; Digital Equipment)
6. L (page 147; Mobile and Portable Radios)
7. I (page 147; Mobile and Portable Radios)

8. C (pages 148–149; Cellular/Satellite Telephones)
9. A (pages 146–147; Base Station Radios)
10. F (pages 149–150; Other Communications Equipment)
11. E (pages 148–149; Cellular/Satellite Telephones)
12. D (pages 146–147; Base Station Radios)
13. B (page 121; Words of Wisdom)

Multiple Choice

1. B (pages 122–126; Verbal Communication)
2. A (page 147; Mobile and Portable Radios)
3. D (pages 128–129; Communicating With Children)
4. A (page 131; Communicating With Non–English-Speaking Patients)
5. B (page 148; Digital Equipment)
6. C (page 132; Patient Care Handover)
7. C (pages 149–150; Other Communications Equipment)
8. D (pages 150–151; Radio Communications)
9. B (pages 151–153; Responding to the Scene)
10. B (page 153; Communicating With Medical Control and Hospitals)
11. A (page 154; Giving the Patient Report)

12. B (pages 154–155; The Role of Medical Control)
13. C (pages 129–130; Communicating With Patients Who Are Deaf or Hard of Hearing)
14. D (page 123; Table 4-3 Therapeutic Communication Techniques)
15. A (page 154; Giving the Patient Report)
16. A (pages 154–155; The Role of Medical Control)
17. A (pages 122–126; Verbal Communication)
18. D (pages 120–122; Nonverbal Communication)
19. B (pages 137–138; Types of Forms)
20. C (pages 142–143; Reporting Errors)
21. C (pages 130–131; Communicating With Visually Impaired Patients)
22. D (page 146; Special Reporting Situations)

True/False

1. T (pages 146–147; Base Station Radios)
2. T (pages 122–126; Verbal Communication)
3. F (page 120; Age, Culture, and Personal Experience)
4. F (page 131; Communicating With Non–English-Speaking Patients)
5. F (page 143; Documenting Refusal of Care)

6. T (pages 142–143; Reporting Errors)
7. F (pages 147–148; Repeater-Based Systems)
8. T (pages 128–129; Communicating With Children)
9. T (pages 151–153; Responding to the Scene)
10. T (pages 134–137; Patient Care Report)

Fill-in-the-Blank

1. narrative (pages 137–138; Types of Forms)
2. transmitter, receiver (pages 146–147; Base Station Radios)
3. dedicated line (page 147; Base Station Radios)
4. Noise (page 121; Physical Factors)
5. litigation (page 143; Documenting Refusal of Care)
6. Pagers (page 152; Responding to the Scene)
7. importance (page 151; Responding to the Scene)
8. medical control (page 153; Communicating With Medical Control and Hospitals)
9. channel (page 146; Base Station Radios)
10. Closed-ended questions (page 122; Verbal Communication)
11. repeat (page 156; Calling Medical Control)
12. standing orders (page 156; Maintenance of Radio Equipment)
13. tone, volume (page 120; Age, Culture, and Personal Experience)
14. honest (page 129; Communicating With Children)
15. interpreter (page 131; Communicating With Non–English-Speaking Patients)
16. standard procedure (page 135; Patient Care Report)
17. Competent (page 143; Documenting Refusal of Care)

Critical Thinking

Multiple Choice

1. C (page 143; Documenting Refusal of Care)
2. D (pages 138–141; Standardized Narrative Formats)
3. A (pages 142–143; Reporting Errors)
4. D (pages 142–143; Reporting Errors)
5. C (page 143; Documenting Refusal of Care)

Short Answer

1.
   1. Allocating specific radio frequencies for use by EMS providers
   2. Licensing base stations and assigning appropriate radio call signs for those stations
   3. Establishing licensing standards and operating specifications for radio equipment used by EMS providers
   4. Establishing limitations for transmitter power output
   5. Monitoring radio operations (pages 146–147; Radio Communications)
2.
   1. Make and keep eye contact with your patient at all times.
   2. Provide your name and use the patient's proper name.
   3. Tell the patient the truth.
   4. Use language that the patient can understand.
   5. Be careful what you say about the patient to others.
   6. Be aware of your body language.
   7. Always speak slowly, clearly, and distinctly.
   8. If the patient is hard of hearing, face the person so that he or she can read your lips.
   9. Allow time for the patient to answer or respond to your questions.
   10. Act and speak in a calm, confident manner while caring for the patient. (pages 122–126; Verbal Communication)
3.
   1. Continuity of care
   2. Legal documentation
   3. Education
   4. Administrative information

5. Essential research record

6. Evaluation and continuous quality improvement (pages 134–137; Patient Care Report)

4. 1. Handwritten forms with checkboxes and a narrative section

2. Electronic PCRs (ePCRs) written using a tablet, laptop, or similar device (pages 137–138; Patient Care Report)

Ambulance Calls

1. Dispatch the closest ambulance for an emergency response. Call for assistance from the fire department and local law enforcement. Try to calm down the caller to obtain additional information. If the caller is still of no help, ask her to get someone else to the phone. Relay any additional information to the responding units.

2. You should determine whether anyone on scene can translate for you. (Children will often speak both English and Spanish.) If no one on scene can translate, you should contact a department translator. Every department should have a group of translators for different languages common to your community or an electronic translation device. (Ideally, you should speak languages commonly heard in your area.) If neither of these options is available, you should attempt as much nonverbal communication as possible, obtain baseline vital signs, and perform a primary assessment to determine the nature of the problem. If the patient appears to refuse your help, you are in a tough situation. You cannot leave without knowing what the medical emergency is (if any), and you cannot obtain an informed refusal if clear communication does not occur. Consider asking for law enforcement assistance as they have access to translation services as well.

3. Attempt to locate any identification that he may have on his person. If this is not possible or you cannot locate any forms of identification, you should notify law enforcement officers. The child should undergo a medical examination to ensure that no injuries or other medical emergencies are present. Take care to communicate in a nonintimidating manner (taking care in level/tone of voice and posture) and attempt to establish trust with the patient.

Fill-in-the-Patient Care Report

EMS Patient Care Report (PCR)			
Date: ~~Today's date~~	**Incident No.:** 2011–8898	**Nature of Call:** Dirtbike crash/ trauma	**Location:** 18553 Old Redwood Highway
Dispatched: 1721	**En Route:** 1721	**At Scene:** 1728	**Transport:** 1735	**At Hospital:** 1741	**In Service:** 1755

Patient Information

Age: 19 years	**Allergies:** Unknown
Sex: Male	**Medications:** Unknown
Weight (in kg [lb]): 73 kg (161 lb)	**Past Medical History:** Unknown
	Chief Complaint: Partial amputation of left foot

Vital Signs

Time: 1736	**BP:** 104/66	**Pulse:** 102	**Respirations:** 18 Unlabored	**SpO$_2$:** 97%
Time: 1741	**BP:** 110/72	**Pulse:** 90	**Respirations:** 14 Unlabored	**SpO$_2$:** 99%

EMS Treatment
(circle all that apply)

Oxygen @ _15_ L/min via (circle one): NC (NRM) BVM	Assisted Ventilation	Airway Adjunct	CPR
Defibrillation	(Bleeding Control)	(Bandaging)	(Splinting)	(Other: Shock Treatment)

Narrative

Responded to 9-1-1 dispatch to a motocross park for a dirtbike crash. Arrived to find the patient, a 19-year-old man, lying supine on the ground and in obvious pain from near amputation of his left foot below the ankle. Patient had patent airway and adequate breathing, and I controlled the bleeding at the injury site with direct pressure. Patient was placed on high-flow oxygen therapy, secured to the backboard utilizing all appropriate spinal precautions, and loaded into ambulance. First set of vitals indicated possible onset of hypoperfusion, so I covered the patient with a blanket. Called report to the receiving facility and obtained a second set of vitals, which showed improvement when compared to the first. Patient was transported without incident and appropriately turned over to the trauma center staff after I provided a complete verbal report.**End of Report**

Medical Terminology

General Knowledge

Matching

1. D (pages 165–167; Anatomy of a Medical Term)
2. F (pages 165–167; Anatomy of a Medical Term)
3. J (pages 170–171; Superior and Inferior)
4. G (page 171; Proximal and Distal)
5. C (page 172; Ventral and Dorsal)
6. A (page 172; Palmar and Plantar)
7. B (page 172; Movement Terms)
8. I (page 173; Prone and Supine)
9. E (page 172; Movement Terms)
10. H (page 172; Ventral and Dorsal)
11. C (pages 165–166; Prefixes)
12. G (page 166; Table 5-2 Common Prefixes in EMS)
13. A (pages 168–169; Table 5-4 Common Number Prefixes)
14. E (pages 168–169; Table 5-4 Common Number Prefixes)
15. F (pages 165–166; Prefixes)
16. D (page 166; Table 5-2 Common Prefixes in EMS)
17. B (page 166; Table 5-2 Common Prefixes in EMS)
18. F (page 167; Table 5-3 Common Suffixes in EMS)
19. C (page 167; Table 5-3 Common Suffixes in EMS)
20. B (page 167; Table 5-3 Common Suffixes in EMS)
21. E (page 167; Table 5-3 Common Suffixes in EMS)
22. G (page 167; Table 5-3 Common Suffixes in EMS)
23. A (page 167; Table 5-3 Common Suffixes in EMS)
24. D (page 167; Table 5-3 Common Suffixes in EMS)

Multiple Choice

1. B (page 171; Lateral and Medial)
2. D (page 166; Table 5-2 Common Prefixes in EMS)
3. C (pages 180–185; Table 5-12 Common Abbreviations)
4. B (pages 176–178; Table 5-9 Common Word Roots and Combining Forms, page 180; Table 5-11 Common Suffixes)
5. A (page 173; Prone and Supine)
6. C (pages 176–178; Table 5-9 Common Word Roots and Combining Forms, page 180; Common Suffixes in Medical Terminology)
7. B (pages 180–185; Table 5-12 Common Abbreviations)
8. D (pages 180–185; Table 5-12 Common Abbreviations)
9. A (pages 180–185; Table 5-12 Common Abbreviations)
10. C (pages 176–178; Table 5-9 Common Word Roots and Combining Forms, page 180; Common Suffixes in Medical Terminology)

True/False

1. T (pages 165–166; Prefixes)
2. F (page 171; Proximal and Distal)
3. T (pages 180–185; Table 5-12 Common Abbreviations)
4. T (page 167; Table 5-3 Common Suffixes in Medical Terminology)
5. F (page 165; Word Roots)
6. T (pages 165–167; Anatomy of a Medical Term)
7. F (page 168; Plural Endings)
8. F (page 171; Proximal and Distal)
9. T (pages 180–185; Table 5-12 Common Abbreviations)
10. F (page 180; Table 5-11 Common Suffixes)

Fill-in-the-Blank

1. Superficial (page 171; Superficial and Deep)
2. superior (page 170; Superior and Inferior)
3. plantar (page 172; Palmar and Plantar)
4. quadrants (pages 172–173; Other Directional Terms)
5. Adduction (page 172; Movement Terms)
6. medial (page 171; Lateral and Medial)
7. Fowler position (pages 173–174; Fowler Position)
8. suffix (page 166; Breaking Terms Apart)
9. prone (page 173; Prone and Supine)
10. Abbreviations (page 174; Abbreviations and Symbols)

Labeling

1. Directional Terms (page 171; Figure 5-1)

   A. Distal

   B. Proximal

   C. Anterior (front)

   D. Posterior (rear)

   E. Patient's right

   F. Midline

   G. Medial

   H. Lateral

   I. Patient's left

   J. Superior (nearer the head)

   K. Inferior (nearer the feet)

2. Movement Terms (page 172; Common Direction, Movement, and Position Terms)

   A. Flexion

   B. Extension

   C. Abduction

   D. Adduction

Critical Thinking

Multiple Choice

1. C   (page 174; Breaking Terms Apart)
2. B   (page 170; Table 5-6 Prefixes That Describe Position)
3. D   (pages 176–178; Table 5-9 Common Word Roots and Combining Forms, page 180; Table 5-11 Common Suffixes)
4. C   (pages 180–185; Table 5-12 Common Abbreviations)

Short Answer

1. • Flexion: bending of a joint

   • Extension: straightening of a joint

   • Adduction: motion toward the midline

   • Abduction: motion away from the midline (page 172; Movement Terms)

2. 1. Singular words that end in "a" change to "ae" when plural.

   2. Singular words that end in "is" change to "es" when plural.

   3. Singular words that end in "ex" or "ix" change to "ices."

   4. Singular words that end in "on" or "um" change to "a."

   5. Singular words that end in "us" change to "i." (page 168; Plural Endings)

3.
1. Word root
2. Prefix
3. Suffix
4. Combining vowels (page 165; Anatomy of a Medical Term)

4.
- Cardi/o
- Gastr/o
- Hepat/o
- Arthr/o
- Oste/o
- Pulmon/o (pages 166–167; Combining Vowels)

Fill-in-the-Patient Care Report

EMS Patient Care Report (PCR)				
Date: Today's date	Incident No.: 2016-153	Nature of Call: MCA		Location: 152 East Bramble St.
Dispatched: 1200	En Route: 1202	At Scene: 1210	Transport: 1220	At Hospital: 1223	In Service: 1235

Patient Information	
Age: 53 years Sex: Male Weight (in kg [lb]):	Allergies: None known Medications: Metformin, Lisinopril, Omeprazole Past Medical History: HTN, NIDDM, GERD, appendectomy Chief Complaint: Chest pain

Vital Signs				
Time: 1215	BP: 148/92	Pulse: 82/regular	Respirations: 16	SpO$_2$: 98% on O$_2$

EMS Treatment (circle all that apply)				
Oxygen @ 15 L/min via (circle one): NC (NRM) BVM	Assisted Ventilation	Airway Adjunct		CPR
Defibrillation	Bleeding Control	Bandaging	Splinting	Other:

Narrative
Dispatched to a residential home for a 53-year-old male with chest pain. Arrived on scene and was greeted by wife, who informed the crew the patient experienced chest pain while mowing the lawn. On entering the residence, the patient was located in the living room, sitting on the couch. He appeared in respiratory distress. He complained of chest pain and shortness of breath. Patient was awake and able to communicate with crew. He was placed on high-flow oxygen via a nonrebreathing mask while the initial assessment was performed. ALS was summoned due to patient experiencing chest pain. Vital signs were obtained, and a secondary focused exam was performed. Lungs were clear and equal bilaterally. Abdomen was nontender in all four quadrants. Pulses were equal bilaterally in all extremities. The patient was secured to the litter in a semi-Fowler position. He was transported to the unit and secured. The patient was transported to the hospital located 2 minutes from his home. ALS was canceled due to the short ETA to the hospital. On arrival at the hospital, the patient stated he was beginning to feel better. Care was transferred to the ED staff. A verbal report was given to the nursing staff. Unit restocked and back in service without incident.**End of Report**

The Human Body

General Knowledge

Matching

1. G (page 213; Capillaries)
2. E (pages 190–191; Topographic Anatomy)
3. J (pages 190–191; The Planes of the Body)
4. O (pages 192–193; Joints)
5. C (pages 206–207; Ventilation)
6. M (pages 206–207; Ventilation)
7. A (pages 224–226; The Integumentary System (Skin): Anatomy)
8. F (pages 232–233; The Urinary System: Anatomy and Physiology)
9. D (page 190; Pathophysiology)
10. B (page 192; Table 6-2 Support Structures Within the Skeletal System)
11. I (pages 192–193; Joints)
12. N (pages 203–204; Respiration)
13. K (pages 206–207; Ventilation)
14. H (pages 206–207; Ventilation)
15. L (page 209; Normal Heartbeat)
16. B (page 197; Ankle and Foot)
17. B (page 196; The Lower Extremities)
18. A (page 195; Upper Extremities)
19. B (page 196; The Lower Extremities)
20. B (page 197; Ankle and Foot)
21. A (page 195; Upper Extremities)

22. A (page 195; Upper Extremities)
23. A (pages 197–198; The Musculoskeletal System: Anatomy)
24. B (pages 197–198; The Musculoskeletal System: Anatomy)
25. A (pages 197–198; The Musculoskeletal System: Anatomy)
26. A (pages 197–198; The Musculoskeletal System: Anatomy)
27. C (pages 197–198; The Musculoskeletal System: Anatomy)
28. C (pages 208–209; The Heart)
29. A (pages 197–198; The Musculoskeletal System: Anatomy)
30. C (pages 197–198; The Musculoskeletal System: Anatomy)
31. A (pages 222–223; Spinal Cord)
32. C (pages 220–224; The Nervous System: Anatomy and Physiology)
33. E (pages 223–224; Sensory Nerves)
34. B (page 224; Motor Nerves)
35. F (pages 220–221; Brain)
36. D (pages 220–224; The Nervous System: Anatomy and Physiology)

Multiple Choice

1. C (page 239; Table 6-14 Types of Shock)
2. B (page 234; The Female Reproductive System and Organs)

3. B (pages 198–200; The Upper Airway)
4. B (pages 230–232; The Endocrine System: Anatomy and Physiology)

5. D   (pages 211–213; Arteries)

6. D   (page 229; Bile Ducts)

7. B   (pages 232–233; The Urinary System: Anatomy and Physiology)

8. C   (page 228; Pancreas)

True/False

1. F   (pages 211–213; Arteries)

2. F   (pages 192–193; Joints)

3. T   (page 195; Upper Extremities, page 197; Ankle and Foot)

4. F   (pages 215–217; Circulation)

5. F   (pages 194–195; The Thorax)

6. F   (page 207; Factors That Impair Respiration)

7. T   (page 215; The Spleen)

Fill-in-the-Blank

1. seven (page 193; The Spinal Column)

2. mandible (page 193; The Skull)

3. five (pages 200–201; The Lower Airway)

4. 12 (pages 193–194; The Spinal Column)

5. 33 (pages 193–194; The Spinal Column)

6. talus, fibula, tibia (page 196; The Lower Extremities)

7. frontal, parietal, temporal, occipital (page 193; Brain)

8. interstitial (page 217; The Function of Blood)

9. ventilation (page 203; The Respiratory System: Physiology)

10. V/Q (page 237; Ventilation/Perfusion Mismatch)

Labeling

1. The Skull (page 194; Figure 6-6)

   A. Parietal bone

   B. Frontal bone

   C. Maxilla

   D. Temporal bone

   E. Nasal bones

   F. Zygomatic bone

   G. Maxillae

   H. Foramen magnum

   I. Occipital bone

   J. Mandible

2. The Spinal Column (page 194; Figure 6-7)

   A. Cerebrum

   B. Foramen magnum

   C. Brainstem

   D. Cerebellum

   E. Cervical nerves

   F. Cervical vertebrae

   G. Thoracic nerves

   H. Thoracic vertebrae

   I. Lumbar vertebrae

   J. Lumbosacral nerves

   K. Sacral vertebrae

   L. Coccygeal vertebrae

3. The Thorax (page 195; Figure 6-8)

   A. Sternal notch

   B. Manubrium

   C. Sternum

   D. Body

   E. Xiphoid process

   F. Anterior ribs

   G. Costal arch

4. The Shoulder Girdle (page 195; Figure 6-9)

A. Sternoclavicular joint

B. Clavicle

C. Acromioclavicular (A/C) joint

D. Humerus

E. Sternum

F. Scapula

G. Glenohumeral (shoulder) joint

5. The Wrist and Hand (page 195; Figure 6-10)

A. Index

B. Long

C. Ring

D. Small

E. Phalanges

F. Thumb

G. Metacarpals

H. Carpometacarpal joint

I. Carpals

J. Radius

K. Ulna

6. The Pelvis (page 196; Figure 6-11)

A. Inferior vena cava

B. Descending aorta

C. Iliac crest

D. Ilium

E. Sacrum

F. Pubis

G. Acetabulum

H. Pubic symphysis

I. Ischial tuberosity

J. Femoral artery

K. Ischium

L. Femoral vein

7. The Lower Extremity (page 196; Figure 6-12)

A. Pelvis

B. Femoral head

C. Greater trochanter

D. Hip

E. Lesser trochanter

F. Femur

G. Thigh

H. Patella (knee cap)

I. Knee

J. Fibula

K. Leg

L. Tibia (shin bone)

M. Ankle

N. Tarsals

O. Foot

P. Metatarsals

Q. Phalanges

8. The Foot (page 197; Figure 6-13 A)

A. Achilles tendon

B. Medial malleolus

C. Talus

D. Navicular

E. Medial cuneiform

F. Phalanges

G. Metatarsal

H. Calcaneus

9. The Respiratory System (page 200; Figure 6-16)

    A. Upper airway

    B. Nasopharynx

    C. Nasal air passage

    D. Pharynx

    E. Oropharynx

    F. Mouth

    G. Epiglottis

    H. Larynx

    I. Trachea

    J. Apex of the lung

    K. Bronchioles

    L. Lower airway

    M. Carina

    N. Main bronchi

    O. Base of the lung

    P. Diaphragm

    Q. Alveoli

10. The Circulatory System (page 208; Figure 6-25)

    A. Tissue cells

    B. Systemic (body) capillaries

    C. Venule

    D. Arteriole

    E. Vein

    F. Aorta

    G. Artery

    H. Pulmonary (lung) capillaries

    I. Right atrium

    J. Heart

    K. Left atrium

    L. Right ventricle

    M. Left ventricle

11. Central and Peripheral Pulses (page 213; Figure 6-29)

    A. Superficial temporal

    B. External maxillary

    C. Carotid

    D. Brachial

    E. Ulnar

    F. Radial

    G. Femoral

    H. Posterior tibial

    I. Dorsalis pedis

12. The Brain (page 221; Figure 6-34)

    A. Cerebrum

    B. Brainstem

    C. Cerebellum

13. Anatomy of the Skin (page 224; Figure 6-36)

    A. Hair

    B. Pore

    C. Epidermis

    D. Germinal layer of epidermis

    E. Sebaceous gland

    F. Arrector pilli muscle

    G. Dermis

    H. Nerve (sensory)

    I. Sweat gland

    J. Hair follicle

    K. Blood vessel

    L. Subcutaneous fat

    M. Fascia

    N. Subcutaneous tissue

    O. Muscle

14. The Male Reproductive System (page 234; Figure 6-43)

A. Ureter

B. Urinary bladder

C. Vasa deferentia

D. Prostate gland

E. Pubic bone

F. Prostate gland

G. Urethra

H. Urethra

I. Epididymis

J. Testis

K. Penis

L. Glans penis

M. Scrotum

15. The Female Reproductive System (page 235; Figure 6-44)

A. Uterine (fallopian) tube

B. Uterus

C. Ovary

D. Cervix

E. Vagina

Critical Thinking

Multiple Choice

1. C (pages 196–197; The Lower Extremities)
2. A (pages 193–194; The Spinal Column)
3. A (pages 226–228; Organs and Vascular Structures)
4. C (page 239; Table 6-14)
5. B (pages 211–213; Arteries)

Short Answer

1. 1. Plasma: A sticky, yellow fluid that carries the blood cells and nutrients.

    2. Red blood cells: Give blood its red color and carry oxygen

    3. White blood cells: Play a role in the body's immune defense mechanism against infection

    4. Platelets: Essential in the formation of blood clots.

    5. Protein molecules: Help control the movement of water into and out of circulation, among other functions. (pages 214–215; Blood Composition)

2. 1. Cervical spine: 7 vertebrae

    2. Thoracic spine: 12 vertebrae

    3. Lumbar spine: 5 vertebrae

    4. Sacrum: 5 vertebrae

    5. Coccyx: 4 vertebrae (pages 193–194; The Spinal Column)

3. • **RUQ:** liver, gallbladder, large intestine, small intestine

    • **LUQ:** stomach, spleen, large intestine, small intestine

    • **RLQ:** large intestine, small intestine, appendix, ascending colon

    • **LLQ:** large intestine, small intestine (pages 226–228; Organs and Vascular Structures)

4. **1.** Superior and inferior vena cava

   2. Right atrium

   3. Right ventricle

   4. Pulmonary artery

   5. Lungs

   6. Pulmonary vein

   7. Left atrium

   8. Left ventricle

   9. Aorta (page 209; Circulation)

Ambulance Calls

1. Liver, gallbladder, small intestine, large intestine, pancreas, diaphragm, right lung if the pathway is up, right kidney depending on length of knife. You could also have involvement of the other four quadrants based on the direction of travel of the blade.

2. Sternum, ribs, heart, aorta, pulmonary arteries, superior vena cava, inferior vena cava, lungs, pleura, esophagus, diaphragm

3. Humerus, ribs, scapula, clavicle, acromioclavicular joint, glenohumeral joint, sternoclavicular joint

Fill-in-the-Patient Care Report

EMS Patient Care Report (PCR)			
Date: Today's date	**Incident No.:** 2011-0000	**Nature of Call:** Assault	**Location:** Alpha St. and 15th Ave.
Dispatched: 2312	**En Route:** 2312	**At Scene:** 2329	**Transport:** 2341 **At Hospital:** 2354 **In Service:** 0009

Patient Information	
Age: 38 years **Sex:** Female **Weight (in kg [lb]):** 52 kg (115 lb)	**Allergies:** Unknown **Medications:** Unknown **Past Medical History:** Unknown **Chief Complaint:** Generalized pain

Vital Signs				
Time: 2343	**BP:** 108/56	**Pulse:** 96	**Respirations:** 16 GTV/labored	**SpO$_2$:** 96%
Time: 2349	**BP:** 104/54	**Pulse:** 104	**Respirations:** 18 adequate tidal volume/labored	**SpO$_2$:** 95%

EMS Treatment
(circle all that apply)

Oxygen @ _15_ L/min via (circle one): NC (NRM) BVM		Assisted Ventilation	Airway Adjunct	CPR
Defibrillation	Bleeding Control	Bandaging	(Splinting)	(Other: Shock Treatment)

Narrative

Dispatched to 9-1-1 scene for assault victim. Arrived to find 38-year-old woman lying on the sidewalk, guarding her torso and moaning. Police officer on scene advised that the patient was assaulted by several people. Confirmed airway, breathing, and adequate circulation. Properly secured patient to long backboard after initiating oxygen therapy via a nonrebreathing mask. Once en route to the trauma center, baseline vitals were obtained, indicating possible onset of hypoperfusion. Patient found to have contusions to both upper extremities, left lateral chest, anterior of both lower extremities, as well as abdominal rigidity and guarding. Subsequent vitals indicated continuing trend of possible hypoperfusion. Treated patient for shock and contacted receiving facility to give verbal report. Arrived at the trauma center and properly transferred patient to their care, providing a full verbal report to attending physician.**End of Report**

CHAPTER

7 Life Span Development

General Knowledge

Matching

1. L (page 258; Toddlers (1 to 3 Years) and Preschoolers (3 to 6 Years))
2. J (page 254; Neonates (Birth to 1 Month) and Infants (1 Month to 1 Year) Psychosocial Changes)
3. A (page 266; Renal System)
4. E (pages 258–260; Toddlers (1 to 3 Years) and Preschoolers (3 to 6 Years))
5. B (page 255; Cardiovascular System)
6. N (pages 260–261; School-Age Children (6 to 12 Years))
7. K (pages 260–261; School-Age Children (6 to 12 Years) Psychosocial Changes)
8. C (page 263; Early Adults (19 to 40 Years))
9. H (pages 256–257; Neonates (Birth to 1 Month) and Infants (1 Month to 1 Year) Nervous System)
10. I (pages 260–261; School-Age Children (6 to 12 Years) Psychosocial Changes)
11. M (pages 256–257; Neonates (Birth to 1 Month) and Infants (1 Month to 1 Year) Nervous System)
12. D (pages 256–257; Neonates (Birth to 1 Month) and Infants (1 Month to 1 Year) Nervous System)
13. F (pages 257–258; Neonates (Birth to 1 Month) and Infants (1 Month to 1 Year) Psychosocial Changes)
14. G (pages 263–264; Middle Adults (41 to 60 Years))

Multiple Choice

1. B (page 266; Older Adults (61 Years and Older) Renal System)
2. C (pages 261–262; Adolescents (12 to 18 Years))
3. A (pages 260–261; School-Age Children (6 to 12 Years) Psychosocial Changes)
4. D (pages 266–267; Older Adults (61 Years and Older) Nervous System)
5. D (page 261; Adolescents (12 to 18 Years) Physical Changes)
6. C (pages 254–258; Neonates (Birth to 1 Month) and Infants (1 Month to 1 Year))
7. B (pages 264–267; Older Adults (61 Years and Older) Physical Changes)
8. B (pages 256–257; Neonates (Birth to 1 Month) and Infants (1 Month to 1 Year) Nervous System)
9. C (pages 265–266; Older Adults (61 Years and Older) Respiratory System)
10. B (pages 257–258; Neonates (Birth to 1 Month) and Infants (1 Month to 1 Year) Psychosocial Changes)
11. C (pages 264–265; Older Adults (61 Years and Older) Cardiovascular System)
12. A (pages 258–260; Toddlers (1 to 3 Years) and Preschoolers (3 to 6 Years))
13. A (page 264; Middle Adults (41 to 60 Years) Psychosocial Changes)
14. B (pages 256–257; Neonates (Birth to 1 Month) and Infants (1 Month to 1 Year) Nervous System)

True/False

1. F (pages 267–268; Older Adults (61 Years and Older) Psychosocial Changes)
2. F (pages 254–258; Neonates (Birth to 1 Month) and Infants (1 Month to 1 Year))
3. T (page 254; Table 7-1 Vital Signs at Various Ages)
4. T (page 266; Older Adults (61 Years and Older) Endocrine System)
5. T (page 267; Older Adults (61 Years and Older) Sensory Changes)
6. F (page 262; Adolescents (12 to 18 Years) Psychosocial Changes)
7. F (page 260; Toddlers (1 to 3 Years) and Preschoolers (3 to 6 Years) Psychosocial Changes)
8. T (pages 257–258; Neonates (Birth to 1 Month) and Infants (1 Month to 1 Year) Immune System)
9. T (page 257; Noticeable Characteristics at Various Ages)
10. F (page 262; Adolescents (12 to 18 Years) Psychosocial Changes)

Fill-in-the-Blank

1. Early, 40 (page 263; Early Adults (19 to 40 Years))
2. 90, 150; 20, 30 (page 254; Table 7-1 Vital Signs at Various Ages)
3. cancer (pages 263–264; Middle Adults (41 to 60 Years) Physical Changes)
4. hearing, vision (page 267; Older Adults (61 Years and Older) Sensory Changes)
5. identity (page 262; Adolescents (12 to 18 Years) Psychosocial Changes)
6. neonate, 8, 25 (page 254; Neonates (Birth to 1 Month) and Infants (1 Month to 1 Year) Physical Changes)
7. fragile, barotrauma (pages 255–256; Neonates (Birth to 1 Month) and Infants (1 Month to 1 Year) Pulmonary System)
8. 18, effect (pages 259–260; Toddlers (1 to 3 Years) and Preschoolers (3 to 6 Years) Psychosocial Changes)
9. nutritional, older (page 266; Older Adults (61 Years and Older) Digestive System)
10. mental (pages 266–267; Older Adults (61 Years and Older) Nervous System)

Critical Thinking

Multiple Choice

1. A (page 254; Table 7-1 Vital Signs at Various Ages)
2. A (pages 260–261; School-Age Children (6 to 12 Years) Psychosocial Changes)
3. B (page 254; Table 7-1 Vital Signs at Various Ages)

Short Answer

1. As people age, the size of the airway increases, and the surface area of the alveoli decreases. The natural elasticity of the lungs also decreases, forcing individuals to increasingly use the muscles between their ribs, called intercostal muscles, to breathe. As the elasticity of the lungs decreases, the overall strength of the intercostal muscles and diaphragm also decreases. (pages 265–266; Older Adults (61 Years and Older) Respiratory System)

2. Conventional reasoning means that children are looking for approval from their peers and society. (pages 260–261; School-Age Children (6 to 12 Years) Psychosocial Changes)

3. "Trust versus mistrust" refers to a stage of development from birth to about 18 months of age that involves an infant's needs being met by his or her parents or caregivers. When the parents or caregivers provide an organized, routine environment, the infant gains trust in those individuals. If the environment is not perceived as secure by the infant, a sense of mistrust will develop. (pages 257–258; Neonates (Birth to 1 Month) and Infants (1 Month to 1 Year) Psychosocial Changes)

4. Atherosclerosis most commonly affects coronary vessels. Cholesterol and calcium build up inside the walls of blood vessels, forming plaque. The accumulation of plaque eventually leads to a partial or complete blockage of blood flow. More than 60% of people older than 65 years have atherosclerotic disease. This can lead to decreased blood supply to the organs of the body. (pages 264–265; Older Adults (61 Years and Older) Cardiovascular System)

5. • Neonate (0 to 1 month)

   • Infant (1 month to 1 year)

   • Toddler (1 to 3 years)

   • Preschool age (3 to 6 years)

   • School age (6 to 12 years)

   • Adolescent (12 to 18 years)

   • Early adult (19 to 40 years)

   • Middle adult (41 to 60 years)

   • Late adult (61 and older) (various pages; Section Headings)

Ambulance Calls

1. You should be concerned about intracranial bleeding with this patient because he is at an age where brain shrinkage has likely occurred, and the hematoma suggests that he hit his head after falling, which could have ruptured some of the bridging blood vessels.

2. The first thing that must be remembered is that our daily experiences as EMTs can "color" our responses. This means that you can begin to see similarities between calls where none actually exist. It is very important to treat each call as a new and different situation and not to make assumptions without very clear reasons. In this particular situation, you should not try to speak to the child alone. Children between the ages of 10 and 18 months are at the pinnacle of the separation anxiety stage, and removing the child from the parents will likely cause her to become noncommunicative and very upset. In this situation, you should keep the child with her parents, and if you truly suspect some type of abuse, you should report it afterward based on your local guidelines.

3. The best way to help this patient is to separate him from the other students before asking him about his injuries. Adolescents are very focused on their public image and are easily embarrassed. Falling off the stage in front of his peers would have embarrassed this teen enough, and publicly admitting to a subsequent injury would make it even worse for him.

Fill-in-the-Patient Care Report

EMS Patient Care Report (PCR)			
Date: Today's date	**Incident No.:** 2011-9999	**Nature of Call:** Respiratory distress	**Location:** 16654 Geary St.

Dispatched: 0345	**En Route:** 0348	**At Scene:** 0359	**Transport:** 0410	**At Hospital:** 0417	**In Service:** 0435

Patient Information					

Age: 93 years **Sex:** Female **Weight (in kg [lb]):** 44 kg (97 lb)			**Allergies:** Penicillin **Medications:** Blood pressure **Past Medical History:** Three MIs **Chief Complaint:** Respiratory distress		

Vital Signs				
Time: 0409	**BP:** N/A	**Pulse:** 110	**Respirations:** N/A	**SpO$_2$:** 95%

EMS Treatment
(circle all that apply)

Oxygen @ _15_ L/min via (circle one): NC NRM (BVM)		(Assisted Ventilation)	Airway Adjunct	CPR
Defibrillation	Bleeding Control	Bandaging	Splinting	Other:

Narrative

Dispatched on a 9-1-1 call for a respiratory distress patient. Arrived to find the patient, a 93-year-old woman, in the tripod position and clearly struggling to breathe. Just as patient contact was made, patient went into respiratory arrest, and bag-mask ventilations were immediately initiated. Patient was moved to the gurney and loaded into the ambulance for transport. Because of ongoing interventions, no BP was taken, the pulse was 110 irregular, and there was a consistent SpO$_2$ reading of 95% while en route to the receiving facility. No ALS units were available per dispatch. Patient report to the receiving facility was relayed through the dispatch center, and ventilations were continued during entire transport. At the receiving facility, patient care was properly transferred to the facility staff, and a full verbal report was provided.**End of Report**

CHAPTER

8 Lifting and Moving Patients

General Knowledge

Matching

1. C (page 302; Extremity Lift)
2. J (pages 310–311; Flexible Stretchers)
3. H (pages 287–288; Moving a Patient With a Stair Chair)
4. E (pages 311–312; Basket Stretchers)
5. A (pages 305–306; Using a Scoop Stretcher)
6. I (pages 306–307; Backboards)
7. F (pages 300–301; Direct Ground Lift)
8. B (page 310; Portable/Folding Stretchers)
9. D (pages 290–291; The Wheeled Ambulance Stretcher)
10. G (page 307; Bariatrics)

Multiple Choice

1. D (pages 277–280; Body Mechanics)
2. C (page 295; Urgent Moves)
3. C (page 277; Anatomy Review)
4. C (page 277; Anatomy Review)
5. B (page 277; Anatomy Review)
6. A (page 277; Anatomy Review)
7. B (pages 287–288; Moving a Patient With a Stair Chair)
8. A (pages 284–287; Lifting and Carrying a Patient on a Backboard or Stretcher)
9. D (page 276; Backboards)
10. D (pages 291–293; Directions and Commands)
11. D (page 309; Bariatric Stretchers)
12. B (pages 287–288; Moving a Patient With a Stair Chair)
13. A (pages 280–282; Principles of Safe Reaching and Pulling)
14. A (pages 280–282; Principles of Safe Reaching and Pulling)
15. D (pages 280–282; Principles of Safe Reaching and Pulling)
16. B (pages 284–287; Lifting and Carrying a Patient on a Backboard or Stretcher)
17. A (pages 294–295; Emergency Moves)
18. B (pages 294–295; Emergency Moves)
19. C (pages 294–295; Emergency Moves)
20. B (page 277; Anatomy Review)
21. A (pages 295–300; Urgent Moves)
22. C (pages 306–307; Other Carries)
23. A (pages 311–312; Basket Stretchers)
24. B (page 307; Geriatrics)
25. B (page 307; Bariatrics)
26. D (page 276; Backboards)
27. B (pages 294–295; Emergency Moves)
28. A (pages 284–287; Lifting and Carrying a Patient on a Backboard or Stretcher)
29. D (pages 304–305; Draw Sheet Method)

True/False

1. T (page 310; Portable/Folding Stretchers)
2. T (page 277; Anatomy Review)
3. F (pages 282–284; Patient Weight)
4. F (pages 282–284; Principles of Safe Lifting and Carrying)
5. T (pages 294–295; Emergency Moves)
6. F (pages 284–287; Lifting and Carrying a Patient on a Backboard or Stretcher)
7. F (pages 295–300; Rapid Extrication Technique)
8. F (pages 291–293; Directions and Commands)

9. T   (page 307; Bariatrics)
10. T   (page 312; Neonatal Isolettes)
11. T   (pages 310–311; Flexible Stretchers)

12. T   (page 309; Pneumatic and Electronic Powered Wheeled Stretchers)
13. F   (page 307; Bariatrics)

Fill-in-the-Blank

1. body mechanics (page 277; Anatomy Review)
2. upright (page 278; Anatomy Review)
3. power lift (pages 279–280; Anatomy Review)
4. palm (pages 279–280; Anatomy Review)
5. locked-in (page 283; Table 8-1 Guidelines for Carrying a Patient on a Stretcher)
6. sideways (pages 280–282; Principles of Safe Reaching and Pulling)
7. locked (pages 284–287; Lifting and Carrying a Patient on a Backboard or Stretcher)
8. diamond (pages 284–287; Lifting and Carrying a Patient on a Backboard or Stretcher)

9. movement (pages 290–291; Loading a Wheeled Stretcher Into an Ambulance)
10. spine movement (pages 295–300; Rapid Extrication Technique)
11. direct ground lift (pages 300–301; Direct Ground Lift)
12. extremity lift (page 302; Extremity Lift)
13. fluid resistant (pages 290–291; The Wheeled Ambulance Stretcher)
14. decontaminate (page 312; Decontamination)

Critical Thinking

Short Answer

1. **1.** **Emergency clothes drag**

  2. Blanket drag

  3. Arm drag

  4. Arm-to-arm drag

  5. Firefighter's drag

  6. Front cradle

  7. One-person walking assist

  8. Firefighter's carry

  9. Pack strap (page 294; Figure 8-14, page 296; Figure 8-16)

2. **1.** The vehicle or scene is unsafe.

  2. Explosives or other hazardous materials are on the scene.

  3. There is a fire or a danger of fire.

  4. The patient cannot be properly assessed before being removed from the vehicle.

  5. The patient has a life-threatening condition that requires immediate transport to the hospital.

  6. The patient blocks the EMT's access to another seriously injured patient. (page 296; Table 8-3 Situations in Which to Use the Rapid Extrication Technique)

3. **1.** Make sure there are enough providers for sufficient lifting power.

  2. Follow the manufacturer's directions for safe and proper use of the stretcher.

  3. Make sure that all stretchers and patients are fully secured before you move the ambulance. (page 291; Table 8-2 Guidelines for Loading the Stretcher Into the Ambulance)

4. 1. Estimate the weight of both the patient and the associated equipment to be lifted and gauge the limitations of the team's abilities.

2. Coordinate your movements with those of the other team members while constantly communicating with them.

3. Do not twist your body as you are carrying the patient.

4. Keep the weight that you are carrying as close to your body as possible while keeping your back in a locked-in position.

5. Do not bend at the waist; this could hyperextend your back. Instead, flex at the hips and bend at the knees. (page 283; Table 8-1 Guidelines for Carrying a Patient on a Stretcher)

5. Always keep your back in a straight, upright position and lift without twisting. (page 277; Anatomy Review)

Ambulance Calls

1. Immobilize the patient on a long backboard, apply high-flow oxygen, and consider the use of a basket stretcher. Use a minimum of four people to carry the patient back up the ledge. Plan the route, and brief your helpers before moving the patient. Clarify whether you will move on "three" or count to three, then move. Coordinate the move until the patient is loaded into the ambulance.

2. **One of the most critical steps in caring for this patient is realizing that it will require additional help and calling for that help as early as possible.** It is highly unlikely that you will be able to move this patient, especially without significantly hurting yourself or your partner. You can attempt to move the patient, but if you cannot successfully do so, you will have to open his airway, in his current position. Do the best you can until additional personnel arrive and the patient can be moved.

3. Patients whose conditions will be exacerbated by physical activity should not walk to the stretcher or ambulance. If a patient's condition is such that it is not medically necessary that you carry him or her, it is safer for the patient to walk on his or her own power to the ambulance. However, this patient should not/cannot walk. This produces a safety issue for you and your partner, especially given the fact that there is no elevator. Fortunately, this patient can sit upright; thus, the use of a stair chair would be appropriate in this situation. Regardless, you should ask for more personnel, given the patient's large size. Back injuries are very common in EMS. For providers to avoid these injuries, correct lifting techniques should be used, and assistance should be requested whenever the patient is large or in a position not conducive to correct lifting procedures.

Skills

Skill Drills

Skill Drill 8-1: Performing the Power Lift

1. Lock your back in a **slight** curve. **Spread** and bend your legs. Grasp the backboard, palms up and just in front of you. **Balance** and **center** the weight between your arms.

2. Position your feet, **straddle** the object, and **distribute** your weight evenly. Lift by **straightening** your legs, keeping your back locked in. (pages 279–280; Skill Drill 8-1 Performing the Power Lift)

Skill Drill 8-2: Performing the Diamond Carry

1. Position yourselves facing the patient.

2. The providers at each side turn the head-end hand palm down and release the other hand.

3. The providers at each side turn toward the foot end. The provider at the foot end turns to face forward. (page 285; Skill Drill 8-2 Performing the Diamond Carry)

Skill Drill 8-3: Performing the One-Handed Carry

1. **Face** each other and use both **hands**.

2. Lift the backboard to **carrying height**.

3. **Turn** in the direction you will walk, and **switch** to using one hand. (page 286; Skill Drill 8-3 Performing the One-Handed Carry)

Skill Drill 8-7: Performing the Rapid Extrication Technique

1. The first provider provides in-line manual support of the head and cervical spine.

2. The second provider gives commands, applies a cervical collar, and performs the primary assessment.

3. The second provider supports the torso. The third provider frees the patient's legs from the pedals and moves the legs together, without moving the pelvis or spine.

4. The second provider and the third provider rotate the patient as a unit in several short, coordinated moves. The first provider (relieved by the fourth provider as needed) supports the patient's head and neck during rotation (and later steps).

5. The first (or fourth) provider places the backboard on the seat against the patient's buttocks. (Use of a backboard may depend on local protocols.)

6. The third provider moves to an effective position for sliding the patient. The second and third providers slide the patient along the backboard in coordinated, 8- to 12-inch (20- to 30-cm) moves until the patient's hips rest on the backboard.

7. The third provider exits the vehicle, moves to the backboard opposite the second provider, and they continue to slide the patient until the patient is fully on the board.

8. The first (or fourth) provider continues to stabilize the head and neck while the second provider and the third provider carry the patient away from the vehicle and onto the prepared stretcher. (pages 297–298; Skill Drill 8-7 Performing the Rapid Extrication Technique)

Skill Drill 8-9: Extremity Lift

1. The patient's hands are **crossed** over the chest. Grasp the patient's wrists or **forearms** and pull the patient to a **sitting** position.

2. Your partner moves to a position between the patient's **legs**, facing in the **same** direction as the patient, and places his or her hands under the **knees**.

3. Rise to a **crouching** position. On **command**, lift and begin to move. (page 303; Skill Drill 8-9 Performing the Extremity Lift)

Skill Drill 8-10: Direct Carry

1. Position the stretcher **parallel** to the bed. Secure the **stretcher** to prevent movement. Face the patient while standing between the **bed** and the **stretcher**. Position your arms under the patient's **neck** and **shoulders**. Your partner should position his or her hands under the patient's **knees**.

2. Lift the patient from the bed in a smooth, **coordinated** fashion.

3. Slowly carry the patient to the **stretcher**.

4. **Gently** lower the patient onto the stretcher and secure with **straps**. (page 304; Performing the Direct Carry)

CHAPTER

9 The Team Approach to Health Care

General Knowledge

Matching

1. D (page 323; Dependent, Independent, and Interdependent Groups)
2. A (page 323; Dependent, Independent, and Interdependent Groups)
3. B (page 325; Supportive and Coordinated Leadership)
4. C (page 325; Supportive and Coordinated Leadership)
5. F (pages 321–323; Types of Teams)
6. E (pages 322–323; Groups)

Multiple Choice

1. B (pages 322–323; Groups)
2. C (pages 325–326; Crew Resource Management)
3. A (pages 322–323; Groups)
4. D (page 331; Troubleshooting Team Conflicts)
5. C (page 321; An Era of Team Health Care)
6. C (page 321; Community Paramedicine and Mobile Integrated Healthcare Teams)
7. D (page 323; Clear Roles and Responsibilities)
8. D (page 323; Diverse and Competent Skill Sets)
9. D (page 328; Where BLS Care Ends and ALS Care Begins)
10. C (page 323; Dependent)
11. D (pages 326–328; Transfer of Patient Care)
12. B (pages 325–326; Crew Resource Management)
13. D (pages 328–329; Assisting With ALS Skills)
14. C (page 322; Special Teams)

True/False

1. F (pages 321–322; Regular Teams)
2. F (page 322; Temporary Teams)
3. T (page 323; Diverse and Competent Skill Sets)
4. T (page 328; Where BLS Care Ends and ALS Care Begins)
5. F (page 331; Troubleshooting Team Conflicts)
6. T (page 328; BLS and ALS Providers Working Together)
7. T (pages 320–321; Introduction)

Fill-in-the-Blank

1. group (pages 322–323; Groups)
2. train, work (pages 321–322; Regular Teams)
3. Crew resource management (pages 325–326; Crew Resource Management)
4. interdependent group (page 323; Interdependent)
5. team leader (page 325; Supportive and Coordinated Leadership)
6. Community paramedicine (page 321; Community Paramedicine and Mobile Integrated Healthcare Teams)

Critical Thinking

Short Answer

1. 1. The patient comes first.
   2. Do not engage.
   3. Keep your cool.
   4. Separate the person from the issue.
   5. Choose your battles. (page 331; Troubleshooting Team Conflicts)

2. 1. A common goal
   2. An image of themselves as "a group"
   3. A sense of continuity of the group
   4. A set of shared values
   5. Different roles within the group (pages 322–323; Groups)

Ambulance Calls

1. Do not be afraid to inform the paramedic that the leads have not been appropriately attached. You can save valuable time by simply relaying what you have seen. Sometimes, EMTs can feel intimidated by the presence of paramedics and become afraid to speak out when they see something that doesn't appear right. Do not underestimate your ability to help because sometimes you may notice things that the paramedic does not. Everyone has the same goal of patient care, and it is pertinent to point out those things that may interfere with this goal.

2. If successful intubation has occurred, you will hear equal, bilateral breath sounds and no sounds over the epigastrium. This endotracheal tube should be removed, and the patient should be ventilated with high-flow oxygen via a bag-mask device and the placement of an oral airway. Secondary placement devices should be utilized when assessing placement of the ET tube. Direct visualization of the ET tube passing through the cords along with the use of a waveform end-tidal capnography device to ensure that successful placement has been accomplished. If endotracheal intubation is not possible, consider the use of supraglottic airways such as the i-gel airway device, King LT airway, or laryngeal mask airway. Always follow local protocols.

3. You should immediately suggest slowing the IV to a TKO rate, raise the patient's head, and apply high-flow oxygen (or increase the current L/min). You may also suggest considering the use of CPAP if the patient is alert enough to follow orders. Notify the receiving facility of the error. Healthy adults can handle the sudden influx of intravenous fluids without detrimental effects, but individuals who have diseased or otherwise weakened hearts, lungs, or kidneys do not possess the ability to cope with the fluid overload. To avoid this occurrence, check and double-check the drip chamber/flow rate to prevent accidental fluid boluses. Continuously monitor the patient.

CHAPTER

10 Patient Assessment

General Knowledge

Matching

1. P (pages 348–349; Determine Number of Patients)
2. Q (page 359; Skin Color)
3. M (page 398; Head, Neck, and Cervical Spine)
4. T (page 357; Pulse Rate)
5. B (page 359; Skin Color)
6. S (page 342; Introduction)
7. L (pages 355–357; Assess Breathing)
8. A (pages 385–387; Breath Sounds)
9. O (pages 345–346; Determine Mechanism of Injury/Nature of Illness)
10. R (pages 410–413; Vital Vocabulary)
11. G (page 359; Skin Color)
12. E (pages 352–353; Assess Level of Consciousness)
13. F (pages 368–369; OPQRST)
14. I (pages 357–358; Assess Pulse)
15. K (pages 410–413; Vital Vocabulary)
16. C (pages 355–357; Assess Breathing)

17. D (page 359; Skin Color)
18. J (pages 410–413; Vital Vocabulary)
19. H (pages 410–413; Vital Vocabulary)
20. N (pages 398–399; Chest)
21. I (pages 368–369; OPQRST)
22. L (pages 368–369; OPQRST)
23. C (pages 368–369; OPQRST)
24. E (page 370; Obtain SAMPLE History)
25. H (page 370; Obtain SAMPLE History)
26. K (pages 368–369; OPQRST)
27. F (page 370; Obtain SAMPLE History)
28. B (page 370; Obtain SAMPLE History)
29. J (pages 368–369; OPQRST)
30. G (pages 368–369; OPQRST)
31. A (page 370; Obtain SAMPLE History)
32. D (page 370; Obtain SAMPLE History)

Multiple Choice

1. C (page 341 Patient Assessment Flow Chart, section on Scene Size-up)
2. A (pages 371–372; Sexual History)
3. B (pages 345–346; Determine Mechanism of Injury/Nature of Illness)
4. D (page 360; Capillary Refill)
5. B (page 385; Depth of Breathing)
6. A (pages 377–378; Secondary Assessment)
7. C (page 351; Form a General Impression)
8. B (pages 350–351; Primary Assessment)
9. C (pages 363–365; Determine Priority of Patient Care and Transport)
10. B (pages 352–353; Assess Level of Consciousness)
11. B (page 384; Respiratory Rate)
12. D (pages 357–358; Assess Pulse)
13. A (page 359; Skin Color)

14. C (pages 357–358; Assess Pulse)
15. D (page 387; Pulse Rate)
16. D (page 359; Skin Color)
17. C (pages 345–346; Determine Mechanism of Injury/Nature of Illness)
18. C (page 352; Assess and Control External Bleeding)
19. A (pages 345–346; Determine Mechanism of Injury/Nature of Illness)
20. C (pages 352–353; Assess Level of Consciousness)
21. B (pages 361–363; Performing a Rapid Exam to Identify Life Threats)
22. C (pages 394–396; Pupils)
23. D (pages 355–357; Assess Breathing)
24. A (page 354; Assess the Airway)
25. B (pages 385–387; Breath Sounds)
26. C (page 371; Physical Abuse or Violence)

27. B   (page 375; Language Barriers)
28. C   (pages 401–402; Pulse Oximetry)
29. D   (pages 388–392; Blood Pressure)
30. A   (pages 388–392; Blood Pressure)
31. B   (page 399; Abdomen)
32. B   (page 398; Head, Neck, and Cervical Spine)
33. A   (pages 363–365; Determine Priority of Patient Care and Transport)
34. B   (pages 355–357; Assess Breathing)

35. A   (pages 357–358; Assess Pulse)
36. B   (page 359; Skin Color)
37. C   (pages 388–392; Blood Pressure)
38. B   (page 405; Reassessment)
39. A   (page 342; Introduction)
40. D   (pages 359–360; Skin Temperature)
41. A   (page 376; Visual Impairments)
42. C   (page 375; Language Barriers)

True/False

1. F   (pages 352–353; Assess Level of Consciousness)
2. F   (page 406; Reassess Patient)
3. T   (pages 400–401; Extremities)
4. F   (pages 357–358; Assess Pulse)
5. T   (page 351; Form a General Impression)
6. T   (page 398; Head, Neck, and Cervical Spine)
7. F   (pages 398–399; Chest)
8. F   (page 399; Abdomen)
9. T   (page 406; Recheck Interventions)
10. T   (pages 344–345; Ensure Scene Safety)
11. F   (pages 352–353; Assess Level of Consciousness)
12. T   (pages 394–396; Pupils)
13. F   (pages 394–396; Pupils)
14. F   (pages 355–357; Assess Breathing)
15. T   (pages 383–384; Respiratory System)
16. T   (pages 363–365; Determine Priority of Patient Care and Transport)

17. T   (pages 363–365; Determine Priority of Patient Care and Transport)
18. T   (pages 367–368; Investigate the Chief Complaint (History of Present Illness))
19. F   (page 374; Alcohol and Drugs)
20. T   (page 371; Physical Abuse or Violence)
21. T   (page 371; Sexual History)
22. F   (page 372; Overly Talkative)
23. T   (pages 372–373; Anxiety)
24. F   (pages 373–374; Anger and Hostility)
25. T   (page 374; Alcohol and Drugs)
26. T   (page 374; Crying)
27. F   (page 374; Depression)
28. T   (pages 361–363; Performing a Rapid Exam to Identify Life Threats)
29. T   (pages 400–401; Extremities)

Fill-in-the-Blank

1. sign (page 342; Introduction)
2. Standard precautions (pages 347–348; Take Standard Precautions)
3. incident command system (page 348; Determine Number of Patients)
4. Advanced life support (page 349; Consider Additional/Specialized Resources)
5. primary assessment (pages 350–351; Primary Assessment)
6. general impression (page 351; Form a General Impression)
7. Perfusion (page 412; Vital Vocabulary)
8. Orientation (pages 352–353; Assess Level of Consciousness)
9. constrict (pages 294–296; Pupils)
10. stridor (pages 383–384; Respiratory System)
11. jaw-thrust maneuver (page 355; Unresponsive Patients)
12. exhalation (pages 383–384; Respiratory System)

13. airway (page 354; Assess the Airway)
14. suction (page 355; Unresponsive Patients)
15. respiratory infection (page 356; Quality of Breathing)
16. Nasal flaring (page 356; Assess Breathing)
17. CPR (page 358; Assess Pulse)
18. Tachycardia (page 388; Pulse Rate)
19. conjunctiva (page 359; Skin Color)
20. hypoperfusion (pages 359–360; Skin Temperature)
21. diaphoretic (page 360; Skin Moisture)
22. 2 (page 360; Capillary Refill)
23. coagulate (page 361; Assess and Control External Bleeding)
24. 90 (page 361; Performing a Rapid Exam to Identify Life Threats)
25. Golden Hour (pages 363–365; Determine Priority of Patient Care and Transport)
26. life threats (pages 350–351; Primary Assessment)
27. History taking (pages 366–367; History Taking)

28. open-ended (page 367; Investigate the Chief Complaint (History of Present Illness))

29. SAMPLE (page 369; Obtain SAMPLE History)

30. Pertinent negatives (page 369; Identify Pertinent Negatives)

31. Blood glucose (pages 402–404; Blood Glucometry)

32. Palpation (page 391; Secondary Assessment)

33. Capnography (page 402; Capnography)

34. Diastolic pressure (page 386; Blood Pressure)

35. neurologic (page 394; Neurologic System)

Critical Thinking

Short Answer

1. To identify and initiate treatment of immediate or potential life threats (pages 350–351; Primary Assessment)

2. Age, sex, race, level of distress, and overall appearance (page 351; Form a General Impression)

3. A—Airway; B—Breathing; C—Circulation (pages 361–363; Identify and Treat Life Threats)

4. Orientation to person, place, time, and event. Person (name) evaluates long-term memory. Place and time evaluate intermediate-term memory. Event evaluates short-term memory. (pages 352–353; Assess Level of Consciousness)

5. 1. Is the patient breathing?

  2. Is the patient breathing adequately?

  3. Is the patient hypoxic? (pages 355–357; Assess Breathing)

6. D—Deformities

  C—Contusions

  A—Abrasions

  P—Punctures/penetrations

  B—Burns

  T—Tenderness

  L—Lacerations

  S—Swelling (page 362; Table 10-3 The DCAP-BTLS Mnemonic)

7. 1. Does the scene pose a threat to you, your patient, or others?

  2. How many patients are there?

  3. Do we have the resources to respond to their conditions? (page 349; Consider Additional/Specialized Resources)

8. Pupils equal and round, regular in size, react to light (page 394; Pupils)

9. A sign is a condition that can be seen, heard, felt, smelled, or measured (objective). A symptom is something that the patient reports to you as a problem or feeling (subjective). (page 342; Introduction)

10. 1. Is there pain associated with urination?

  2. Do you have any discharge, sores, or an increase in urination?

  3. Do you have burning or difficulty voiding?

  4. Has there been any trauma?

  5. Have you had recent sexual encounters? (page 371; Sexual History)

Ambulance Calls

1. Maintain cervical spine control and immediately manage the airway by suction and oxygen. Conduct a rapid survey and transport the patient to the nearest appropriate facility. This patient is a priority transport based on his mechanism of injury, level of consciousness, and airway compromise. Damage to the vehicle indicates possible occult injuries.

2. This patient is having a very serious asthma attack. Accessory muscle use (nasal flaring, tracheal tugging, suprasternal and intercostal muscle retractions), work of breathing, wheezing, and one-to two-word responses all point to the seriousness of his attack. You should transport immediately.

3. The mechanism of injury is significant for this patient. Not only did he fall down a flight of wooden stairs, but he landed on a cement floor. His head injury is likely more significant than the bruising and laceration you can see. He could also have skull fractures, contusions, or intracranial bleeding. With any significant trauma to the head comes the likelihood of cervical spine fractures. You should also question the mechanism of his fall because medical conditions can sometimes precipitate injuries. Full cervical spine precautions must be taken, along with application of high-flow oxygen and prompt transport.

Skills

Skill Drills

Skill Drill 10-1: Performing a Rapid Exam to Identify Life Threats (pages 362–363)

1. Assess the head. Have your partner maintain in-line stabilization if indicated.

2. Assess the neck.

3. Assess the chest. Listen to breath sounds on both sides of the chest.

4. Assess the abdomen.

5. Assess the pelvis. If there is no pain, gently compress the pelvis downward and inward to look for tenderness and instability.

6. Assess all four extremities. Assess pulse and motor and sensory function.

7. Assess the back. If spinal immobilization is indicated, do so with minimal movement to the patient's spine by log rolling the patient in one motion.

Skill Drill 10-3: Obtaining Blood Pressure by Auscultation (page 391)

1. Follow standard precautions. Check for a dialysis fistula, central line, previous mastectomy, and injury to the arm. If any are present, use the brachial artery on the other arm. Apply the cuff snugly. The lower border of the cuff should be about 1 inch (2.5 cm) above the antecubital space.

2. Support the exposed arm at the level of the heart. Palpate the brachial artery.

3. Place the stethoscope over the brachial artery, and grasp the ball-pump and turn-valve.

4. Close the valve, and pump to 30 mm Hg above the point at which you stop hearing pulse sounds. Note the systolic and diastolic pressures as you let air escape slowly.

5. Open the valve, and quickly release remaining air. (pages 360–361; Secondary Assessment)

CHAPTER

Airway Management

General Knowledge

Matching

1. C (pages 424–425; Inhalation)
2. I (pages 425–426; Exhalation)
3. H (pages 420–423; Anatomy of the Lower Airway)
4. G (pages 420–423; Anatomy of the Lower Airway)
5. K (page 426; Regulation of Ventilation)
6. E (page 425; Table 11-2 Ventilation Terminology)
7. A (pages 420–423; Anatomy of the Lower Airway)
8. F (pages 424–425; Inhalation)
9. L (page 423; Table 11-1 Ventilation, Oxygenation, and Respiration)
10. D (page 420; Larynx)
11. J (page 426; Regulation of Ventilation)
12. B (pages 432–434; Recognizing Abnormal Breathing)

Multiple Choice

1. D (pages 427–428; External Respiration)
2. B (page 457; Words of Wisdom Oxygen-Delivery Devices)
3. B (page 432; Table 11-3 Normal Respiratory Rate Ranges)
4. B (pages 432–434; Recognizing Abnormal Breathing)
5. A (page 426; Regulation of Ventilation)
6. A (pages 446–449; Oropharyngeal Airways)
7. C (pages 446–449; Oropharyngeal Airways)
8. D (pages 464–468; Bag-Mask Device Technique)
9. C (page 468; Words of Wisdom: Indications That Artificial Ventilation is Adequate)
10. C (pages 442–446; Suctioning)
11. D (pages 463–468; The Bag-Mask Device)
12. C (page 428; Figure 11-13)
13. D (pages 439–440; Opening the Airway)
14. B (pages 432–434; Recognizing Abnormal Breathing)
15. B (pages 431–432; Assessment of Respiration)

True/False

1. F (page 449; Nasopharyngeal Airways)
2. T (page 457; Words of Wisdom: Oxygen-Delivery Devices)
3. F (pages 446–449; Oropharyngeal Airways)
4. F (page 453; Safety Considerations)
5. F (pages 453–454; Pin-Indexing System)

Fill-in-the-Blank

1. vocal cords (page 420; Anatomy of the Upper Airway)
2. higher (pages 425–426; Exhalation)
3. 21, 78 (page 427; External Respiration)
4. carbon dioxide (page 426; Regulation of Ventilation)
5. diaphragm, intercostal muscles (page 424; Physiology of Breathing)
6. positive, pressure (page 469; Continuous Positive Airway Pressure)
7. hypoxia (page 426; Regulation of Ventilation)
8. Passive ventilation (pages 467–468; Passive Ventilation)

Labeling

1. Upper and Lower Airways (page 419, Figure 11-1)

   A. Upper airway

   B. Nasopharynx

   C. Nasal air passage

   D. Pharynx

   E. Oropharynx

   F. Mouth

   G. Epiglottis

   H. Larynx

   I. Trachea

   J. Apex of the lung

   K. Bronchioles

   L. Lower airway

   M. Carina

   N. Main bronchus

   O. Pulmonary capillaries

   P. Base of the lung

   Q. Diaphragm

   R. Alveoli

2. Oral Cavity (page 420, Figure 11-3)

   A. Hard palate

   B. Soft palate

   C. Entrance to auditory tube

   D. Nasal cavity

   E. Upper lip

   F. Tongue

   G. Nasopharynx

   H. Gingiva

   I. Uvula

   J. Oropharynx

   K. Epiglottis

   L. Laryngopharynx

   M. Hyoid bone

3. Thoracic Cavity (page 423, Figure 11-8)

   A. Trachea

   B. Vena cava

   C. Aorta

   D. Bronchus

   E. Heart

   F. Lung

   G. Diaphragm

Critical Thinking

Multiple Choice

1. B   (pages 441–442; Jaw-Thrust Maneuver)
2. D   (pages 442–443; Suctioning)
3. C   (pages 446–449; Oropharyngeal Airways)

4. D   (page 467; Gastric Distention)
5. A   (page 462; Words of Wisdom: Ventilation Rates)

Short Answer

1. 1. A patient who is in respiratory arrest or with agonal respirations

   2. The patient is hypoventilating.

   3. The patient is unable to speak.

   4. The patient cannot protect his or her own airway.

5. The patient has a systolic blood pressure less than 90 mm Hg.

6. Active GI bleeding with nausea or vomiting present.

7. The patient has experienced facial trauma.

8. The patient has signs of cardiogenic shock.

9. The patient cannot sit upright.

10. The CPAP mask cannot be positioned or fitted correctly to the patient's face.

11. The patient is unable to tolerate the mask.

12. Signs and symptoms of a pneumothorax or chest trauma

13. A patient who has a tracheostomy

14. Active gastrointestinal bleeding or vomiting

15. The patient is unable to follow verbal commands. (page 470; Contraindications)

2. • Adults: 12 to 20 breaths/min

   • Children: 12 to 40 breaths/min

   • Infants: 30 to 60 breaths/min (page 462; Words of Wisdom: Ventilation Rates)

3. Give slow, gentle breaths over 1 second (enough to see the chest rise). (page 467; Gastric Distention)

4. 1. Respiratory rate of less than 12 breaths/min or greater than 20 breaths/min in the presence of shortness of breath

    2. Irregular rhythm

    3. Diminished, absent, or noisy breath sounds

    4. Reduced flow of expired air at the nose and mouth

    5. Unequal or inadequate chest expansion

    6. Increased effort of breathing

    7. Shallow depth

    8. Pale, cyanotic, or cool (clammy) skin

    9. Skin pulling in around the ribs during inspiration (pages 432–434; Recognizing Abnormal Breathing)

5. They are the secondary muscles of respiration. They are not used in normal breathing. They include the sternocleidomastoid (neck) muscles, chest pectoralis major muscles, and abdominal muscles. (pages 432–434; Recognizing Abnormal Breathing)

6. When the patient has experienced severe trauma to the head or face (page 449; Nasopharyngeal Airways)

7. 1. Select the proper-sized airway and apply a water-soluble lubricant.

    2. Place the airway in the larger nostril with the curvature following the curve of the floor of the nose.

    3. Advance the airway gently.

    4. Continue until the flange rests against the skin. (page 449; Nasopharyngeal Airways)

8. Tonsil tips are best because they have a large diameter and do not collapse. In addition, they are curved, which allows easy, rapid placement. (pages 442–446; Suctioning)

Ambulance Calls

1. Maintain cervical spine stabilization. Immediately open the airway with the jaw-thrust maneuver. Suction to remove the obstruction. Assess the airway for breathing (rate, rhythm, quality), and provide oxygen via a nonrebreathing mask or bag-mask device. Continue initial assessment, rapid extrication, and rapid transport.

2. You should reposition the head and attempt to reventilate the patient. If you are unsuccessful in your second attempt, you must take action to clear her airway. If you fail to clear her airway, she will likely go into cardiac arrest as well. Choking victims have been known to walk away from others without indicating that they are choking, and when this occurs in a restaurant setting, many of these people will go into a bathroom. If you find a patient in a restroom who cannot be ventilated, they likely have a foreign body airway obstruction (FBAO), most often as a result of ingested food.

3. The most common cause of airway obstruction in an unconscious patient is the tongue. The patient's husband told you that he helped her to the ground without injury, so it is safe to open her airway using a head tilt–chin lift maneuver. If you were unsure of the presence of trauma, this position would not be used. Instead, you would use the jaw-thrust maneuver to manage her airway. In either case, you must continually monitor her condition and be prepared for vomitus.

Fill-in-the-Patient Care Report

EMS Patient Care Report (PCR)

Date: Today's date	Incident No.: 2011-0000	Nature of Call: Possible overdose		Location: Market Street High School	
Dispatched: 1530	**En Route:** 1530	**At Scene:** 1543	**Transport:** 1556	**At Hospital:** 1608	**In Service:** 1625

Patient Information

Age: 14 years	Allergies: Unknown
Sex: Female	Medications: Unknown
Weight (in kg [lb]): 50 kg (110 lb)	Past Medical History: Unknown
	Chief Complaint: Unresponsive

Vital Signs

Time: 1545	BP: 124/86	Pulse: 112/regular	Respirations: 12 shallow/ inadequate tidal volume	SpO$_2$: 93%

EMS Treatment
(circle all that apply)

Oxygen @ _15_ L/min via (circle one): NC NRM (BVM)	(Assisted Ventilation)	(Airway Adjunct: OPA)	CPR
Defibrillation	Bleeding Control	Bandaging	Splinting	Other:

Narrative

Responded to 9-1-1 call for possible drug overdose at Market Street High School. Arrived and was directed to an unresponsive 14-year-old girl on the floor of a restroom and was advised that patient had previous "troubles" with drugs, although no physical evidence was observed in the patient's immediate surroundings. Patient presented with no response to painful stimulus; cyanosis around lips and fingernails; and shallow, snoring respirations. Patient's respirations were immediately assisted with a BVM and 100% oxygen, and she was loaded into the ambulance, where a firefighter rode along to assist. Vital signs, when compared to the baseline set, indicated that assisted ventilations and oxygen therapy were improving patient's SpO$_2$ levels. While en route, the receiving facility was updated with patient condition. On arrival, she was transferred appropriately to the care of the ED staff, and a full verbal report was provided to the charge RN.**End of Report**

Skills

Skill Drills

Skill Drill 11-2: Positioning the Unconscious Patient (page 440)

1. Support the **head** while your partner straightens the patient's legs.
2. Have your partner place his or her **hand** on the patient's far **shoulder** and hip.
3. **Roll** the patient as a unit, with the EMT at the patient's **head** calling the count to begin the move.
4. **Open** and **assess** the patient's airway and **breathing** status.

Skill Drill 11-4: Inserting an Oral Airway (page 447)

1. Size the **airway** by measuring from the patient's **earlobe** to the corner of the **mouth**.
2. Open the patient's **mouth** with the cross-finger technique. Hold the **airway** upside down with your other hand. Insert the airway with the tip facing the **roof** of the mouth.
3. **Rotate** the airway **180°**. Insert the airway until the **flange** rests on the patient's lips and teeth. In this position, the airway will hold the **tongue** forward.

Skill Drill 11-7: Placing an Oxygen Cylinder Into Service (page 445)

1. Using an oxygen **wrench**, turn the valve **counterclockwise** to slowly "crack" the cylinder.

1. Attach the regulator/flowmeter to the **valve** stem using the two pin-**indexing** holes, and make sure that the **washer** is in place over the larger hole.
2. Align the **regulator** so that the pins fit snugly into the correct holes on the **valve** stem, and hand tighten the **regulator**.
3. Attach the **oxygen** connective tubing to the **flowmeter**.

Skill Drill 11-8: Performing One-Rescuer Bag-Mask Ventilations (page 465)

1. Assemble the necessary equipment and position yourself **above** the patient's **head**. Open the airway using the appropriate maneuver.
2. **Suction** as necessary to clear away any **secretions**. Insert an appropriate basic airway **adjunct**.
3. Select the appropriately sized **mask** and position it properly on the patient's face. Use the **EC-clamp** technique to make a seal. Avoid the fleshy soft tissue of the neck.
4. Squeeze the bag with your free hand. Watch for adequate **chest rise**. Squeeze at the appropriate rate based on the patient's age.

Principles of Pharmacology

General Knowledge

Matching

1. H (pages 498–500; Routes of Administration)
2. I (pages 495–497; How Medications Work)
3. F (pages 495–497; How Medications Work)
4. D (pages 495–497; How Medications Work)
5. G (pages 495–497; How Medications Work)
6. B (pages 495–497; How Medications Work)
7. C (pages 495–497; How Medications Work)
8. E (page 501; Tablets and Capsules)
9. A (page 502; Topical Medications)

Multiple Choice

1. D (pages 495–497; How Medications Work)
2. A (pages 511–512; Nitroglycerin)
3. A (pages 497–498; Medication Names)
4. A (pages 498–500; Routes of Administration)
5. B (page 511; Aspirin)
6. C (page 515; Intranasal Medication—Naloxone)
7. B (pages 515–516; Oxygen)
8. B (page 513; Epinephrine)
9. B (pages 517–518; Medications Administered Using an MDI or Small-Volume Nebulizer)
10. A (pages 511–512; Nitroglycerin)
11. C (pages 498–500; Routes of Administration)
12. C (page 515; Naloxone)
13. C (pages 507, 510; Oral Glucose)
14. A (pages 497–498; Medication Names)
15. B (pages 507, 510; Oral Glucose)
16. B (pages 515–516; Oxygen)

True/False

1. T (pages 515–516; Oxygen)
2. F (pages 507, 510; Oral Glucose)
3. F (page 513; Epinephrine)
4. T (pages 511–512; Nitroglycerin)
5. F (pages 498–500; Routes of Administration)
6. F (pages 498–500; Routes of Administration)
7. F (pages 498–500; Routes of Administration)
8. T (pages 511–512; Nitroglycerin)

Fill-in-the-Blank

1. Glucose (pages 507, 510; Oral Glucose)
2. Epinephrine (page 513; Epinephrine)
3. sublingually (page 512; Administering Nitroglycerin by Tablet)
4. Unintended effects (page 497; How Medications Work)
5. solutions (page 501; Solutions and Suspensions)
6. medication (pages 495–497; How Medications Work)

Critical Thinking

Multiple Choice

1. D (pages 511–512; Nitroglycerin)
2. A (pages 511–512; Nitroglycerin)
3. A (page 513; Epinephrine)

4. A (pages 507, 510; Oral Glucose)
5. B (page 511; Aspirin)

Short Answer

1. 1. Intravenous
    2. Intramuscular
    3. Transcutaneous
    4. Oral
    5. Intraosseous
    6. Inhalation
    7. Sublingual
    8. Subcutaneous
    9. Per rectum
    10. Intranasal (pages 498–500; Routes of Administration)

2. 1. Right patient
    2. Right medication and indication
    3. Right dose
    4. Right route
    5. Right time
    6. Right education
    7. Right to refuse
    8. Right response and evaluation
    9. Right documentation (page 503; Table 12-3 The "Rights" of Medication Administration)

3. 1. Secreted naturally by the adrenal glands
    2. Dilates lung passages
    3. Constricts blood vessels
    4. Increases heart rate and blood pressure (page 513; Epinephrine)

4. 1. Obtain medical direction per local protocol.
    2. Confirm correct medication and expiration date.
    3. Attempt to determine if the patient is allergic to any medications.
    4. Prepare the medication and attach the atomizer.
    5. Place the atomizer in one nostril, pointing up and slightly outward.
    6. Administer a half dose (1 mL maximum) into each nostril.
    7. Reassess the patient and document appropriately. (page 515; Intranasal Medications: Naloxone)

5. 1. Relaxes the muscular walls of the coronary arteries and veins

   2. Results in less blood returning to the heart

   3. Decreases blood pressure

   4. Relaxes arteries throughout the body

   5. Often causes a mild headache and/or burning under the tongue after administration (pages 511–512; Nitroglycerin)

6. To avoid misdirecting the spay of the MDI and ensure inhalation of all medication (pages 517–518; Medications Administered Using an MDI or Small-Volume Nebulizer)

Ambulance Calls

1. This patient is in serious trouble. The history of the events combined with his level of consciousness, stridor, and hypotension are obvious signs of an anaphylactic reaction. You must immediately administer epinephrine in order to counteract the effects of the insect stings (ie, histamine release). If available, ALS providers should be requested. If not available, transport to the nearest appropriate facility should occur without delay. With the presence of multiple stings, this patient will likely need repeat doses of epinephrine as well as the administration of antihistamines, breathing treatments, and possibly advanced airway maneuvers. Your partner should apply high-flow oxygen and remove any remaining stingers in the neck or face by scraping them from the skin. Your prompt action is essential to patient survival.

2. This patient is most likely suffering from hypoglycemia. Although this patient is confused, he is able to talk and swallow. Some states allow EMTs to perform blood glucose tests, and this would provide information regarding this patient's blood glucose level. If your local protocols do not allow for this skill, you can gather much information about this patient through his physical signs and medical history (all indicative of low blood sugar). You should administer (at least) one tube of oral glucose and reassess his mentation and vital signs. Provide treatment and transport according to local protocols.

3. Place the patient in a position of comfort. Call for an ALS unit to assist. Give 100% oxygen via a nonrebreathing mask. Check blood pressure! Check the expiration date on the nitroglycerin. Contact medical control for permission to assist patient with one nitroglycerin tablet, sublingual. Monitor vital signs. Provide rapid transport.

Fill-in-the-Patient Care Report

EMS Patient Care Report (PCR)			
Date: Today's date	**Incident No.:** 2010-345	**Nature of Call:** Respiratory distress	**Location:** Northern Park
Dispatched: N/A	**En Route:** N/A	**At Scene:** 1300	**Transport:** 1308	**At Hospital:** 1318	**In Service:** 1340

Patient Information	
Age: 38 years **Sex:** Female **Weight (in kg [lb]):** 45 kg (100 lb)	**Allergies:** Unknown **Medications:** Metered-dose inhaler for asthma **Past Medical History:** Asthma **Chief Complaint:** Respiratory distress

Vital Signs				
Time: 1308	**BP:** 142/98	**Pulse:** 110 regular	**Respirations:** 28 labored	**SpO₂:** 88%
Time: 1313	**BP:** 138/90	**Pulse:** 102 regular	**Respirations:** 24 labored	**SpO₂:** 92%
Time: 1318	**BP:** 132/88	**Pulse:** 96 regular	**Respirations:** 20 GTV	**SpO₂:** 96%

EMS Treatment (circle all that apply)				
Oxygen @ _15_ L/min via (circle one): NC (NRM) BVM	**Assisted Ventilation**	**Airway Adjunct**	**CPR**
Defibrillation	**Bleeding Control**	**Bandaging**	**Splinting**	**Other:**

Narrative
Summoned by civilian on scene for a respiratory distress. Arrived at patient's location to find a 38-year-old female on a park bench in the tripod position and struggling to breathe. Additionally, I observed a bluish hue around the patient's mouth and fingernails and accessory muscle use in her neck. A bystander handed me a metered-dose inhaler prescribed for asthma and told me that the patient had dropped it. The patient took the inhaler and inhaled one full puff of the device. The patient was then placed on high-concentration oxygen via a nonrebreathing mask and prepared for transport. The patient was already beginning to show signs of improvement (bluish color fading, better tidal volume) as I obtained the first set of vitals and began transport to the emergency department. During transport, I was able to initiate reassessments, obtaining two more full sets of vital signs, which tended to show that the patient was improving as a result of the inhaler use and the oxygen therapy. While en route, I provided the receiving facility with a patient report, and the transport was uneventful. Once at the emergency department, the patient was properly transferred to their care, and a full verbal report was provided.**End of Report**

Shock

General Knowledge

Matching

1. B (page 531; Introduction)
2. G (pages 531–534; Perfusion)
3. H (pages 531–534; Perfusion)
4. C (pages 531–534; Perfusion)
5. E (pages 531–534; Perfusion)

6. A (pages 538–539; Anaphylactic Shock)
7. F (page 537; Septic Shock)
8. I (page 539; Psychogenic Shock)
9. D (page 540; The Progression of Shock)

Multiple Choice

1. A (page 531; Introduction)
2. B (pages 531–534; Perfusion)
3. B (pages 531–534; Perfusion)
4. C (pages 531–534; Perfusion)
5. D (pages 543–545; Treating Cardiogenic Shock)
6. D (pages 536–537; Obstructive Shock)
7. D (page 534; Table 13-1 Causes of Shock)
8. C (pages 531–534; Perfusion)
9. B (pages 534–536; Cardiogenic Shock)
10. A (pages 537–538; Neurogenic Shock)

11. D (page 537; Septic Shock)
12. A (pages 537–538; Neurogenic Shock)
13. B (page 539; Hypovolemic Shock)
14. A (page 540; The Progression of Shock)
15. A (pages 538–539; Anaphylactic Shock)
16. A (pages 534–539; Types of Shock)
17. B (page 542; Secondary Assessment)
18. B (pages 534–536; Cardiogenic Shock)
19. B (page 539; Psychogenic Shock)

True/False

1. T (pages 538–539; Anaphylactic Shock)
2. F (pages 534–536; Cardiogenic Shock)
3. T (page 531; Introduction)
4. F (page 540; The Progression of Shock)
5. F (page 540; The Progression of Shock)

6. T (page 546; Treating Anaphylactic Shock)
7. T (page 537; Septic Shock)
8. F (pages 531–534; Perfusion)
9. F (page 534; Causes of Shock)
10. F (page 540; The Progression of Shock)

Fill-in-the-Blank

1. Shock (page 531; Introduction)
2. contraction (page 533; Perfusion)
3. tolerant (pages 531–534; Perfusion)
4. contraction (page 533; Perfusion)
5. platelets, plasma (page 533; Perfusion)
6. shock (hypoperfusion) (page 531; Introduction)

7. Sphincters, contract, dilate (page 533; Perfusion)
8. Diastolic, systolic (page 533; Perfusion)
9. complications (page 548; Treating Shock in Older Patients)
10. involuntary (page 532; Perfusion)

Critical Thinking

Multiple Choice

1. A (pages 534–536; Cardiogenic Shock)
2. C (pages 537–538; Neurogenic Shock)
3. C (page 537; Septic Shock)
4. B (page 540; The Progression of Shock)
5. D (page 543; Emergency Medical Care for Shock)

Short Answer

1. • **Causes:** Extreme, life-threatening allergic reaction

   • **Signs/Symptoms:** Can develop within seconds, mild itching/rash, burning skin, vascular dilation, generalized edema, profound coma, rapid death

   • **Treatment:** Manage airway, assist ventilations, administer high-flow oxygen, determine cause, assist with administration of epinephrine, transport promptly, consider ALS (pages 538–539; Anaphylactic Shock, page 546; Treating Anaphylactic Shock)

2. • **Causes:** Inadequate heart function, disease of muscle tissue, impaired electrical system, disease or injury

   • **Signs/Symptoms:** Chest pain; irregular pulse; weak pulse; low blood pressure; cyanosis (lips, under nails); cool, clammy skin; anxiety; rales; pulmonary edema

   • **Treatment:** Position comfortably, administer high-flow oxygen, assist ventilations, transport promptly, consider ALS (pages 534–538; Cardiogenic Shock, pages 543–545; Treating Cardiogenic Shock)

3. • **Causes:** Loss of blood or fluid

   • **Signs/Symptoms:** Rapid, weak pulse; low blood pressure; change in mental status; cyanosis (lips, under nails); cool, clammy skin; increased respiratory rate

   • **Treatment:** Secure airway, assist ventilations, administer high-flow oxygen, control external bleeding, keep warm, transport promptly, consider ALS (page 539; Hypovolemic Shock, pages 547–548; Treating Hypovolemic Shock)

4. • **Causes:** Damaged cervical spine, which causes widespread blood vessel dilation

   • **Signs/Symptoms:** Bradycardia (slow pulse), low blood pressure, signs of neck injury

   • **Treatment:** Secure airway, spinal stabilization, assist ventilations, administer high-flow oxygen, preserve body heat, transport promptly, consider ALS (pages 537–538; Neurogenic Shock, page 546; Treating Neurogenic Shock)

5. • **Causes:** Temporary, generalized vascular dilation; anxiety; bad news; sight of injury/blood; prospect of medical treatment; severe pain; illness; tiredness

   • **Signs/Symptoms:** Rapid pulse, normal or low blood pressure

   • **Treatment:** Determine duration of unconsciousness, position the patient supine, record initial vital signs and mental status, suspect head injury if patient is confused or slow to regain consciousness, transport promptly (page 539; Psychogenic Shock, pages 546–547; Treating Psychogenic Shock)

6. • **Causes:** Severe bacterial infection

   • **Signs/Symptoms:** Warm skin or fever, tachycardia, low blood pressure

   • **Treatment:** Transport promptly, administer oxygen, assist ventilation, keep warm, consider ALS (page 537; Septic Shock, page 546; Treating Septic Shock)

7. **1.** Pump failure

   2. Blood or fluid loss from blood vessels

   3. Poor vessel function (blood vessels dilate) (page 534; Figure 13-3)

8. Falling blood pressure; labored or irregular breathing; ashen, mottled, or cyanotic skin; thready or absent peripheral pulses; dull eyes or dilated pupils; poor urinary output (page 540; Table 13-3 Progression of Shock)

Ambulance Calls

1. When assessing the victim of a fall, you must take into consideration not only the patient's complaints and obvious injuries but also the mechanism of injury, including the height of the fall, the surface on which he or she landed, the position in which he or she landed, and any medical and/or previous traumatic injuries that could exacerbate the injuries. This patient landed on a hard surface, most likely a wooden floor, and now presents with numbness and tingling of his lower body. These are all indicators of spinal cord injury. Assume spinal fractures are present; ensure that you assess pulse, motor, and sensation of all extremities prior to placing him in full spinal precautions; and reassess again after he is stabilized. Be alert for signs of neurogenic shock. Document your findings and continue this assessment en route to the hospital.

2. This patient is in shock, and it seems to be related to an infectious organism (septic shock). In this case, although he has not lost blood volume through hemorrhage, his vessels, or "container," have become too large, making his available blood volume inadequate. Immediate transport is required. The patient should be given high-flow oxygen. Consider ALS.

3. Treat this patient for anaphylactic shock. Apply high-flow oxygen while inquiring if the patient has an EpiPen. Based on local protocols, obtain orders and administer the EpiPen, if available. Monitor the patient's vital signs. Rapid transport is required. Consider ALS.

Fill-in-the-Patient Care Report

EMS Patient Care Report (PCR)				
Date: Today's date	**Incident No.:** 2010-123	**Nature of Call:** MCA		**Location:** Highway 62 at Exit 19
Dispatched: 0200	**En Route:** 0200	**At Scene:** 0205	**Transport:** 0213	**At Hospital:** 0218	**In Service:** 0233

Patient Information	
Age: 18 years	**Allergies:** Unknown
Sex: Male	**Medications:** Unknown
Weight (in kg [lb]): 65 kg (143 lb)	**Past Medical History:** Unknown
	Chief Complaint: Unable to move legs

Vital Signs				
Time: 0213	**BP:** 98/62	**Pulse:** 110/weak	**Respirations:** 18/shallow—adequate tidal volume	**SpO$_2$:** 94% on O$_2$

EMS Treatment
(circle all that apply)

Oxygen @ _15_ L/min via (circle one): NC (NRM) BVM	Assisted Ventilation	Airway Adjunct	CPR
Defibrillation	**Bleeding Control**	**Bandaging**	(Splinting)	(Other: Shock Treatment)

Narrative

Summoned by highway patrol for a motorcyclist down on Highway 62 at exit 19. Arrived to find an 18-year-old man supine on the highway, complaining of inability to move his legs and feeling "odd." Patient was alert, had a patent airway, and although his breathing was rapid and shallow, it seemed to be producing adequate oxygenation. Initiated spinal stabilization and high-flow oxygen therapy via a nonrebreathing mask prior to applying cervical collar and immobilizing patient to a long backboard. Once en route to the trauma center, I obtained vitals showing hypotension; increased heart rate; rapid breathing; decreased O$_2$ sat with high-flow oxygen; and pale, cool, moist skin. Removed patient's clothing to check for injuries and found that his lower extremities were cooler than his torso and that the skin on his legs was dry. Immediately upgraded transport to lights and siren, treated patient for shock, and called verbal report to the receiving facility. Arrived at the trauma center prior to obtaining a second set of vitals, and the patient was properly transferred to their care. A full verbal report was provided.**End of Report**

Assessment Review

1. A (page 541; Scene Size-up)
2. A (page 541; Primary Assessment)
3. B (page 542; History Taking)
4. B (page 546; Emergency Medical Care for Shock)
5. C (page 542; Secondary Assessment)

BLS Resuscitation

General Knowledge

Matching

1. G (pages 575–576; Mechanical Piston Device)
2. E (page 587; Foreign Body Airway Obstruction in an Adult)
3. C (pages 557–559; Elements of BLS)
4. D (pages 557–559; Elements of BLS)
5. A (pages 557–559; Elements of BLS)

6. F (page 569; Gastric Distention)
7. J (page 576; Impedance Threshold Device)
8. I (pages 566–567; Opening the Airway in Adults)
9. B (pages 566–567; Opening the Airway in Adults)
10. H (pages 567–568; Recovery Position)

Multiple Choice

1. D (pages 557–559; Elements of BLS)
2. B (pages 557–559; Elements of BLS)
3. B (pages 591–593; Removing a Foreign Body Airway Obstruction in Infants: Responsive Infants)
4. A (pages 562–563; Positioning the Patient)
5. D (page 577; Infant and Child CPR)
6. A (page 577; Infant and Child CPR)
7. C (pages 584–586; When Not to Start CPR)
8. C (pages 586–587; When to Stop CPR)
9. A (pages 593–594; Cardiac Arrest in Pregnancy)
10. B (pages 566–567; Opening the Airway in Adults)
11. C (page 569; Gastric Distention)
12. B (page 569; Stoma Ventilation)
13. A (pages 567–568; Recovery Position)
14. D (page 563; Check for Breathing and a Pulse)

15. A (page 563; Provide External Chest Compressions)
16. D (pages 563–566; Proper Hand Position and Compression Technique)
17. B (page 563; Check for Breathing and a Pulse)
18. C (page 578; Infant and Child CPR: Check for Breathing and a Pulse)
19. C (page 578; Infant and Child CPR: Check for Breathing and a Pulse)
20. C (pages 588–589; Foreign Body Airway Obstruction in Adults: Responsive Patients)
21. B (pages 589–590; Foreign Body Airway Obstruction in Adults: Unresponsive Patients)
22. D (page 588; Chest Thrusts)
23. C (page 587; Mild Airway Obstruction)

True/False

1. T (pages 560–561; Assessing the Need for BLS)
2. F (pages 560–561; Assessing the Need for BLS)
3. T (pages 560–561; Assessing the Need for BLS)
4. F (pages 567–568; Recovery Position)
5. T (page 568; Provide Artificial Ventilations)
6. T (pages 584–586; When Not to Start CPR)
7. T (pages 559–560; The Components of CPR)
8. F (pages 569–571; One-Rescuer Adult CPR)
9. F (pages 563–566; Proper Hand Position and Compression Technique)

10. T (page 583; Infant and Child CPR: Provide Rescue Breathing)
11. F (pages 594–595; Grief Support for Family Members and Loved Ones)
12. T (page 562; AED Usage in Children)
13. T (pages 563–566; Proper Hand Position and Compression Technique)
14. T (pages 571–572; Two-Rescuer Adult CPR)
15. T (pages 584–586; When Not to Start CPR)

Fill-in-the-Blank

1. 4, 6 (page 557; Elements of BLS)
2. wet, skin (page 562; Wet Patients)
3. chest compressions (page 560; Assessing the Need for BLS)
4. pacemaker (page 562; Pacemakers and Implanted Defibrillators)
5. Advance directives (page 585; When Not to Start CPR)
6. firm, flat (pages 562–563; Positioning the Patient)
7. airway (pages 566–567; Opening the Airway and Providing Artificial Ventilation)
8. automated external defibrillator (page 561; Automated External Defibrillation)
9. carotid (page 563; Check for Breathing and a Pulse)
10. mechanical piston device (pages 575–576; Mechanical Piston Device)

Critical Thinking

Short Answer

Complete this section with short written answers using the space provided.

1. 1. Rigor mortis, or stiffening of the body after death

   2. Dependent lividity (livor mortis), a discoloration of the skin due to pooling of blood

   3. Putrefaction or decomposition of the body

   4. Evidence of nonsurvivable injury, such as decapitation (pages 584–586; When Not to Start CPR)

2. 1. Recognition and activation of EMS

   2. Immediate, high-quality CPR

   3. Rapid defibrillation

   4. Basic and advanced EMS

   5. Advanced life support and postarrest care

   6. Recovery (pages 559–560; The Components of CPR)

3. 1. Injury, both blunt and penetrating

   2. Infections of the respiratory tract or another organ system

   3. A foreign body airway obstruction

   4. Submersion (drowning)

   5. Electrocution

   6. Poisoning or drug overdose

   7. Sudden infant death syndrome (SIDS) (page 577; Infant and Child CPR)

4. To perform the head tilt–chin lift maneuver, make sure the patient is supine. Place one hand on the patient's forehead and apply firm backward pressure with your palm to tilt the head back. Next, place the tips of your fingers of your other hand under the lower jaw near the bony part of the chin. Lift the chin upward, bringing the entire lower jaw with it, helping to tilt the head back. (page 566; Figure 14-11)

5. To perform the jaw-thrust maneuver, place your fingers behind the angle of the lower jaw on both sides and move the jaw upward. Keep the head in a neutral position. If the mouth remains closed, use your thumbs to pull the patient's lower jaw down to allow breathing. (pages 566–567; Opening the Airway in Adults)

6. Take standard precautions. Once you have determined that the patient is unresponsive, call for additional help. Check for breathing and a carotid pulse for no more than 10 seconds. Ensure that the patient is on a firm, flat surface in a supine position. Place your hands in the proper position. Give 30 compressions at a rate of 100 to 120 per minute for an adult. Using a rhythmic motion, apply pressure vertically from your shoulders down through both arms to depress the sternum 2 inches to 2.4 inches (5 cm to 6 cm) in an adult, then rise up gently and fully. Count the compressions aloud. (pages 569–571; One-Rescuer Adult CPR)

7. Rescuer one should finish the cycle of 30 compressions while a second rescuer moves to the opposite side of the chest and moves into position to begin compressions. Rescuer one delivers two ventilations, and then rescuer two should take over compressing by administering 30 compressions. (page 571; Switching Positions)

8. Standing: Stand behind the patient and wrap your arms around his or her abdomen. Make a fist with one hand, then grasp the fist with the other hand. Place the thumb side of the fist against the patient's abdomen between the umbilicus and the xiphoid process. Press your fist into the patient's abdomen in quick inward and upward thrusts until the object is expelled or the patient becomes unconscious. (page 588; Abdominal-Thrust Maneuver)

9. Standing: Stand behind the patient and wrap your arms under the armpits and around the patient's chest. Make a fist with one hand, then grasp the fist with the other hand. Place the thumb side of the fist against the patient's sternum. Press your fist into the patient's chest and perform backward thrusts until the object is expelled or the patient becomes unconscious.

   Supine: Kneel next to the patient. Place your hands as you would to deliver chest compressions. Deliver 30 chest compressions, open the airway, and look in the mouth. If the object is visible, remove it. If not, continue the cycle of chest compressions and opening the airway. (page 588; Chest Thrusts)

10. 1. Hold the infant face down, with the body resting on your forearm. Support the infant's jaw and face with your hand and keep the head lower than the body.

    2. Deliver five back slaps between the shoulder blades, using the heel of your hand.

    3. Place your free hand behind the infant's head/back and turn the infant faceup.

    4. Give five quick chest thrusts on the sternum using two fingers.

    5. Check the airway. If the object is visible, then remove it. (page 593; Unresponsive Infants)

Ambulance Calls

1. Question the family about the last time they spoke with her. Explain that she has been down too long for CPR to be effective. Comfort family members. Notify your dispatcher to alert the supervisor and either law enforcement, the coroner, or a funeral home according to local protocols.

2. With the FDA's approval of AEDs for home use, it will become more common to see them being used by the lay provider. Simply purchasing an AED does not ensure appropriate usage during real-life events. Training by knowledgeable, skilled instructors is needed to minimize confusion and inappropriate AED use. Remove the AED and explain to them that AEDs are meant to be used only when a person is not breathing and has no pulse. Emphasize that it is appropriate to have the AED nearby in the event that a person goes into cardiorespiratory arrest, but that it is not to be applied until then. After the patient has been transported to the hospital, tell the friends and family that you appreciate their willingness to be prepared for emergencies and that you would like to see them be successful in their usage of their AED. If you or your department offers CPR/AED courses, offer to train them and/or point them in the right direction to receive the appropriate training.

3. Given the scene, you must assume that there is the likelihood for trauma. This means that you must assess and maintain his airway without manipulating his spine. Use the jaw-thrust maneuver and apply full cervical spine precautions. Also, consider possible causes of his unconscious state, including any scene hazards and potential medical conditions.

Skills

Skill Drills

Skill Drill 14-1: Performing Chest Compressions (page 564)

1. Take standard precautions. Place the **heel** of one hand on the **center** of the chest.
2. Place the **heel** of your other hand over the first **hand**.
3. With your arms straight, lock your **elbows**, and position your shoulders directly over your hands. Depress the sternum at a rate of **100** to **120** compressions per minute and to a depth of **2 inches** to **2.4 inches (5 cm to 6 cm)** using a direct downward movement. Allow the chest to return to its normal position; do not lean on the chest between compressions. **Compression** and relaxation should be of equal duration.

Skill Drill 14-2: Performing One-Rescuer Adult CPR (page 570)

1. Take standard precautions. Establish unresponsiveness and call for help. Use your cell phone if needed.
2. Check for breathing and a carotid pulse for no more than 10 seconds.
3. If breathing and pulse are absent, begin CPR until an AED is available. Give 30 chest compressions at a rate of 100 to 120 per minute.
4. Open the airway according to your suspicion of spinal injury.

5. Give two ventilations of 1 second each and observe for visible chest rise. Continue cycles of 30 chest compressions and two ventilations until additional personnel arrive or the patient starts to move. (page 527; One-Rescuer Adult CPR)

Skill Drill 14-3: Performing Two-Rescuer Adult CPR (page 572)

1. Take standard **precautions**. Establish **unresponsiveness** and take positions.
2. Check for breathing and a **carotid** pulse.
3. Begin CPR, starting with **chest compressions**. Give 30 chest compressions at a rate of **100** to **120** per minute. If the AED is available, then apply it and follow the voice prompts.
4. **Open** the airway according to your suspicion of spinal injury.
5. Give **two ventilations** of 1 second each and observe **visible chest rise**. Continue cycles of 30 chest compressions and two ventilations (switch roles every five cycles [2 minutes]) until ALS providers take over or the patient starts to move. Reanalyze the patient's cardiac rhythm with the AED every 2 minutes and deliver a shock if indicated. (page 528; Two-Rescuer Adult CPR)

CHAPTER

15

Medical Overview

General Knowledge

Matching (all answers can be found in Table 15-1 Common Medical Emergencies)

1. A		**11.** A	
2. G		**12.** D	
3. B		**13.** H	
4. I		**14.** B	
5. A		**15.** G	
6. F		**16.** D	
7. K		**17.** K	
8. C		**18.** D	
9. J		**19.** I	
10. E		**20.** C	

Multiple Choice

1. C	(pages 606–607; Scene Size-up)	
2. B	(pages 606–607; Scene Size-up)	
3. C	(pages 608–609; History Taking)	
4. B	(pages 608–609; History Taking)	
5. C	(pages 609–610; Secondary Assessment)	
6. B	(pages 609–610; Secondary Assessment)	
7. D	(pages 611–612; Type of Transport)	
8. C	(page 613; Destination Selection)	
9. B	(pages 614–615; HIV Infection)	
10. B	(pages 614–615; HIV Infection)	

11. C	(page 620; Ebola)	
12. C	(page 617; Table 15-2 Characteristics of Hepatitis)	
13. C	(page 617; Table 15-2 Characteristics of Hepatitis)	
14. A	(pages 618–619; Tuberculosis)	
15. D	(pages 619–620; Methicillin-Resistant *Staphylococcus aureus*)	
16. B	(pages 613–614; Epidemic and Pandemic Considerations)	

True/False

1. T	(pages 605–606; Patient Assessment)	
2. T	(pages 607–608; Primary Assessment)	
3. T	(pages 613–614; Epidemic and Pandemic Considerations)	
4. T	(pages 608–609; History Taking)	
5. F	(pages 609–610; Secondary Assessment)	
6. T	(pages 611–612; Type of Transport)	
7. T	(pages 614–615; HIV Infection)	
8. F	(pages 614–615; HIV Infection)	
9. T	(page 620; MERS-CoV)	
10. T	(pages 615–617; Hepatitis)	
11. F	(pages 614–615; HIV Infection)	

12. T	(pages 618–619; Tuberculosis)	
13. T	(pages 619–620; Methicillin-Resistant *Staphylococcus aureus*)	
14. F	(page 619; Whooping Cough)	
15. T	(page 618; Meningitis)	
16. F	(page 614; Influenza)	
17. T	(pages 609–610; Secondary Assessment)	
18. F	(pages 608–609; History Taking)	
19. T	(page 613; Destination Selection)	
20. T	(pages 611–612; Type of Transport)	
21. F	(page 614; Herpes Simplex)	

Fill-in-the-Blank

1. Hematologic emergencies (page 605; Types of Medical Emergencies)
2. Tunnel vision (page 606; Patient Assessment)
3. AVPU (page 607; Primary Assessment)
4. 5, 15 (page 611; Reassessment)
5. medical control (page 611; Management, Transport, and Destination)
6. AED (page 611; Management, Transport, and Destination)
7. High-priority (pages 611–612; Type of Transport)
8. ground, air (page 612; Type of Transport)
9. infectious disease (page 613; Infectious Diseases)
10. Hepatitis (page 615; Hepatitis)
11. Hepatitis A (page 616; Hepatitis)
12. track marks (page 610; Secondary Assessment)
13. Virulence (pages 616–617; Hepatitis)
14. Tuberculosis (pages 618–619; Tuberculosis)
15. meningitis (page 618; Meningitis)

Fill-in-the-Table (page 615; Words of Wisdom: Causes of Infectious Disease)

Causes of Infectious Disease		
Type of Organism	**Description**	**Example**
Bacteria	**Grow and reproduce outside the human cell in the appropriate temperature and with the appropriate nutrients**	*Salmonella*
Viruses	Smaller than bacteria; multiply only inside a host and die when exposed to the environment	**Human immunodeficiency virus**
Fungi	**Similar to bacteria in that they require the appropriate nutrients and organic material to grow**	**Mold**
Protozoa (parasites)	**One-celled microscopic organisms, some of which cause disease**	Amoebas
Helminths (parasites)	Invertebrates with long, flexible, rounded, or flattened bodies	**Worms**

Critical Thinking

Short Answer

Complete this section with short written answers using the space provided.

1.
   1. The patient's blood is splashed or sprayed into your eyes, nose, or mouth or into an open sore or cut; even microscopic openings in the skin are a possible source.
   2. You have blood from an infected patient on your hands and then touch your own eyes, nose, mouth, or an open sore or cut.
   3. A needle used to inject the patient breaks your skin.
   4. Broken glass at a motor vehicle collision or other incident may penetrate your glove (and skin), which may have already been covered with blood from an infected patient. (pages 614–615; HIV Infection)

2.
   1. Scene size-up
   2. Primary assessment
   3. History taking
   4. Secondary assessment
   5. Reassessment (pages 605–606; Patient Assessment)

3. **1.** Unresponsive/altered mental status

   2. Airway/breathing problems

   3. Circulatory problems, such as severe bleeding or signs of shock (pages 611–612; Type of Transport)

4. **1.** Where did you recently travel?

   2. Did you receive any vaccinations before your trip?

   3. Were you exposed to any infectious diseases?

   4. Is there anyone else in your travel party who is sick?

   5. What types of food did you eat?

   6. What was your source of drinking water? (pages 620–621; Travel Medicine)

Ambulance Calls

1. It seems likely that this patient could be suffering from tuberculosis. You and your crew should apply protection immediately. You should place an N95 or HEPA mask on yourself and other crew members and a surgical mask on the patient. Although a surgical mask on the patient provides minimal protection, it provides a visual reminder to all who are involved in the patient's care of the possibility of an airborne communicable disease. The surgical mask should still allow for the placement of a nasal cannula for oxygen. Proper notification to the receiving hospital should be made so that isolation precautions can be in place when the patient arrives. Although the risk of contracting the illness is minimal to you and the crew, everyone should alert their management and follow their exposure-control plan. All crew members potentially exposed should receive a tuberculin skin test and follow up with a designated health care facility.

2. You should begin by verifying the chief complaint of chest pain. Ask the patient what she was doing when the pain began and whether anything potentially caused it. Does anything make the pain better or worse? Inquire as to the quality of the pain. Ask the patient to describe the pain, and determine if the pain is constant or intermittent. Where in her chest is the pain? Have the patient point to the painful area and determine whether the pain is localized to that area or if it radiates to other areas. Ask the patient to rate her pain on a scale from 1 to 10. Explain to her that 0 means no pain and that 10 means the worst pain. This will give you a baseline for reassessment after you begin treatment. Inquire as to how long she's had the pain. Is it just this incident, or has she had previous episodes?

CHAPTER

16 | Respiratory Emergencies

General Knowledge

Matching

1. N (pages 628–629; Anatomy of the Respiratory System)
2. D (pages 638–639; Acute Pulmonary Edema)
3. H (page 635; Epiglottitis)
4. J (page 639; Chronic Obstructive Pulmonary Disease)
5. L (pages 644–645; Pleural Effusion)
6. O (pages 637–638; Tuberculosis)
7. G (page 628; Introduction)
8. E (page 636; Pneumonia)
9. M (pages 633–634; Causes of Dyspnea)
10. A (page 639; Chronic Obstructive Pulmonary Disease)
11. K (pages 646–647; Hyperventilation)
12. F (pages 642–644; Asthma, Hay Fever, and Anaphylaxis)
13. I (pages 645–646; Pulmonary Embolism)
14. B (pages 642–644; Asthma, Hay Fever, and Anaphylaxis)
15. C (page 644; Spontaneous Pneumothorax)

Multiple Choice

1. C (page 645; Pulmonary Edema)
2. C (pages 629–631; Physiology of Respiration)
3. B (pages 652–653; Questioning a Patient With Difficulty Breathing)
4. C (pages 629–631; Physiology of Respiration)
5. B (pages 629–631; Physiology of Respiration)
6. C (pages 634–635; Croup)
7. C (pages 629–631; Physiology of Respiration)
8. A (pages 633–634; Causes of Dyspnea)
9. B (page 636; Pneumonia)
10. A (pages 638–639; Acute Pulmonary Edema)
11. C (pages 638–639; Acute Pulmonary Edema)
12. A (page 639; Chronic Obstructive Pulmonary Disease)
13. B (pages 666–667; Cystic Fibrosis)
14. B (page 641; Comparison of COPD and Congestive Heart Failure)
15. A (page 644; Spontaneous Pneumothorax)
16. C (pages 642–643; Asthma)
17. B (pages 642–643; Asthma)
18. A (pages 643–644; Anaphylactic Reactions)
19. C (pages 644–645; Pleural Effusion)
20. A (page 664; Obstruction of the Airway)
21. B (pages 646–647; Hyperventilation)
22. C (page 631; Signs and Symptoms of Inadequate Breathing)
23. D (page 656; Emergency Medical Care)
24. A (pages 629–631; Physiology of Respiration)
25. A (page 663; Treatment of Specific Conditions: COPD)
26. B (page 631; Signs and Symptoms of Inadequate Breathing)
27. B (pages 655–656; Reassessment)
28. D (pages 652–653; Questioning a Patient With Difficulty Breathing)
29. C (page 658; Respiratory Inhalation Medications)
30. B (page 657; Metered-Dose Inhaler and Small-Volume Nebulizer: Indications)
31. D (pages 638–639; Acute Pulmonary Edema)
32. C (pages 663–664; Treatment of Specific Conditions: Asthma)
33. B (page 637; Influenza Type A)
34. C (pages 653–655; Secondary Assessment)
35. A (pages 642–644; Asthma, Hay Fever, and Anaphylaxis)

True/False

1. F (page 639; Chronic Obstructive Pulmonary Disease)
2. T (page 644; Spontaneous Pneumothorax)
3. F (pages 642–644; Asthma, Hay Fever, and Anaphylaxis: Anaphylactic Reactions)
4. F (pages 644–645; Pleural Effusion)
5. T (pages 647–648; Carbon Monoxide Poisoning)
6. T (pages 638–639; Acute Pulmonary Edema)
7. F (pages 646–647; Hyperventilation)
8. T (page 639; Chronic Obstructive Pulmonary Disease)
9. T (page 639; Chronic Obstructive Pulmonary Disease)
10. T (pages 666–667; Cystic Fibrosis)
11. T (page 648; Scene Size-up)
12. T (pages 653–655; Secondary Assessment)
13. F (pages 631–633; Carbon Dioxide Retention and Hypoxic Drive)
14. T (page 658; Metered-Dose Inhaler and Small-Volume Nebulizer: Side Effects)
15. F (pages 646–647; Hyperventilation)
16. T (page 635; Epiglottitis)
17. T (pages 635–636; Respiratory Syncytial Virus)
18. F (page 661; Skill Drill 16-2 Assisting a Patient With a Small-Volume Nebulizer)
19. T (pages 650–651; Assessing Breath Sounds)
20. T (pages 645–646; Pulmonary Embolism)

Fill-in-the-Blank

1. carbon dioxide (pages 629–631; Physiology of Respiration)
2. oxygen (pages 631–633; Carbon Dioxide Retention and Hypoxic Drive)
3. Oxygen (pages 629–631; Physiology of Respiration)
4. alveoli (page 629; Physiology of Respiration)
5. N95 respirator (page 634; Tuberculosis)
6. tracheostomy (page 665; Tracheostomy Dysfunction)
7. Carbon monoxide (pages 647–648; Carbon Monoxide Poisoning)
8. stridor (page 651; Assessing Breath Sounds)
9. Rales or crackles (pages 650–651; Assessing Breath Sounds)
10. SAMPLE, OPQRST (pages 652–653; Questioning a Patient With Difficulty Breathing)
11. Hay fever (page 643; Hay Fever (Allergic Rhinitis))
12. inhaler, nebulizer (page 656; Metered-Dose Inhaler and Small-Volume Nebulizer)
13. Pertussis (whooping cough) (pages 636–637; Whooping Cough)
14. Rhonchi (page 651; Assessing Breath Sounds)
15. emphysema (page 639; Chronic Obstructive Pulmonary Disease)

Labeling

1. Obstruction, Scarring, and Dilation of the Alveolar Sac (page 640; Figure 16-7)

   A. Bronchiole

   B. Inflammation or infection

   C. Obstruction

   D. Mucus

   E. Infection

   F. Alveolus

   G. Trapped air

   H. Dilated alveolus

Critical Thinking

Short Answer

1. 1. Normal rate
   2. Regular pattern of inhalation and exhalation
   3. Clear and equal lung sounds on both sides of the chest
   4. Regular and equal chest rise and fall
   5. Adequate depth
   6. Unlabored; without adventitious breath sounds (page 631; Table 16-1 Signs of Normal Breathing)

2. 1. Asthma
   2. Chronic obstructive pulmonary disease
   3. Congestive heart failure/pulmonary edema
   4. Pneumonia
   5. Bronchitis
   6. Anaphylaxis (page 632; Table 16-3 Signs and Symptoms Seen in Various Respiratory Conditions)

3. 1. Patient is unable to coordinate administration and inhalation.
   2. Inhaler is not prescribed for patient.
   3. You did not obtain permission from medical control or local protocol.
   4. Patient has already met maximum prescribed dose before your arrival.
   5. Medication is expired.
   6. There are other contraindications specific to the medication. (page 657; Metered-Dose Inhaler and Small-Volume Nebulizer: Indications and Contraindications)

4. An ongoing irritation of the respiratory tract; excess mucus production obstructs small airways and alveoli. Protective mechanisms are impaired. Repeated episodes of irritation and pneumonia can cause scarring and alveolar damage, leading to COPD. (page 639; Chronic Obstructive Pulmonary Disease)

5. Obstruction with secretions, mucus, foreign bodies, and/or airway swelling; Bleeding; Leaking; Dislodgement; Infection (page 665; Tracheostomy Dysfunction)

6. A condition characterized by a chronically high blood level of carbon dioxide in which the respiratory center no longer responds to high blood levels of carbon dioxide. In these patients, low blood oxygen causes the respiratory center to respond and stimulate respiration. If the arterial level of oxygen is then raised, as happens when the patient is given additional oxygen, there is no longer any stimulus to breathe; both the high carbon dioxide and low oxygen drives are lost. (pages 631–633; Carbon Dioxide Retention and Hypoxic Drive)

7. 1. Is the air going in?
   2. Does the chest rise and fall with each breath?
   3. Is the rate adequate for the age of your patient? (pages 648–650; Assessing ABCs in Respiratory Patients)

Ambulance Calls

1. This child has all the classics signs of epiglottitis. You should do nothing to excite or frighten the child because doing so will likely cause his airway to spasm and close. Remember to use nonthreatening body language (place yourself below his eye level), give the child distance (until you establish trust), and perform any exam using a full-body scan. This is a true emergency that requires immediate transport to the hospital, but you must do so tactfully. Use parents to assist with patient care efforts, such as applying humidified oxygen (blow-by or mask).

2. This patient's chief complaint, age, weight, smoking, and birth control use all place her at risk of pulmonary embolism (PE). PE patients most often experience a sudden onset of shortness of breath that they describe as sharp and worsening with inspiration. You should provide high-flow oxygen, obtain vital signs, and perform a secondary assessment en route to the hospital (including auscultation of lung sounds). Provide prompt transport to the nearest appropriate facility.

3. Place the patient in a position of comfort. Provide high-flow oxygen via a nonrebreathing mask and monitor his vital signs. This patient requires rapid transport to the nearest appropriate facility.

4. This patient is likely experiencing pulmonary edema associated with his cardiac history. Place the patient in a sitting-up position and administer 100% oxygen through a nonrebreathing mask. Suction the frothy secretions from the patient's airway, as necessary. Consider CPAP for this patient, and be prepared to provide full ventilatory support for this patient should he deteriorate. This patient requires prompt transport to the nearest appropriate facility.

Skills

Skill Drills

Skill Drill 16-1: Assisting a Patient With a Metered-Dose Inhaler (page 650)

1. Check to make sure you have the correct medication for the correct patient. Check the expiration date. Ensure inhaler is at room temperature or **warmer**.

2. Remove oxygen mask. Hand inhaler to patient. Instruct about breathing and **lip seal**.

3. Instruct patient to press inhaler and inhale one puff. Instruct about **breath holding**.

4. Reapply **oxygen**. After a few **breaths**, have patient repeat **dose** if order or protocol allows.

Skill Drill 16-2: Assisting a Patient With a Small-Volume Nebulizer (page 651)

1. Check to make sure you have the correct medication for the correct patient. Check the expiration date. Confirm you have the correct patient and correct dose.

2. Pour the medication into the container on the nebulizer. In some cases, sterile saline may be added (about 3 mL) to achieve the optimum volume of fluid for the nebulized application.

3. Attach the medication container to the nebulizer, mouthpiece, and tubing. Attach oxygen tubing to the oxygen tank. Set the flowmeter at 6 L/min.

4. Instruct the patient on how to breathe.

Assessment Review

1. D (pages 653–654; Secondary Assessment)
2. B (pages 646–647; Hyperventilation)
3. A (pages 648–651; Primary Assessment)
4. B (pages 655–656; Reassessment)
5. D (pages 655–656; Reassessment)

Emergency Care Summary (pages 609–617; Emergency Medical Care, Treatment of Specific Conditions)

General Management of Respiratory Emergencies
Managing life threats to the patient's **ABCs** and ensuring the delivery of high-flow oxygen are the primary concerns with any respiratory emergency. Patients breathing at a rate of less than **12** breaths/min or greater than **20** breaths/min should receive **high-flow oxygen**. Continually assess the patient's mental status, and provide emotional support as needed. Transport in a position of comfort. For all respiratory emergencies, make sure you have taken the appropriate standard precautions, including the use of an **N95 respirator** in a patient with suspected tuberculosis.

Upper or Lower Airway Infection
Dyspnea from an upper airway infection may be from **croup** or **epiglottitis**. Patients should receive **humified** oxygen if available. Patients who are sitting forward, seem lethargic, or are drooling may have **epiglottitis**. Do not force the patient to lie down or attempt to suction or insert an **oropharyngeal** airway because this may cause a spasm and a complete airway obstruction. Transport should be rapid.
Lower airway infections may be from the common cold, bronchitis, or **pneumonia**. Patients need supplemental oxygen, monitoring of vital signs, and transport to the hospital.

Asthma, Hay Fever, and Anaphylaxis
Not all wheezing is the result of asthma! Obtain a thorough **history** from the patient or family. If the patient is wheezing and has asthma, assist with the patient's prescribed **inhaler** or administer a small-volume nebulizer containing **albuterol**. Provide supplemental oxygen and provide ventilatory support as needed. Patients whose asthma progresses to **status asthmaticus** require immediate transportation. Be prepared to assist their ventilations because they may become too exhausted to breathe.
Hay fever usually requires only support and transport, but if the condition has worsened from generalized cold symptoms, the patient may require supplemental oxygen and **airway** support.
Anaphylaxis is a true emergency that requires rapid intervention and **transport**. Airway, oxygen, and ventilatory support are paramount. Determine if the patient has a prescribed **epinephrine**. Transport promptly. Reassess the patient's condition en route to the hospital.

Pneumothorax
A pneumothorax may occur spontaneously or may be the result of a **traumatic event**. Place the patient in a position of comfort, and support the **ABCs**. Provide prompt transport, monitor the patient carefully, and be prepared to assist ventilations and provide **cardiopulmonary resuscitation** if necessary.

Obstruction of the Airway
Managing an airway obstruction is a priority. Use age-appropriate **basic** life support foreign body airway obstruction **maneuvers** to clear the airway. Administer supplemental oxygen, and transport the patient to the closest hospital. Some patients do not want to go to a hospital after the obstruction is cleared. Encourage them to be transported for evaluation of possible **injury** to the airway.

Hyperventilation
Gather a thorough **history**, and attempt to determine the **underlying cause** because the hyperventilation may be the result of a serious problem. Do not have the patient breathe into a **paper bag**; this maneuver could make things worse. Instead, **reassure** the patient, administer supplemental oxygen, and provide prompt transport to the hospital.

Cardiovascular Emergencies

General Knowledge

Matching

1.	L	(pages 677–679; Anatomy and Physiology)
2.	C	(pages 679–684; Circulation)
3.	O	(pages 677–679; Anatomy and Physiology)
4.	G	(pages 679–684; Circulation)
5.	N	(pages 677–679; Anatomy and Physiology)
6.	K	(page 679; Circulation)
7.	H	(pages 677–679; Anatomy and Physiology)
8.	M	(pages 677–679; Anatomy and Physiology)
9.	B	(pages 684–685; Atherosclerosis)
10.	D	(pages 687–688; Sudden Death)
11.	F	(page 684; Pathophysiology)
12.	I	(pages 684–685; Atherosclerosis)
13.	J	(pages 687–688; Sudden Death)
14.	A	(pages 687–688; Sudden Death)
15.	E	(pages 687–688; Sudden Death)
16.	P	(pages 684–685; Atherosclerosis)
17.	G	(page 684; Pathophysiology)
18.	E	(pages 684–685; Atherosclerosis)
19.	F	(pages 685–686; Angina Pectoris)
20.	C	(page 688; Cardiogenic Shock)
21.	A	(pages 688–690; Congestive Heart Failure)
22.	D	(pages 690–692; Hypertensive Emergencies)
23.	B	(pages 690–692; Hypertensive Emergencies)

Multiple Choice

1.	C	(pages 677–679; Anatomy and Physiology)
2.	D	(pages 677–679; Anatomy and Physiology)
3.	A	(pages 677–679; Anatomy and Physiology)
4.	B	(pages 677–679; Anatomy and Physiology)
5.	A	(pages 677–679; Anatomy and Physiology)
6.	B	(pages 679–684; Circulation)
7.	C	(pages 679–684; Circulation)
8.	A	(pages 677–679; Anatomy and Physiology)
9.	C	(pages 679–684; Circulation)
10.	A	(pages 684–685; Atherosclerosis)
11.	B	(pages 684–685; Atherosclerosis)
12.	B	(page 684; Pathophysiology)
13.	D	(pages 684–685; Atherosclerosis)
14.	B	(pages 685–686; Angina Pectoris)
15.	A	(pages 685–686; Angina Pectoris)
16.	B	(pages 690–692; Hypertensive Emergencies)
17.	C	(pages 685–686; Angina Pectoris)
18.	C	(pages 686–688; Acute Myocardial Infarction)
19.	C	(pages 686–688; Acute Myocardial Infarction)
20.	A	(pages 688–690; Congestive Heart Failure)
21.	B	(page 688; Cardiogenic Shock)
22.	D	(pages 687–688; Sudden Death)
23.	A	(pages 687–688; Sudden Death)
24.	A	(pages 688–690; Congestive Heart Failure)
25.	D	(page 689; Table 17-1)
26.	B	(pages 688–690; Congestive Heart Failure)
27.	C	(page 687; Physical Findings of AMI and Cardiac Compromise)
28.	C	(pages 692–693; Primary Assessment)
29.	B	(page 691; Table 17-2 OPQRST Mnemonic for Assessing Pain)
30.	C	(page 691; Table 17-2 OPQRST Mnemonic for Assessing Pain)
31.	A	(page 689; Table 17-1)
32.	B	(pages 696–697; Emergency Medical Care for Chest Pain or Discomfort)
33.	C	(pages 696–697; Emergency Medical Care for Chest Pain or Discomfort)
34.	B	(pages 703–704; Heart Surgeries and Cardiac Assistive Devices)

35. A (pages 703–704; Heart Surgeries and Cardiac Assistive Devices)

36. C (pages 705–707; Automated External Defibrillators)

37. C (pages 705–707; Automated External Defibrillators)

38. B (pages 705–707; Automated External Defibrillators)

39. C (page 705; Figure 17-15)

40. A (page 707; Rationale for Early Defibrillation)

41. D (page 692; Scene Size-up)

42. A (pages 692–693; Primary Assessment)

43. D (pages 711–712; Skill Drill 17-3 Using an AED)

44. C (pages 711–712; Skill Drill 17-3 Using an AED)

45. C (pages 714–715; Cardiac Arrest During Transport)

True/False

1. F (pages 677–679; Anatomy and Physiology)

2. F (pages 679–684; Circulation)

3. T (pages 684–685; Atherosclerosis)

4. F (pages 684–685; Atherosclerosis)

5. T (pages 685–686; Angina Pectoris)

6. F (pages 685–686; Angina Pectoris)

7. T (pages 697–699; Administering Nitroglycerin)

8. T (pages 708–710; AED Maintenance)

9. T (pages 685–686; Angina Pectoris)

10. F (pages 679–684; Circulation)

11. T (page 706; Special Populations)

12. T (page 706; Special Populations)

13. F (pages 690–692; Hypertensive Emergencies)

14. T (pages 686–687; The Pain of AMI)

15. T (page 694; History Taking)

Fill-in-the-Blank

1. septum (page 677; Anatomy and Physiology)

2. aorta (page 677; Anatomy and Physiology)

3. right (page 679; Circulation)

4. atrioventricular (page 678; Anatomy and Physiology)

5. dilation (page 679; Circulation)

6. Red blood (page 678; Anatomy and Physiology)

7. Diastolic (page 680; Circulation)

8. four (page 677; Anatomy and Physiology)

9. left (page 678; Anatomy and Physiology)

10. CPAP (page 692; Primary Assessment)

11. dependent edema (page 690; Congestive Heart Failure)

12. 180 mm Hg (page 691; Hypertensive Emergencies)

13. pulmonary veins (page 690; Congestive Heart Failure)

14. 90 mm Hg (page 689; Table 17-1)

15. inferior (page 687; Physical Findings of AMI and Cardiac Compromise)

Labeling

1. Right and Left Sides of the Heart (page 678; Figure 17-2 A and B)

   A. Superior vena cava (oxygen-poor blood from head and upper body)

   B. Left pulmonary artery (blood to left lung)

   C. Right pulmonary artery (blood to right lung)

   D. Right atrium

   E. Inferior vena cava (oxygen-poor blood from lower body)

   F. Right ventricle

   G. Oxygen-rich blood to head and upper body

   H. Right pulmonary veins (oxygen-rich blood from right lung)

   I. Left pulmonary veins (oxygen-rich blood from left lung)

   J. Left atrium

   K. Left ventricle

   L. Oxygen-rich blood to lower body

2. Electrical Conduction System (page 678; Figure 17-3)

   A. Atrioventricular (AV) node

   B. Bundle of His

   C. SA node

   D. Left bundle branch

   E. Internodal pathways

   F. Left posterior fascicle

   G. Right bundle branch

   H. Purkinje fibers

   I. Left anterior fascicle

3. Pulse Points (page 683; Figure 17-7 A–F)

   A. Carotid

   B. Femoral

   C. Brachial

   D. Radial

   E. Posterior tibial

   F. Dorsalis pedis

Critical Thinking

Short Answer

1. • In an AMI, the onset of pain is gradual, with additional symptoms. The pain is typically described as a tightness or pressure. The severity of pain increases with time and may wax and wane. The pain is usually substernal and very rarely radiates to the back. Peripheral pulses are equal.

   • With a dissecting aneurysm, the onset of pain is abrupt, without additional symptoms. The pain is typically described as sharp or tearing. The severity of pain is at its maximum from the onset and does not abate once started. The pain can be located in the chest, with radiation to the back, between the shoulder blades. There can be a blood pressure discrepancy between the arms or a decrease in a femoral or carotid pulse. (page 691; Table 17-2 AMI Versus Dissecting Aortic Aneurysm)

2. 1. Failure of the machine to not shock fine ventricular fibrillation

   2. Applying the AED to a patient who is moving, squirming, or being transported

   3. Turning off the AED before analysis or shock is complete (pages 708–710; AED Maintenance)

3. 1. If the patient regains a pulse

   2. After six to nine shocks have been delivered

   3. If the machine gives three consecutive "no shock" messages (page 714; After Automated External Device Shocks)

4. 1. Be aware of the surface the patient is lying on. Wet and metal surfaces may conduct electricity, making defibrillation of the patient dangerous to EMTs.

   2. What is the age of the patient? Use pediatric AED pads when appropriate.

   3. Does the patient have a medication patch in the area where the AED pads will be placed? If so, remove the medication patch, wipe the area clean, and then attach the AED pad.

4. Does the patient have an implantable pacemaker or internal defibrillator in the same area where the AED pads will be located? If so, place the AED pad below the pacemaker or defibrillator, or place the pads in anterior and posterior positions. (page 716; Safety Tips)

5. Stable angina is characterized by pain in the chest of coronary origin that is relieved by rest or nitroglycerin. Unstable angina is characterized by pain in the chest of coronary origin that occurs in response to progressively less exercise or fewer stimuli than ordinarily required to produce angina. If untreated, it can lead to AMI. (pages 685–686; Angina Pectoris)

6. 1. It may or may not be caused by exertion, but it can occur at any time.

   2. It does not resolve in a few minutes.

   3. It may or may not be relieved by rest or nitroglycerin. (pages 686–687; The Pain of AMI)

7. 1. Sudden death

   2. Cardiogenic shock

   3. Congestive heart failure (CHF) (pages 687–688; Consequences of AMI)

8. 1. Sudden onset of weakness, nausea, or sweating without an obvious cause

   2. Chest pain, discomfort, or pressure that is often crushing or squeezing and that does not change with each breath

   3. Pain, discomfort, or pressure in the lower jaw, arms, back, abdomen, or neck

   4. Irregular heartbeat with syncope

   5. Shortness of breath, or dyspnea

   6. Nausea/vomiting

   7. Pink, frothy sputum

   8. Sudden death (page 686; Signs and Symptoms of AMI)

9. 1. Take vital signs, and give oxygen via a nonrebreathing mask with an oxygen flow of 10 to 15 L/min. Medical control may order the use of CPAP.

   2. Allow the patient to remain sitting in an upright position with the legs down.

   3. Be reassuring; many patients with CHF are quite anxious because they cannot breathe.

   4. Patients who have had problems with CHF before will usually have specific medications for its treatment. Gather these medications and take them to the hospital.

   5. Nitroglycerin may be of value if the patient's systolic blood pressure is greater than 100 mm Hg. If the patient has been prescribed nitroglycerin, and medical control or standing orders advise you to do so, you can administer it sublingually.

   6. Prompt transport to the emergency department is essential. (page 689; Table 17-1)

Ambulance Calls

1. The patient is feeling better, so it is likely that he was experiencing an episode of angina; however, because you cannot rule out an AMI, this patient should be strongly encouraged to go to the hospital for evaluation. Place the patient in a position of comfort. Provide oxygen therapy, if appropriate. Monitor his vital signs and provide normal transport. If the patient continues to have chest pain, reassess and consider administering an additional nitroglycerin tablet, if local protocol permits. In addition to BLS care, this patient will also benefit from ALS care; therefore, an attempt to rendezvous with an ALS unit should be made.

2. Denial is one of the biggest indicators of heart attack. Although this patient is considered "younger" and otherwise healthy, he is having signs and symptoms of a myocardial infarction. It may take some convincing of the need for treatment and transport, but you must be clear on the potential consequences of his refusal of care (informed refusal). If he initially refuses, explain what physical

signs you see that lead you to believe he is likely having a heart attack, express genuine concern for his well-being, and allow him to speak directly with medical control. More often than not, when patients hear the same or similar information from a physician, it has a different effect. If he allows you to examine, treat, and transport him, apply oxygen (if appropriate), transport promptly, and follow local protocols.

3. This patient could be having a heart attack. A common symptom that women (especially postmenopausal women) experience when having a heart attack is the sudden onset of generalized weakness. Although chest pain is a common indicator of heart attack, if a patient is not experiencing pain or pressure, it does not necessarily mean that he or she is not experiencing a cardiac event. It is important to note that heart disease is the number-one killer of women in the United States, taking more lives than cancer and killing more women than men every year. If your patient exhibits any combination of the "associated symptoms" of heart attack, such as nausea; vomiting; shortness of breath; pain or numbness in the neck, jaw, back, or arm(s); or cool, pale, sweaty skin, you should suspect the possibility of a heart attack. You should apply oxygen (if appropriate), obtain vital signs, allow the patient to maintain a position of comfort, and provide immediate transport to the nearest appropriate facility.

Fill-in-the-Patient Care Report

EMS Patient Care Report (PCR)

Date: Today's date	Incident No.: 011543	Nature of Call: Chest pain	Location: 1574 S. Main St.

Dispatched: 1901	En Route: 1901	At Scene: 1909	Transport: 1921	At Hospital: 1926	In Service: 1935

Patient Information

Age: 58 years Sex: Male Weight (in kg [lb]): Unknown	Allergies: Aspirin Medications: Lisinopril, nitroglycerin, metformin, and metoprolol Past Medical History: Hypertension, angina, and diabetes Chief Complaint: Chest tightness

Vital Signs

Time: 1914	BP: 136/88	Pulse: 88	Respirations: 22	SpO$_2$: 99%
Time: 1921	BP: 122/74	Pulse: 84	Respirations: 18	SpO$_2$: 98%

EMS Treatment
(circle all that apply)

Oxygen @ 15 L/min via (circle one): NC NRM BVM	Assisted Ventilation	Airway Adjunct	CPR
Defibrillation	Bleeding Control	Bandaging	Splinting	Other:

Narrative

9-1-1 dispatch for 58-year-old man complaining of chest pain. Arrived on scene and was met by the patient's wife at the front door, who stated that the patient has been experiencing chest pain for approximately 30 minutes with no relief from two nitroglycerin tablets. We were directed to the living room, where we found our patient sitting up on the couch, with some obvious shortness of breath. Patient stated that he was sitting on the couch when he began to feel "incredible constant pressure" in his chest. Patient stated that he initially thought it was his angina but reported that "this feels different." Patient currently rates pain as a 5/10. Oxygen was applied at 15 L/min via a nonrebreathing mask. Primary and secondary assessment performed, along with vital signs. Per local protocol, because the patient's systolic blood pressure was above 100 mm Hg, one tablet of nitroglycerin was administered sublingually to the patient. The patient was secured to a stretcher and taken to unit. Patient was transported to local facility. Reassessment of patient indicated his pain was now a 4/10. On arrival at facility, patient was stable. Care was transferred to ED staff. Verbal report was given to staff. No further incidents. Unit cleaned and restocked. Crew went available and returned to station.**End of Report**

Skills

Skill Drills

Skill Drill 17-1: Administration of Nitroglycerin (page 698)

1. Obtain an order from **medical control**. Take the patient's blood pressure. Administer **nitroglycerin** only if the **systolic** blood pressure is greater than 100 mm Hg.

2. Check the medication and expiration date. Ask the patient about the last dose he or she took and its **effects**. Make sure that the patient understands the route of **administration**. Prepare to have the patient lie down to prevent **fainting**.

3. Ask the patient to lift his or her **tongue**. Place the tablet or spray the dose under the **tongue** (while wearing gloves), or have the patient do so. Have the patient keep his or her mouth **closed** with the tablet or spray under the tongue until it is dissolved and absorbed. Caution the patient against **chewing** or swallowing the tablet.

4. Recheck the blood pressure within **5** minutes. Record each medication and the time of administration. Reevaluate the **chest pain** and blood pressure, and repeat treatment, if necessary.

Skill Drill 17-3: Using an AED (pages 711–712)

1. Take standard precautions. Determine scene safety. Question bystanders. Determine responsiveness. Assess compression effectiveness if CPR is already in progress. If the patient is unresponsive and CPR has not been started yet, begin providing chest compressions and rescue breaths at a rate of 30 compressions to two breaths and a rate of 100 to 120 compressions per minute, continuing until an AED arrives and is ready for use.

2. Turn on the AED. Apply the AED pads to the chest and attach the pads to the AED.

3. Push the Analyze button, if there is one, and wait for the AED to determine whether a shockable rhythm is present. Stop CRP when the AED instructs you to.

4. If a shock is advised, state aloud, "Clear the patient," and ensure that no one is touching the patient. Reconfirm that no one is touching the patient and push the Shock button. Continue CPR for five cycles (2 minutes) after the shock is delivered.

5. After five cycles (2 minutes) of CPR, pause CPR and allow the AED to analyze the rhythm. If shock is advised, clear the patient, push the Shock button, and immediately resume CPR compressions. If no shock is advised, immediately resume CPR compressions, and be sure to switch rescuers. Repeat the cycle of five cycles (2 minutes) of CPR, one shock (if indicated), and 2 minutes of CPR. Transport, and contact medical control as needed.

Assessment Review

1. B   (pages 676–677; Introduction)
2. A   (pages 693–695; History Taking)
3. D   (pages 692–693; Primary Assessment)
4. C   (pages 693–695; History Taking)
5. B   (pages 703–704; Heart Surgeries and Cardiac Assistive Devices)

Neurologic Emergencies

General Knowledge

Matching

1. M (pages 729–730; Hemorrhagic Stroke)
2. N (page 730; Left Hemisphere)
3. D (pages 732–733; Seizures)
4. O (pages 724–725; Anatomy and Physiology)
5. K (pages 724–725; Anatomy and Physiology)
6. E (pages 724–725; Anatomy and Physiology)
7. H (page 735; The Postictal State)
8. B (pages 725–726; Pathophysiology, page 736; Hypoglycemia)
9. F (pages 734–735; The Importance of Recognizing Seizures)
10. L (pages 747–748; Stroke)
11. A (page 735; The Postictal State)
12. C (pages 732–733; Seizures)
13. I (pages 732–733; Seizures)
14. J (pages 747–748; Stroke)
15. G (page 730; Transient Ischemic Attack)

Multiple Choice

1. D (pages 732–733; Seizures)
2. A (pages 724–725; Anatomy and Physiology)
3. A (pages 724–725; Anatomy and Physiology)
4. C (page 736; Causes of Altered Mental Status)
5. C (pages 728–729; Ischemic Stroke)
6. A (pages 729–730; Hemorrhagic Stroke)
7. B (pages 729–730; Hemorrhagic Stroke)
8. B (pages 728–729; Ischemic Stroke)
9. D (page 730; Transient Ischemic Attack)
10. A (page 736; Hypoglycemia)
11. D (pages 725–726; Pathophysiology)
12. A (pages 734–735; The Importance of Recognizing Seizures)
13. D (page 733; Table 18-2 Common Causes of Seizures)
14. C (page 736; Causes of Altered Mental Status)
15. B (page 736; Hypoglycemia)
16. C (page 733; Causes of Seizures)
17. C (pages 726–727; Headache)
18. A (pages 726–727; Headache)
19. B (pages 3729–730; Hemorrhagic Stroke)
20. D (pages 726–727; Headache)
21. A (page 731; Conditions That May Mimic Stroke)
22. B (pages 738–739; Primary Assessment)
23. C (page 730; Transient Ischemic Attack)
24. C (pages 738–739; Primary Assessment)
25. B (pages 741–744; Stroke Assessment)
26. D (pages 741–744; Stroke Assessment)
27. B (page 730; Left Hemisphere)
28. A (pages 728–729; Ischemic Stroke)
29. D (pages 745–747; Emergency Medical Care)

True/False

1. T (page 735; The Postictal State)
2. T (pages 725–726; Pathophysiology)
3. T (page 733; Causes of Seizures)
4. F (page 735; The Postictal State)
5. T (pages 726–727; Headache)
6. F (pages 724–725; Anatomy and Physiology)
7. T (pages 726–727; Headache)
8. T (pages 728–729; Ischemic Stroke)
9. F (pages 728–729; Ischemic Stroke)
10. T (pages 730–731; Right Hemisphere)
11. F (pages 729–730; Hemorrhagic Stroke)
12. F (pages 732–733; Seizures)

13. T (pages 734–735; The Importance of Recognizing Seizures)

14. T (page 736; Hypoglycemia)

15. T (page 736; Hypoglycemia)

16. T (page 737; Other Causes of Altered Mental Status)

17. T (pages 737–738; Patient Assessment)

18. F (pages 744–745; Reassessment)

19. F (pages 744–745; Reassessment)

20. T (pages 741–744; Stroke Assessment)

Fill-in-the-Blank

1. 12 (page 725; Anatomy and Physiology)

2. cerebellum (page 725; Anatomy and Physiology)

3. ischemic, hemorrhagic (page 728; Types of Stroke)

4. oxygen, glucose, temperature (pages 725–726; Pathophysiology)

5. carbon monoxide poisoning (page 726; Headache)

6. focal-onset aware (page 732; Seizures)

7. opposite (page 725; Anatomy and Physiology)

8. temporal (page 732; Seizures)

9. Incontinence (page 732; Seizures)

10. epileptic seizures (page 733; Causes of Seizures)

11. postictal state (page 735; The Postictal State)

12. hemiparesis (page 735; The Postictal State)

13. foreign body obstruction (page 738; Primary Assessment)

14. Glasgow Coma Scale (page 745; Stroke Assessment)

15. Thrombolytic therapy (page 748; Stroke)

Labeling

1. Brain (page 725; Figure 18-1)

  A. Cerebrum

  B. Skull

  C. Brainstem

  D. Cerebellum

  E. Spinal cord

2. Spinal Cord (page 726; Figure 18-2)

  A. Cerebrum

  B. Cerebellum

  C. Brainstem

  D. Foramen magnum

  E. Spinal cord

  F. Spinal nerves

Critical Thinking

Short Answer

1. **1.** Facial droop—Ask patient to show teeth or smile.

  Normal: Both sides of the face move equally well.

  Abnormal: One side of the face does not move as well as the other.

  2. Arm drift—Ask patient to close eyes and hold arms out with palms up.

  Normal: Both arms move the same, or both arms do not move.

  Abnormal: One arm does not move, or one arm drifts down compared to the other side.

  3. Speech—Ask patient to say, "The sky is blue in Cincinnati."

  Normal: Patient uses correct words with no slurring.

  Abnormal: Patient slurs words, uses inappropriate words, or is unable to speak. (page 742; Table 18-4 Cincinnati Prehospital Stroke Scale)

2. New therapies for stroke are available but must be used as soon as possible after the start of symptoms. You should minimize time on the scene, and notify the receiving hospital as soon as possible. (pages 747–748; Stroke)

3. A period of time after a seizure, generally lasting from 5 to 30 minutes, in which a patient is unresponsive at first and gradually regains consciousness. The postictal state is over when the patient regains a complete return of his or her normal level of consciousness. The patient will likely appear dazed, confused, and fatigued. (page 735; The Postictal State)

4. A focal seizure begins in one part of the brain and is classified as aware or impaired-awareness. In a focal-onset aware seizure, there is no change in mental status. Patients may complain of numbness, weakness, or dizziness. The patient may report sensory disturbances. A focal-onset aware seizure may also cause twitching of the muscles and extremities that may spread slowly from one part of the body to another, but it is not characterized by the dramatic, severe twitching and muscle movements seen in a generalized seizure. In a focal-onset impaired-awareness seizure, the patient has an altered mental status and does not interact normally with his or her environment. This type of seizure results from abnormal discharges from the temporal lobe of the brain. Other characteristics may be lip smacking, eye blinking, and isolated convulsions or jerking of the body or one part of the body, such as an arm. (pages 732–733; Seizures)

5. 1. Hypoglycemia

   2. Postictal state

   3. Subdural or epidural bleeding (page 731; Conditions That May Mimic Stroke)

6. A. Eye Opening—4—Patient is looking at you.

    Verbal—4—Patient is confused about the date/year.

    Motor—5—Patient does not respond to commands, localized to pain.

    Total: 13

  B. Eye Opening—2—Patient opens eyes to painful stimulus.

    Verbal—2—Patient uses incomprehensible sounds.

    Motor—4—Patient withdraws to pain.

    Total: 8

  C. Eye Opening—1—Patient does not open eyes to any stimuli.

    Verbal—1—Patient has no verbal response.

    Motor—1—Patient does not move extremities to any stimuli.

    Total: 3

  D. Eye Opening—4—Patient is looking at you.

    Verbal—5—Patient is able to have an oriented conversation.

    Motor—6—Patient is able to follow commands.

    Total: 15 (page 745; Table 18-7 Glasgow Coma Scale)

Ambulance Calls

1. Given these signs, your patient is likely experiencing a left hemispheric stroke. Any problems related to his ability to understand or use language will be frustrating for both you and the patient. After performing your primary assessment, the Cincinnati Prehospital Stroke Scale can provide valuable information regarding the presence of a stroke. This assessment measures abnormalities in speech and the presence of facial droop and arm drift. Stroke is a true emergency that requires prompt transport. You should apply oxygen to maintain an SpO_2 of at least 94% and take care during transport to prevent injury of affected body parts because the patient will not be able to protect them on his own. It is helpful to place the patient on the affected side and elevate his head approximately 6 inches (15 cm) to facilitate swallowing. Be sure to relate your positive findings of stroke to the hospital to avoid any unnecessary delays in patient care on arrival to the emergency department.

2. Maintain the airway—assist ventilations with high-flow oxygen, if needed. Consider placement of an oral or nasal airway.

   Suction, if necessary, or position lateral recumbent to clear secretions.

   Check glucose level.

   Provide rapid transport.

3. This patient's signs and symptoms cause you to suspect the presence of a hemorrhagic stroke. You should consider applying oxygen (if appropriate) and provide immediate transport. This patient will be more likely to experience seizure activity than patients suffering from ischemic stroke. There is no way for you to determine the type or extent of her stroke because this can be accomplished only in the hospital. Your job is to recognize the seriousness of the situation, provide supportive measures within your scope of practice, provide prompt transport, and notify the receiving facility.

4. When a patient who experienced a seizure wants to refuse EMS care, the following questions need to be discussed and/or considered:

   1. Is the patient awake and completely oriented after the seizure (Glasgow Coma Scale score of 15)?
   2. Does your assessment show no evidence of trauma or complications from the seizure?
   3. Has the patient ever had a seizure before?
   4. Was this seizure the "usual" seizure in every way (length, activity, recovery)?
   5. Is the patient currently being treated with medications and receiving regular evaluations by a physician?

      If the answer to all of these questions is yes, you may consider agreeing to the patient's refusal for transport if the patient can be released to a responsible person and monitored. However, if the answer is no to any of these questions, you should strongly encourage the patient to be transported and evaluated.

Skills

Assessment Review

1. C (page 742; Table 18-4 Cincinnati Prehospital Stroke Scale)

2. B (page 731; Conditions That May Mimic Stroke)

3. A (pagess 747–748; Stroke)

4. C (page 730; Transient Ischemic)

Gastrointestinal and Urologic Emergencies

General Knowledge

Matching

1. I (pages 765–766; Other Organ Systems)
2. D (pages 758–759; Pathophysiology)
3. E (page 756; Anatomy and Physiology)
4. M (pages 760–761; Ulcers)
5. K (pages 765–766; Other Organ Systems)
6. A (pages 758–759; Pathophysiology)
7. C (pages 768–770; Secondary Assessment)
8. J (pages 764–765; Kidneys)
9. F (pages 758–759; Pathophysiology)
10. B (pages 759–760; Abdominal Pain)
11. G (pages 758–759; Pathophysiology)
12. N (page 758; Urinary System)
13. L (pages 765–766; Other Organ Systems)
14. O (pages 758–759; Pathophysiology)
15. H (pages 758–759; Pathophysiology)
16. F (page 760; Table 19-1 Common Abdominal Conditions)
17. B (page 760; Table 19-1 Common Abdominal Conditions)
18. J (page 760; Table 19-1 Common Abdominal Conditions)
19. I (page 760; Table 19-1 Common Abdominal Conditions)
20. E (page 760; Table 19-1 Common Abdominal Conditions)
21. A (page 760; Table 19-1 Common Abdominal Conditions)
22. D (page 760; Table 19-1 Common Abdominal Conditions)
23. H (page 760; Table 19-1 Common Abdominal Conditions)
24. C (page 760; Table 19-1 Common Abdominal Conditions)
25. G (page 760; Table 19-1 Common Abdominal Conditions)

Multiple Choice

1. B (pages 758–759; Pathophysiology)
2. A (pages 768–770; Secondary Assessment)
3. A (pages 765–766; Other Organ Systems)
4. B (page 763; Mallory-Weiss Tear)
5. D (pages 768–770; Secondary Assessment)
6. A (page 760; Table 19-1 Common Abdominal Conditions)
7. B (page 756; Anatomy and Physiology)
8. C (page 761; Pancreatitis)
9. B (page 761; Gallstones)
10. D (page 760; Table 19-1 Common Abdominal Conditions)
11. B (page 762; Esophageal Varices)
12. A (page 768; History Taking)
13. D (page 760; Table 19-1 Common Abdominal Conditions)
14. A (pages 764–765; Kidneys)
15. A (page 770; Reassessment)
16. C (pages 756–757; The GI System)
17. B (page 758; Urinary System)
18. D (pages 758–759; Pathophysiology)
19. C (page 764; Hemorrhoids)
20. A (pages 763–764; Gastroenteritis)
21. C (page 762; Gastrointestinal Hemorrhage)
22. B (page 762; Esophagitis)
23. C (pages 761–762; Appendicitis)
24. A (pages 768–770; Secondary Assessment)
25. D (pages 771–772; Dialysis Emergencies)

26. C   (pages 756–757; The GI System)
27. B   (page 758; The Urinary System)
28. C   (pages 757–758; Additional Abdominal Organs)

29. D   (page 758; Figure 19-2)
30. C   (pages 756–757; The GI System)

True/False

1. F   (pages 759–760; Abdominal Pain)
2. T   (pages 771–772; Dialysis Emergencies)
3. F   (page 768; History Taking)
4. T   (page 768; History Taking)
5. T   (pages 758–759; Pathophysiology)

6. F   (pages 758–759; Pathophysiology)
7. F   (pages 768–770; Secondary Assessment)
8. T   (pages 765–766; Other Organ Systems)
9. T   (pages 760–764; Causes of Acute Abdomen)
10. F   (page 770; Reassessment)

Labeling

1. Solid Organs (page 756; Figure 19-1 A)

    A. Liver

    B. Spleen

    C. Pancreas

    D. Kidney

    E. Kidney

    F. Ovaries

2. Hollow Organs (page 756; Figure 19-1 B)

    A. Gallbladder

    B. Stomach

    C. Ureter

    D. Small intestine

    E. Large intestine

    F. Fallopian tubes

    G. Urinary bladder

    H. Uterus

3. Urinary System (page 758; Figure 19-2)

    A. Kidney

    B. Ureter

    C. Bladder

    D. Prostate gland

    E. Ureter opening

    F. Urethra

    G. Penis

    H. External urethral opening

Critical Thinking

Short Answer

1. Occurs because of connections between the body's two nervous systems. The abdominal organs are supplied by autonomic nerves that, when irritated, stimulate close-lying sensory (somatic) nerves. (pages 759–760; Abdominal Pain)

2. 1. Has the patient's level of consciousness changed?

    2. Has the patient become more anxious?

    3. Have the skin signs started to change?

    4. Has the pain gotten better or worse?

    5. Has the bleeding become worse or better?

    6. Is current treatment improving the patient's condition?

    7. Has an already-identified problem gotten better or worse?

    8. What is the nature of any newly identified problems? (page 770; Reassessment)

3. Paralysis of muscular contractions in the bowel results in retained gas and feces. Nothing can pass through. (pages 758–759; Pathophysiology)

4. 1. Explain to the patient what you are going to do in terms of assessing the abdomen.

   2. Place the patient in a supine position with the legs drawn up and flexed at the knees to relax the abdominal muscles, unless there is any trauma, in which case the patient will remain supine and stabilized. Determine whether the patient is restless or quiet and whether motion causes pain.

   3. Expose the abdomen and visually assess it. Does the abdomen appear distended (enlarged)? Do you see any pulsating masses? Is there bruising to the abdominal wall? Are there any surgical scars?

   4. Ask the patient where the pain is most intense. Palpate in a clockwise direction, beginning with the quadrant after the one the patient indicates is tender or painful; end with the quadrant that the patient indicates is tender and painful. If the most painful area is palpated first, the patient may guard against further examination, making your assessment more difficult and less reliable.

   5. Remember to be very gentle when palpating the abdomen.

   6. Palpate the four quadrants of the abdomen gently to determine whether each quadrant is tense (guarded) or soft when palpated.

   7. Note whether the pain is localized to a particular quadrant or diffuse (widespread).

   8. Palpate and wait for the patient to respond, looking for a facial grimace or a verbal "ouch." Do not ask the patient "Does it hurt here?" as you palpate.

   9. Determine whether the patient exhibits rebound tenderness.

   10. Determine whether the patient can relax the abdominal wall on command. Guarding and rigidity may be detected. (pages 768–770; Secondary Assessment)

Ambulance Calls

1. Appendicitis is a possibility. Place the patient in a position of comfort. Consider applying oxygen, if appropriate. Keep the patient warm, and be prepared to manage shock. Provide rapid transport. Obtain a SAMPLE history. Document OPQRST. Monitor the patient closely.

2. This patient is likely experiencing a bowel obstruction, secondary to an ileus, that is causing his pain and tenderness. If left untreated, his condition will deteriorate. When assessing his abdomen, explain what you will do, place him with knees slightly toward his abdomen, and gently palpate all four quadrants to determine the presence of rigidity or masses. If a patient points to a specific location of pain, palpate that area last. You must take great care in moving and transporting the patient because it will be particularly painful if he is bumped or jostled. Apply oxygen (if necessary), allow him to find a position of comfort, and move him gently. Do not delay transport to attempt to determine the cause of the abdominal pain.

3. Individuals who have experienced a kidney stone(s) will tell you that it is an extremely painful experience. Provide prompt, gentle transport. Monitor his airway, breathing, and circulation. Be prepared for continued vomiting. Apply low-flow oxygen (which can ease nausea), obtain vital signs, do not give anything by mouth, and keep the patient as comfortable as possible. Be sure to thoroughly document all information regarding the patient's signs and symptoms, as well as any treatment you provide. Always follow local protocols.

Skills

Assessment Review

1. D (pages 767–768; Primary Assessment)
2. A (page 768; History Taking)
3. B (page 768; History Taking)
4. A (pages 768–770; Secondary Assessment)
5. D (page 770; Reassessment)

CHAPTER

20 Endocrine and Hematologic Emergencies

General Knowledge

Matching

1. J (pages 778–780; Endocrine Emergencies: Anatomy and Physiology)
2. A (pages 793–794; Sickle Cell Disease)
3. C (pages 782–784; Diabetes Mellitus Type 1)
4. M (pages 801–802; Vital Vocabulary)
5. O (pages 778–780; Endocrine Emergencies: Anatomy and Physiology)
6. Q (pages 784–785; Symptomatic Hyperglycemia)
7. F (pages 782–784; Diabetes Mellitus Type 1)
8. G (page 795; Thrombophilia)
9. D (pages 782–784; Diabetes Mellitus Type 1)

10. B (pages 793–796; Hematologic Emergencies)
11. P (pages 778–780; Endocrine Emergencies: Anatomy and Physiology)
12. E (pages 782–784; Diabetes Mellitus Type 1)
13. L (pages 780–781; Endocrine Emergencies: Pathophysiology)
14. K (pages 780–781; Endocrine Emergencies: Pathophysiology)
15. H (pages 782–784; Diabetes Mellitus Type 1)
16. N (pages 794–795; Hemophilia)
17. I (page 784; Diabetes Mellitus Type 2)

Multiple Choice

1. A (pages 782–784; Diabetes Mellitus Type 1)
2. A (pages 782–784; Diabetes Mellitus Type 1)
3. D (pages 793–794; Sickle Cell Disease)
4. C (pages 780–781; Endocrine Emergencies: Pathophysiology)
5. C (page 798; Emergency Medical Care for Hematologic Disorders)
6. A (pages 782–784; Diabetes Mellitus Type 1)
7. C (pages 782–784; Diabetes Mellitus Type 1)
8. D (pages 780–781; Endocrine Emergencies: Anatomy and Physiology)
9. D (page 781; Figure 20-3)
10. A (pages 778–780; Endocrine Emergencies: Anatomy and Physiology)
11. B (page 781; Table 20-1 Hyperglycemia Versus Hypoglycemia)
12. D (page 795; Thrombophilia)
13. D (page 784; Table 20-2 Common Oral Medications Used to Treat Type 2 Diabetes)

14. A (page 791; Giving Oral Glucose)
15. A (pages 780–781; Endocrine Emergencies: Anatomy and Physiology)
16. A (pages 782–784; Diabetes Mellitus Type 1)
17. C (pages 782–784; Diabetes Mellitus Type 1)
18. A (page 796; Patient Assessment of Hematologic Disorders: Primary Assessment)
19. B (pages 785–786; Symptomatic Hypoglycemia)
20. D (pages 785–786; Symptomatic Hypoglycemia)
21. C (page 792; The Presentation of Hypoglycemia: Seizures)
22. A (pages 782–784; Diabetes Mellitus Type 1)
23. B (pages 792–793; Misdiagnosis of Neurologic Dysfunction)
24. C (page 796; Primary Assessment)
25. D (page 781; Table 20-1 Hyperglycemia Versus Hypoglycemia)
26. B (pages 796–797; Patient Assessment of Hematologic Disorders: History Taking)

27. D (pages 795–796; Deep Vein Thrombosis)
28. D (page 797; Reassessment)
29. D (pages 785–786; Symptomatic Hypoglycemia)
30. D (pages 788–791; Reassessment)
31. C (pages 785–786; Symptomatic Hypoglycemia)
32. C (pages 785–786; Symptomatic Hypoglycemia)

True/False

1. T (pages 782–784; Diabetes Mellitus Type 1)
2. F (pages 793–794; Pathophysiology: Sickle Cell Disease)
3. T (pages 785–786; Symptomatic Hypoglycemia)
4. T (pages 782–784; Diabetes Mellitus Type 1)
5. F (pages 794–795; Hemophilia)
6. T (pages 780–781; Endocrine Emergencies: Pathophysiology)
7. T (pages 782–784; Diabetes Mellitus Type 1)
8. F (pages 778–780; Endocrine Emergencies: Anatomy and Physiology)
9. F (pages 795–796; Deep Vein Thrombosis)
10. T (pages 780–781; Endocrine Emergencies: Pathophysiology)
11. T (pages 782–784; Diabetes Mellitus Type 1)
12. F (page 793; Blood and Its Parts)
13. T (page 784; Diabetes Mellitus Type 2)

Fill-in-the-Blank

1. diabetes mellitus (pages 793–794; Endocrine Emergencies: Pathophysiology)
2. Thrombophilia (page 795; Thrombophilia)
3. autoimmune (page 782; Diabetes Mellitus Type 1)
4. Mediterranean, sickle cell (page 793; Patient Assessment of Hematologic Disorders: Primary Assessment)
5. impaired (page 780; Endocrine Emergencies: Pathophysiology)
6. HHNS (page 785; Symptomatic Hyperglycemia)
7. Hematology, related (page 793; Hematologic Emergencies)
8. sugar, insulin (page 781; Table 20-1 Hyperglycemia Versus Hypoglycemia)

Fill-in-the-Table (page 781; Table 20-1 Hyperglycemia Versus Hypoglycemia)

	Hyperglycemia	Hypoglycemia
History		
Onset	Gradual (hours to days)	Rapid, within minutes
Skin	Warm and dry	Pale, cool, and moist
Infection	Common	Uncommon
Gastrointestinal Tract		
Thirst	Intense	Absent
Hunger	Present and increasing	Absent
Vomiting/abdominal pain	Common	Uncommon
Respiratory System		
Breathing	With DKA there are rapid, deep (Kussmaul) respirations	Normal; may become shallow or ineffective if hypoglycemia is severe and mental status is depressed
Odor of breath	With DKA there may be a sweet, fruity odor	Normal

Cardiovascular System		
Blood pressure	Normal to low	Normal to low
~~Pulse~~	~~Rapid, weak, and thready~~	~~Rapid and weak~~
Nervous System		
Consciousness	Restlessness, possibly progressing to coma; abnormal or slurred speech; unsteady gait	Irritability, confusion, seizure, or coma; unsteady gait
Treatment		
Response	Gradual, within 6 to 12 hours following medical treatment	Immediate improvement after administration of glucose

Critical Thinking

Multiple Choice

1. B   (pages 782–784; Diabetes Mellitus Type 1)
2. C   (page 791; Giving Oral Glucose)
3. D   (page 791; Giving Oral Glucose)
4. D   (page 791; Giving Oral Glucose)

Short Answer

1. Insulin is a hormone that enables glucose to enter the cells, which is essential for cellular metabolism. (pages 778–780; Endocrine Emergencies: Anatomy and Physiology)

2. 1. Dissolving gel

   2. Chewable tablet

   3. Liquid (page 791; Giving Oral Glucose)

3. Due to the oblong shape of the red blood cells, they are poor oxygen carriers and can become lodged in blood vessels and organs. (page 794; Sickle Cell Disease)

4. A patient who is unconscious or unable to swallow should not be given oral glucose. (page 791; Giving Oral Glucose)

5. A patient with thrombophilia has a tendency to develop clots in the blood vessels. These clots can travel through the circulatory system and become lodged in the lungs, obstructing blood flow and oxygen exchange. (page 795; Thrombophilia, pages 795–796; Deep Vein Thrombosis)

6. 1. Hyperglycemia

   2. Altered mental status, drowsiness, lethargy

   3. Severe dehydration, thirst, dark urine

   4. Visual or sensory deficits

   5. Partial paralysis or muscle weakness

   6. Seizures (pages 784–785; Symptomatic Hyperglycemia)

7. 1. Do you take insulin or any pills that lower your blood sugar?

   2. Do you wear an insulin pump? Is it working properly?

   3. Have you taken your usual dose of insulin (or pills) today?

   4. Have you eaten normally today?

   5. Have you had any illness, unusual amount of activity, or stress? (page 787; Patient Assessment of Diabetes: History Taking)

8. Hypoglycemia; it develops rapidly as opposed to hyperglycemia, which takes longer to develop. (page 785; Symptomatic Hypoglycemia)

Ambulance Calls

1. 1. Turn the patient on her side immediately or use suction to clear the airway.

   2. Insert an oral or nasal airway and support ventilations with a bag-mask device attached to oxygen.

   3. Attempt to obtain a blood glucose level.

   4. Transport the patient rapidly because you should never give anything by mouth to an unresponsive patient.

   5. Monitor the patient closely.

2. The prehospital management of patients suffering from sickle cell crises will commonly include only comfort care and rapid transportation. You may also treat individual symptoms as they arise as per standard protocol. For example, a sickle cell patient presenting with difficulty breathing should receive oxygen therapy or ventilatory assistance if required.

3. You cannot give this patient anything by mouth because he is unconscious and therefore unable to protect his own airway. If available, you should request ALS providers because they can administer intravenous dextrose (glucose). If you have no emergency providers available with this scope of practice within your system, you must transport this patient immediately. You may encounter family members who do not understand why you cannot "just give him some sugar." Hopefully, there will be no delays in explaining his need for transport or the seriousness of his condition. Perform a thorough assessment (including blood glucose testing, if permitted), provide oxygen, monitor his ABCs (using airway adjuncts, positive pressure ventilations, and suctioning, as needed), and provide prompt transport.

Fill-in-the-Patient Care Report

EMS Patient Care Report (PCR)			
Date: Today's date	**Incident No.**: 2011-1234	**Nature of Call**: Laceration	**Location**: 12556 Old Lake House Drive
Dispatched: 1752	**En Route**: 1755	**At Scene**: 1803	**Transport**: 1813	**At Hospital**: 1819	**In Service**: 1839

Patient Information	
Age: 14 years **Sex**: Male **Weight (in kg [lb])**: 60 kg (132 lb)	**Allergies**: Unknown **Medications**: Unknown **Past Medical History**: Hemophilia **Chief Complaint**: Bleeding laceration

Vital Signs				
Time: 1813	**BP**: 108/60	**Pulse**: 98	**Respirations**: 16/GTV	**SpO$_2$**: 96%

EMS Treatment
(circle all that apply)

Oxygen @ _15_ L/min via (circle one): NC (NRM) BVM	Assisted Ventilation	Airway Adjunct	CPR
Defibrillation	(Bleeding Control)	(Bandaging: Tourniquet)	Splinting	(Other: Shock Treatment)

Narrative

9-1-1 dispatch for an arm laceration with uncontrolled bleeding. Arrived on scene and was directed to a second-floor bedroom, where the patient, a 14-year-old boy, was holding pressure on a left forearm laceration. Patient's mother advised that he had hemophilia. Observed steady bleeding and attempted to control with pressure. Initiated oxygen therapy at 15 L/min via a nonrebreathing mask and used the stair chair to move the patient down to the gurney, where he was covered with blankets to conserve body temperature and loaded into the ambulance. Obtained vitals, which indicated that the patient might be hypoperfusing. Because steady pressure didn't stop the bleeding, applied a tourniquet proximal to the laceration, which did stop the bleeding. Monitored the patient while en route to the hospital, continued oxygen therapy, and notified the facility of our impending arrival. Delivered the patient to the trauma department, gave a full report to the charge nurse, transferred patient care, and returned to service after cleaning/decontaminating the ambulance.**End of Report**

Allergy and Anaphylaxis

General Knowledge

Matching

1. D (pages 804–806; Pathophysiology)
2. A (pages 804–806; Pathophysiology)
3. H (pages 804–806; Pathophysiology)
4. E (pages 804–806; Pathophysiology)
5. B (pages 804–806; Pathophysiology)
6. G (pages 804–806; Pathophysiology)
7. C (pages 806–808; Insect Stings)
8. F (pages 806–808; Insect Stings)

Multiple Choice

1. B (page 815; Skill Drill 21-1 Using an EpiPen Auto-Injector)
2. D (page 806; Common Allergens)
3. B (pages 804–806; Pathophysiology)
4. B (pages 806–807; Insect Stings)
5. C (pages 811–812; Reassessment)
6. C (pages 811–812; Reassessment)
7. D (pages 809–810; History Taking)
8. C (page 813; Administering an Epinephrine Auto-Injector)
9. D (page 813; Epinephrine)
10. C (pages 806–807; Insect Stings)
11. A (pages 812–813; Emergency Medical Care of Immunologic Emergencies)
12. D (pages 808–809; Primary Assessment)
13. C (page 806; Common Allergens)
14. A (pages 808–809; Primary Assessment)

True/False

1. T (pages 804–806; Pathophysiology)
2. T (pages 804–806; Pathophysiology)
3. F (pages 804–806; Pathophysiology)
4. T (pages 808–809; Primary Assessment)

Fill-in-the-Blank

1. expiration (pages 804–806; Pathophysiology)
2. urticaria (pages 804–806; Pathophysiology)
3. barbed (page 807; Insect Stings)
4. anaphylaxis (pages 804–806; Pathophysiology)
5. circulatory compromise (page 813; Table 21-2 Epinephrine)
6. blood vessels (page 813; Epinephrine)

Critical Thinking

Multiple Choice

1. C (pages 804–806; Pathophysiology)
2. B (pages 804–806; Pathophysiology)
3. D (pages 813–814; Administering an Epinephrine Auto-Injector)
4. A (page 813; Skill Drill 21-1 Using an EpiPen Auto-Injector)
5. D (pages 813–814; Administering an Epinephrine Auto-Injector)

Short Answer

1. Increased blood pressure, tachycardia, pallor, dizziness, chest pain, headache, nausea, vomiting, anxiety, sweating, and palpitations (page 813; Table 21-2 Epinephrine)

2. 1. Insect bites and stings
    2. Medications
    3. Plants
    4. Food
    5. Chemicals (page 806; Common Allergens)

3. 1. Obtain an order from medical control (or follow protocol or standing orders).
    2. Follow standard precautions.
    3. Make sure the medication was prescribed for that patient.
    4. Check for discoloration or expiration of medication.
    5. Remove the cap and wipe the thigh with alcohol, if possible.
    6. Place the tip of the auto-injector against the lateral part of the thigh.
    7. Push firmly until activation.
    8. Hold the auto-injector in place until the medication is injected (3 seconds).
    9. Remove and dispose.
    10. Rub the area for 10 seconds.
    11. Record the time and dose.
    12. Reassess and record the patient's vital signs.
    13. Consider an additional administration (if possible) in 5 minutes if symptoms do not improve. (pages 813–814; Administering an Epinephrine Auto-Injector)

4. **Respiratory:** Shortness of breath (dyspnea); sneezing or itchy, runny nose; chest or throat tightness; dry cough; hoarseness; rapid, noisy, or labored respirations; wheezing and/or stridor

    Circulatory: Decreased blood pressure (hypotension), increased pulse (tachycardia), pale skin, loss of consciousness and coma (page 810; Table 21-1 Additional Signs and Symptoms of an Allergic Reaction)

Ambulance Calls

1. Based on the information you have, there is no way to determine if the child fell out of the tree or climbed down. You should assume that the child fell, which will require you to consider full spinal precautions. You also have the issue of scene safety because the damaged hive is now lying on the ground next to the patient. You must take care not to receive multiple stings yourself, so proceed with caution. If the child is having a severe allergic reaction, hopefully you will have access to an EpiPen Junior. Provide oxygen (if appropriate) and prompt transport according to local protocols.

2. Obtain a physician's order to administer the EpiPen to the patient (if required by local protocol). Check the EpiPen for clarity, expiration date, and so on. Administer the EpiPen and promptly dispose of the auto-injector. Apply high-flow oxygen and provide rapid transport. Monitor the patient and assess vital signs frequently.

Fill-in-the-Patient Care Report

EMS Patient Care Report (PCR)			
Date: Today's date	**Incident No.:** 2011-0101	**Nature of Call:** Allergic reaction	**Location:** 231 Seaside Parkway
Dispatched: 1734	**En Route:** 1734	**At Scene:** 1742	**Transport:** 1748 **At Hospital:** 1801 **In Service:** 1814

Patient Information	
Age: 37 years **Sex:** Male **Weight (in kg [lb]):** 63 kg (138 lb)	**Allergies:** Possible seafood **Medications:** N/A **Past Medical History:** N/A **Chief Complaint:** Allergic reaction

Vital Signs

Time: 1748	BP: 110/64	Pulse: 116	Respirations: 26 Labored	SpO$_2$: 92%
Time: 1755	BP: 140/94	Pulse: 128	Respirations: 18 Adequate Tidal Volume	SpO$_2$: 96%

EMS Treatment
(circle all that apply)

Oxygen @ _15_ L/min via (circle one): NC (NRM) (BVM)	(Assisted Ventilation)	Airway Adjunct	CPR
Defibrillation	Bleeding Control	Bandaging	Splinting (Other: Shock Treatment)

Narrative

Requested for an emergency response to a seafood restaurant for anaphylactic reaction. Arrived and led to patient—37-year-old man—who presented with generalized swelling of the face, neck, and hands; hives; and difficulty breathing. It was immediately apparent that the patient was becoming hypoxic, so we initiated oxygen therapy and requested an ALS rendezvous. We then began transport of the patient, and initial vitals indicated that the patient was anaphylactic. We began to assist ventilations with a bag-mask device until rendezvous with ALS crew. Paramedic Johnson boarded ambulance and administered epinephrine, and patient responded to treatment quickly. A second set of vitals confirmed reversal of anaphylaxis. We provided a verbal report and ETA to the receiving facility, and the rest of the transport was without incident. On arrival at the facility, the patient was appropriately turned over to the receiving staff after we provided a complete verbal report to the charge nurse.
End of Report

Skills

Skill Drill

Skill Drill 21-1: Using an EpiPen Auto-injector (page 815)

1. Remove the **auto-injector's** safety cap, and quickly wipe the thigh with **antiseptic**, if possible.

2. Place the **tip** of the auto-injector against the **lateral** part of the thigh. Push the auto-injector **firmly** against the thigh until a **click** is heard. Hold it in place until all of the **medication** has been injected (3 seconds).

3. Rub the area for **10** seconds.

Assessment Review

1. A (pages 808–809; Primary Assessment)
2. C (pages 813–814; Administering an Epinephrine Auto-Injector)
3. D (pages 813–814; Administering an Epinephrine Auto-Injector)

Toxicology

General Knowledge

Matching

1. F (pages 822–824; Identifying the Patient and the Poison)
2. H (pages 822–824; Identifying the Patient and the Poison)
3. G (pages 824–830; How Poisons Enter the Body)
4. D (pages 834–843; Specific Poisons)
5. J (pages 842–843; Cholinergic Agents)

6. I (pages 822–824; Identifying the Patient and the Poison)
7. K (pages 834–835; Alcohol)
8. E (page 839; Stimulants)
9. B (pages 836–837; Opiates and Opioids)
10. A (pages 834–835; Alcohol)
11. C (page 842; Anticholinergic Agents)

Multiple Choice

1. B (page 833; Emergency Medical Care)
2. B (pages 822–824; Identifying the Patient and the Poison)
3. C (page 846; Plant Poisoning)
4. C (pages 842–843; Cholinergic Agents)
5. A (pages 822–824; Identifying the Patient and the Poison)
6. A (pages 829–830; Injected Poisons)
7. C (page 833; Emergency Medical Care)
8. B (pages 834–835; Alcohol)
9. C (pages 836–837; Opiates and Opioids)
10. D (pages 837–838; Sedative-Hypnotic Drugs)
11. A (page 842; Anticholinergic Agents)
12. C (pages 839–840; Sympathomimetics)
13. A (pages 842–843; Cholinergic Agents)
14. B (pages 843–845; Food Poisoning)
15. A (pages 838–839; Abused Inhalants)
16. D (pages 839–840; Sympathomimetics)
17. C (pages 840–841; Synthetic Cathionones (Bath Salts))
18. A (page 841; Marijuana)
19. B (pages 839–840; Sympathomimetics)

20. D (pages 826–827; Inhaled Poisons)
21. C (pages 826-827; Inhaled Poisons)
22. B (pages 827–828; Absorbed and Surface Contact Poisons)
23. C (pages 829–830; Injected Poisons)
24. D (page 839; Hydrogen Sulfide)
25. A (pages 829–830; Injected Poisons)
26. B (pages 834–835; Alcohol)
27. D (pages 834–835; Alcohol)
28. A (pages 826–827; Inhaled Poisons)
29. C (pages 826–827; Inhaled Poisons)
30. A (pages 828–829; Ingested Poisons)
31. D (pages 836–837; Opiates and Opioids)
32. A (pages 826–827; Inhaled Poisons)
33. D (pages 836–837; Opiates and Opioids)
34. C (page 833; Emergency Medical Care)
35. C (page 833; Emergency Medical Care)
36. B (page 833; Emergency Medical Care)
37. C (page 833; Emergency Medical Care)
38. B (page 833; Emergency Medical Care)
39. D (page 843; Miscellaneous Drugs)
40. B (page 843; Miscellaneous Drugs))

True/False

1. T (page 833; Emergency Medical Care)
2. F (page 833; Emergency Medical Care)
3. F (page 833; Emergency Medical Care)
4. T (pages 826–827; Inhaled Poisons)
5. F (page 833; Emergency Medical Care)
6. T (page 824; Table 22-1 Typical Signs and Symptoms of Specific Overdoses)

7. T (pages 842–843; Cholinergic Agents)
8. F (pages 834–835; Alcohol)
9. T (page 836; Table 22-2 Common Opioids and Opiates)
10. T (pages 839–840; Sympathomimetics)
11. T (pages 834–835; Alcohol)
12. T (page 846; Plant Poisoning)

Fill-in-the-Blank

1. botulism (pages 843–845; Food Poisoning)
2. Bath salts (pages 840–841; Synthetic Cathionones (Bath Salts))
3. Substance abuse (pages 822–824; Identifying the Patient and the Poison)
4. 15 to 20 (pages 827–828; Absorbed and Surface Contact Poisons)
5. respiratory depression (pages 836–837; Opiates and Opioids)
6. hypoglycemia (pages 834–835; Alcohol)
7. recognize (page 824; Identifying the Patient and the Poison)

8. 1 gram, kilogram (page 833; Emergency Medical Care)
9. outward (pages 827–828; Absorbed and Surface Contact Poisons)
10. ingestion (pages 828–829; Ingested Poisons)
11. delirium tremens (pages 834–835; Alcohol)
12. DuoDote Auto-Injector (pages 842–843; Cholinergic Agents)
13. addiction (pages 834–843; Specific Poisons)
14. Hypovolemia (pages 834–835; Alcohol)

Fill-in-the-Table (page 824; Table 22-1 Typical Signs and Symptoms of Specific Overdoses)

Table 22-1 Typical Signs and Symptoms of Specific Overdoses

Agent	Signs and Symptoms
Opiates (Examples: morphine, codeine) Opioids (Examples: heroin, fentanyl, methadone, oxycodone)	• Hypoventilation or respiratory arrest • **Pinpoint pupils** • Sedation or coma • **Hypotension**
Sympathomimetics (Examples: mephedrone, cocaine, methamphetamine)	• Hypertension • **Tachycardia** • Dilated pupils • Agitation or seizures • **Hyperthermia**
Sedative-hypnotics (Examples: diazepam, secobarbital, flunitrazepam, midazolam)	• **Slurred speech** • Sedation or coma • Hypoventilation • **Hypotension**

Anticholinergics (Examples: atropine, diphenhydramine, chlorpheniramine, doxylamine, *Datura stramonium* [jimson weed])	• **Tachycardia** • **Hyperthermia** • Hypertension • Dilated pupils • **Dry skin and mucous membranes** • Sedation, agitation, seizures, coma, or delirium • **Decreased bowel sounds**

Cholinergics (Examples: organophosphates, pilocarpine, nerve gas)	• Airway compromise
	• SLUDGEM
	  • S **Salivation, sweating**
	  • L **Lacrimation (excessive tearing of the eyes)**
	  • U **Urination**
	  • D **Defecation, drooling, diarrhea**
	  • G **Gastric upset and cramps**
	  • E **Emesis**
	  • M **Muscle twitching, miosis (pinpoint pupils)**

Critical Thinking

Short Answer

1. Activated charcoal adsorbs (binds to) the toxin and keeps it from being absorbed in the gastrointestinal tract. (page 833; Emergency Medical Care)

2. 1. Ingestion
   2. Inhalation
   3. Injection
   4. Absorption (surface contact) (pages 824–830; How Poisons Enter the Body)

3. Hypertension, tachycardia, paranoia, and dilated pupils, along with irritability, agitation, anxiety, restlessness, or seizures (pages 839–840; Sympathomimetics)

4. 1. The organism itself causes the disease.
   2. The organism produces toxins that cause disease. (pages 843–845; Food Poisoning)

5. Symptoms of acetaminophen overdose do not appear until the damage is irreversible, up to a week later. Finding evidence at the scene can save a patient's life. (page 843; Miscellaneous Drugs)

6. They describe patient presentation in cholinergic poisoning (ie, organophosphate insecticides, wild mushrooms).

   DUMBELS: Diarrhea, urination, miosis/muscle weakness, bradycardia/bronchospasm/bronchorrhea, emesis, lacrimation, salivation/seizures/sweating

   SLUDGEM: Salivation/sweating, lacrimation, urination, defecation/drooling/diarrhea, gastric upset/cramps, emesis, muscle twitching/miosis (pages 842–843; Cholinergic Agents)

7. **1.** What substance did you take?

2. When did you take it or become exposed to it?

3. How much did you ingest or were exposed to?

4. How long ago did you take it or were exposed?

5. What actions have been taken? Did it help?

6. How much do you weigh? (pages 822–824; Identifying the Patient and the Poison)

Ambulance Calls

1. You should attempt to identify the substance. Some rat poisons are actually blood-thinning agents or anticoagulants, such as warfarin. You should collect the substance and call the poison control center and/or the hospital emergency department for patient care instructions. Some substances require the administration of activated charcoal, whereas others do not. Perform your initial assessment, start oxygen (if appropriate), and provide prompt transport. Know your local protocols.

2. This patient potentially abuses alcohol and illegal substances. However, you cannot automatically assume that his decrease in mentation is directly related to alcohol intoxication or the influence of other substances. He may have other medical conditions, which may mimic intoxication or even be obscured by it. You should perform a thorough assessment, take his vital signs, monitor his ABCs (because these could change at any time), and transport him to the nearest appropriate medical facility for evaluation. It is also important to be aware of the possibility of used needles when performing assessments and/or removing clothing when visualizing any potential injuries. Protect yourself.

3. Maintain the airway with an adjunct and high-flow oxygen via a bag-mask device or a nonrebreathing mask with 100% oxygen. Monitor vital signs and provide supportive measures and rapid transport. Take the pill bottle along to the emergency department. Be alert for possible vomiting, monitor the patient closely, and be prepared for the possible need for CPR.

Skills

Assessment Review

1. C   (pages 822–824; Identifying the Patient and the Poison)

2. B   (page 842; Anticholinergic Agents)

3. B   (pages 843–845; Food Poisoning)

4. B   (pages 839–840; Sympathomimetics)

5. A   (page 833; Emergency Medical Care)

Behavioral Health Emergencies

General Knowledge

Matching

1. I   (pages 862–863; Acute Psychosis)
2. F   (page 863; Schizophrenia)
3. J   (page 864; Excited Delirium)
4. D   (pages 855–856; Defining a Behavioral Crisis)
5. G   (page 856; The Magnitude of Mental Health Disorders)

6. A   (pages 855–856; Defining a Behavioral Crisis)
7. E   (page 857; Functional)
8. H   (pages 855–856; Defining a Behavioral Crisis)
9. C   (pages 855–856; Defining a Behavioral Crisis)
10. B   (page 857; Organic)

Multiple Choice

1. C   (pages 859–860; History Taking)
2. B   (pages 854–855; Myth and Reality)
3. D   (pages 854–855; Myth and Reality)
4. B   (pages 855–856; Defining a Behavioral Crisis)
5. C   (pages 855–856; Defining a Behavioral Crisis)
6. B   (pages 855–856; Defining a Behavioral Crisis)
7. D   (pages 878–879; Vital Vocabulary)
8. C   (page 857; Organic)
9. B   (page 857; Organic)
10. C   (page 857; Functional)
11. B   (pages 861–862; Reassessment)
12. D   (page 858; Table 23-1 Safety Guidelines for a Behavioral Health Emergency)
13. B   (page 857; Scene Size-up)

14. A   (page 864; Excited Delirium)
15. B   (page 870; Table 23-3 Risk Factors for Suicide)
16. A   (pages 869–871; Suicide)
17. A   (page 864; Excited Delirium)
18. C   (pages 873–874; Medicolegal Considerations)
19. C   (pages 864–865; Risks Associated With Patient Restraint)
20. B   (pages 865–866; The Process of Restraining a Patient)
21. D   (page 857; Scene Size-up)
22. A   (page 857; Scene Size-up)
23. A   (pages 859–860; History Taking)
24. B   (pages 855–856; The Process of Restraining a Patient)

True/False

1. F   (pages 854–855; Myth and Reality)
2. T   (page 857; Organic)
3. F   (pages 865–866; Restraint)
4. F   (page 857; Words of Wisdom)
5. T   (page 858; Table 23-1 Safety Guidelines for a Behavioral Health Emergency)
6. F   (page 869; Suicide)
7. T   (pages 874–875; Special Populations)
8. F   (pages 854–855; Myth and Reality)
9. T   (pages 866–867; Performing Patient Restraint)
10. F   (pages 865–866; The Process of Restraining a Patient)

11. F   (pages 865–866; The Process of Restraining a Patient)
12. T   (pages 865–866; The Process of Restraining a Patient)
13. T   (pages 860–861; Secondary Assessment)
14. T   (pages 858–859; Primary Assessment)
15. F   (pages 871–873; Posttraumatic Stress Disorder and Returning Combat Veterans)
16. T   (pages 871–873; Signs and Symptoms of PTSD)
17. F   (page 874; Limited Legal Authority)

Fill-in-the-Blank

1. Behavior (page 855; Defining a Behavioral Crisis)
2. behavioral health emergency (page 855; Defining a Behavioral Crisis)
3. depression (page 855; Defining a Behavioral Crisis)
4. Organic brain syndrome (page 854; Organic)
5. suicide (page 869; Suicide)
6. schizophrenia (page 863; Schizophrenia)
7. law enforcement (page 858; Table 23-1 Safety Guidelines for a Behavioral Health Emergency)
8. implied consent (page 873; Consent)
9. Dissociative PTSD (page 872; Signs and Symptoms of PTSD)
10. minimum (page 864; Restraint)

Critical Thinking

Short Answer

1. 1. Improper functioning of the central nervous system
   2. Hallucinogens/drugs or alcohol
   3. Significant life changes, symptoms, or illness caused by a mental disorder (pages 859–860; History Taking)

2. 1. The degree of force necessary to keep the patient from injuring self or others
   2. The patient's gender, size, strength, and mental status (including drug-induced states)
   3. The type of abnormal behavior the patient is exhibiting (pages 865–867; The Process of Restraining a Patient)

3. 1. Assess the scene.
   2. Ensure that you have a means of communication.
   3. Know where the exits are.
   4. Don personal protective equipment.
   5. Have a definite plan of action.
   6. Urgently deescalate the patient's level of agitation.
   7. Calmly identify yourself.
   8. Be direct.
   9. Be prepared to spend extra time.
   10. Stay with the patient.
   11. Do not get too close to a potentially volatile patient.
   12. Express interest in the patient's story.
   13. Avoid fighting with the patient.
   14. Be honest and reassuring.
   15. Do not judge. (page 858; Table 23-1 Safety Guidelines for a Behavioral Health Emergency)

4. 1. Depression at any age
   2. Previous suicide attempt
   3. Current expression of wanting to commit suicide or sense of hopelessness
   4. Specific plan for suicide
   5. Family history of suicide
   6. Age older than 40 years, particularly for single, widowed, divorced, alcoholic, or depressed individuals
   7. Recent loss of spouse, significant other, family member, or support system

8. Chronic debilitating illness or recent diagnosis of serious illness

9. Feeling anxious, agitated, angry, reckless, or aggressive

10. Financial setback, loss of job, police arrest, imprisonment, or some sort of social embarrassment

11. Alcohol or substance abuse, particularly with increasing usage

12. Children of an alcoholic or abusive parent

13. Withdrawal from family and friends or a lack of social support, resulting in isolation

14. Significant anniversaries of sentinel events

15. Unusual gathering or new acquisition of things that can cause death, such as purchase of a gun or a large volume of pills (page 870; Table 23-3 Risk Factors for Suicide)

5. A technique used by mental health professionals to gain insight into a patient's thinking. It involves repeating, in question form, what the patient has said, encouraging the patient to expand on the thoughts. (pages 859–860; History Taking)

6. 1. History

   2. Posture

   3. The scene

   4. Vocal activity

   5. Physical activity (pages 868–869; The Potentially Violent Patient)

Ambulance Calls

1. Removing restraints (especially when the patient has a known history of recent violence) is ill-advised and potentially against local protocols. Restraints, although uncomfortable, afford you and your patient a safe environment. You should continually monitor the restraints to ensure that they are not too tight and that no manner of restraints (whether applied initially by you in the field or by hospital personnel for an interfacility transport) affects the patient's ability to breathe. Know your local laws regarding the use of restraints and your local protocols for appropriate use and discontinuation.

2. Although he tells you that he is fine, you cannot simply walk away. Those individuals who contemplate suicide often tell people they are "fine." With information passed along by his sister, you must take action. Because there is no evidence that the patient has tried to harm himself and he did not express directly to you that he intends to, you must use persuasive techniques to gain consent to treatment and transport. If the patient refuses, consider contacting law enforcement for assistance.

3. Be understanding and listen. Explain to the patient that she needs medical care. Monitor vital signs and reassure the patient en route.

Skills

Assessment Review

1. D   (pages 868–869; The Potentially Violent Patient)
2. A   (pages 868–869; The Potentially Violent Patient)
3. C   (pages 868–869; The Potentially Violent Patient)
4. B   (pages 868–869; The Potentially Violent Patient)
5. A   (pages 868–869; The Potentially Violent Patient)

CHAPTER

24 Gynecologic Emergencies

General Knowledge

Matching

1. G (pages 882–883; Anatomy and Physiology)
2. E (pages 882–883; Anatomy and Physiology)
3. K (pages 882–883; Anatomy and Physiology)
4. B (pages 882–883; Anatomy and Physiology)
5. H (pages 882–883; Anatomy and Physiology)
6. A (pages 882–883; Anatomy and Physiology)
7. D (pages 882–883; Anatomy and Physiology)
8. C (page 885; Sexually Transmitted Diseases)
9. F (pages 884–885; Pelvic Inflammatory Disease)
10. J (page 885; Sexually Transmitted Diseases)
11. I (page 885; Sexually Transmitted Diseases)

Multiple Choice

1. D (pages 885–886; Vaginal Bleeding)
2. B (page 885; Sexually Transmitted Diseases)
3. B (pages 890–893; Sexual Assault and Rape)
4. B (pages 882–883; Anatomy and Physiology)
5. D (pages 884–885; Pelvic Inflammatory Disease)
6. A (page 885; Sexually Transmitted Diseases)
7. C (page 885; Sexually Transmitted Diseases)
8. B (page 886; Primary Assessment)
9. C (page 887; History Taking)
10. A (page 885; Sexually Transmitted Diseases)
11. A (pages 890–893; Sexual Assault and Rape)
12. C (pages 890–893; Sexual Assault and Rape)
13. D (pages 890–893; Sexual Assault and Rape)
14. A (pages 890–893; Sexual Assault and Rape)
15. C (pages 890–893; Sexual Assault and Rape)
16. A (pages 890–893; Sexual Assault and Rape)
17. C (pages 890–893; Sexual Assault and Rape)
18. D (pages 890–893; Sexual Assault and Rape)

True/False

1. T (page 885; Sexually Transmitted Diseases)
2. T (page 885; Sexually Transmitted Diseases)
3. F (pages 885–886; Vaginal Bleeding)
4. T (page 886; Primary Assessment)
5. T (page 886; Primary Assessment)
6. F (page 887; History Taking)
7. T (page 887; History Taking)
8. F (pages 887–889; Secondary Assessment)
9. T (pages 887–889; Secondary Assessment)
10. F (page 889; Emergency Medical Care)
11. T (pages 887–889; Secondary Assessment)
12. T (page 889; Words of Wisdom)
13. F (pages 885–886; Vaginal Bleeding)
14. F (pages 890–893; Sexual Assault and Rape)
15. T (page 889; Emergency Medical Care)

Fill-in-the-Blank

1. ovaries (pages 882–883; Anatomy and Physiology)
2. puberty (pages 882–883; Anatomy and Physiology)
3. Pelvic inflammatory disease (page 885; Sexually Transmitted Diseases)
4. Gynecologic emergencies (page 886; Scene Size-up)
5. Ectopic pregnancy, spontaneous abortion (pages 885–886; Vaginal Bleeding)
6. external pads (pages 887–889; Secondary Assessment)
7. Vaginal bleeding (page 889; Reassessment)
8. law enforcement (pages 890–893; Sexual Assault and Rape)
9. gonorrhea (page 885; Sexually Transmitted Diseases)
10. menopause (pages 882–883; Anatomy and Physiology)

Labeling

1. Female Reproductive System (page 882; Figure 24-2)

   A. Uterine (fallopian) tube

   B. Uterus

   C. Ovary

   D. Cervix

   E. Vagina

2. External Genitalia (page 882; Figure 24-1)

   A. Labia minora

   B. Labia majora

   C. Urethra

   D. Vaginal orifice

   E. Perineum

   F. Anus

Critical Thinking

Short Answer

1. Where or in what position is the patient found?

   What is the condition of the residence? Clean, filthy, or wrecked? Is there evidence of a fight?

   Are alcohol, tobacco products, or drug paraphernalia present?

   Are there pictures of loved ones? Is there a noticeable absence of pictures? Does the patient live alone or with other people? (page 886; Scene Size-up)

2. 1. Painful urination

   2. Burning or itching

   3. Yellowish or bloody discharge associated with a foul odor

   4. Blood associated with vaginal intercourse

   5. Cramping and abdominal pain

   6. Nausea and vomiting

   7. Bleeding between menstrual periods (page 885; Sexually Transmitted Diseases)

3. Use external pads to control bleeding. Keep the patient warm, place her in a supine position, and provide her with supplemental oxygen, even if she is not experiencing any difficulty breathing. Provide prompt transport to the hospital, and reassess her vital signs every 5 minutes. (page 889; Emergency Medical Care)

Ambulance Calls

1. The patient is most likely suffering from pelvic inflammatory disease (PID). A patient with PID will complain of abdominal pain. The pain is typically described as "achy" and can be worse with walking. Other symptoms include vaginal discharge, fever and chills, and pain or burning on urination.

   Prehospital treatment is limited to supportive care, and nonemergency transport is usually recommended. Place the patient in a position of comfort and monitor vital signs. Consider oxygen (if appropriate). Keep in mind that although this condition is typically not an emergency, these patients require monitoring for any signs of deterioration.

2. The first issue is the medical treatment of the patient. You should assess and treat life threats and inquire about pain. The second issue focuses on the psychological care of the patient. Many women report feeling violated when subjected to interrogation, so do not cross-examine the patient or pass judgment on her during the assessment. Take the patient's history, and limit any physical examination to a brief survey for life-threatening injuries. Keep in mind that this patient has been through a traumatic experience, and your compassion for her will help to gain the patient's confidence. Limit the number of people involved in the assessment/examination process to protect the patient's privacy and dignity. Remember that you are at a crime scene. Do not cut through any clothing or throw away anything from the scene. Place bloodstained articles in a separate paper bag. You should gently persuade the patient to refrain from cleaning herself, urinating, changing clothes, moving her bowels, or rinsing her mouth because this could potentially destroy evidence.

   When documenting this incident, keep the report concise and record only what the patient stated in her own words. Use quotations marks to indicate that you are reporting the patient's version of the events. Refrain from inserting your own opinion into the documentation. Record all of your observations during the physical exam, including the patient's emotional state, the condition of her clothing, obvious injuries, and so forth.

Fill-in-the-Patient Care Report

EMS Patient Care Report (PCR)			
Date: Today's date	**Incident No.:** 011689	**Nature of Call:** Assault	**Location:** 538 N. 10th Street, Apartment 4-C
Dispatched: 2101	**En Route:** 2103	**At Scene:** 2109	**Transport:** 2120	**At Hospital:** 2131	**In Service:** 2147

Patient Information	
Age: 32 years **Sex:** Female **Weight (in kg [lb]):** Unknown	**Allergies:** None known **Medications:** lispro, Lantus, lisinopril **Past Medical History:** Diabetes **Chief Complaint:** Pain to the nose, face, and groin

Vital Signs				
Time: 2114	**BP:** 144/98	**Pulse:** 102	**Respirations:** 22	**SpO$_2$:** 98%
Time: 2125	**BP:** 148/92	**Pulse:** 108	**Respirations:** 20	**SpO$_2$:** 97%

EMS Treatment (circle all that apply)			
Oxygen @ 2 L/min via (circle one): (NC) NRM BVM	Assisted Ventilation	Airway Adjunct	CPR
Defibrillation	Bleeding Control	Bandaging	Splinting	Other:

Narrative

9-1-1 dispatch for 32-year-old assault victim. Dispatcher advised that police were already on scene. No other information was provided. On arrival, crew was directed by PD through a well-kept apartment into a dark room where we found our patient. The patient had obvious multiple contusions to her face and appeared to be emotionally upset. When inquired about the incident, the patient blurted out that she was "raped by a maintenance worker here at the apartment complex." The patient initially stated that she was unsure if she wanted to go to the hospital. She stated that she did want to "change her clothes" and "take a shower." Both EMS and PD stated to patient that she could potentially disrupt any evidence and that changing her clothes and showering were not advised. The patient complained of pain to the nose, face, and groin. She denied any bleeding. The patient appeared withdrawn and reluctant to speak with EMS. A female EMT was offered to the patient; however, the patient stated "No." No obvious life threats were noted on minimal exam. The patient was asked about the incident; however, she declined to comment. Due to the patient's status and limited injuries, no further examination was performed at this time. The patient was continuously monitored for any signs of hemorrhaging or deterioration. The patient was loaded into the unit and transported to the local facility. A radio report was carried out by partner/driver. On arrival at the facility, the patient was stable, with no change in status noted. Care was transferred to the ED staff. A verbal report was given to the nurse, with patient privacy precautions taken. No further incidents. Unit cleaned and restocked. Crew available.**End of Report**

CHAPTER

25 | Trauma Overview

General Knowledge

Matching

1. H (pages 901–904; Penetrating Trauma)
2. G (page 904; MOI Profiles)
3. F (pages 901–904; Energy and Trauma)
4. E (pages 901–904; Energy and Trauma)

5. C (pages 901–904; Energy and Trauma)
6. A (page 904; Blunt and Penetrating Trauma)
7. D (page 904; Blunt and Penetrating Trauma)
8. B (pages 901–904; Energy and Trauma)

Multiple Choice

1. B (page 901; Introduction)
2. C (pages 901–904; Energy and Trauma)
3. C (pages 901–904; Energy and Trauma)
4. B (pages 901–904; Energy and Trauma)
5. D (pages 911–912 ; Car Versus Motorcycle)
6. B (pages 904–911; Vehicular Crashes)
7. C (pages 904–911; Vehicular Crashes)
8. D (pages 924–926; Type of Transport)
9. C (pages 901–904; Penetrating Trauma)
10. A (pages 904–911; Vehicular Crashes)
11. C (page 901; Introduction)
12. B (pages 904–911; Vehicular Crashes)
13. D (pages 917–918; Tissues at Risk)
14. A (pages 904–911; Vehicular Crashes)
15. A (pages 915–918; Blast Injuries)
16. B (pages 907–909; Frontal Crashes)

17. B (pages 919–920; Golen Principles of Prehospital Trauma Care)
18. B (pages 904–911; Vehicular Crashes)
19. C (pages 910–911; Rollover Crashes)
20. B (pages 912–913; Falls)
21. C (pages 904–911; Vehicular Crashes)
22. A (pages 904–911; Vehicular Crashes)
23. B (pages 904–911; Vehicular Crashes)
24. A (page 901; Introduction)
25. C (page 903; Words of Wisdom)
26. A (page 9; Table 25-2 Key Elements for Trauma Centers)
27. B (pages 911–912; Car Versus Motorcycle)
28. D (pages 917–918; Blast Injuries)
29. D (pages 917–918; Tissues at Risk)
30. C (pages 920–921; Injuries to the Neck and Throat)

True/False

1. T (pages 901–904; Energy and Trauma)
2. F (pages 901–904; Energy and Trauma)
3. F (pages 901–904; Energy and Trauma)
4. T (page 909; Rear-End Crashes)
5. T (page 921; Injuries to the Chest)
6. T (pages 912–913; Falls)
7. T (page 901; Introduction)
8. F (pages 919–920; Golden Principles of Prehospital Trauma Care)

9. T (page 910; Lateral Crashes)
10. F (page 909; Rear-End Crashes)
11. T (page 911; Car Versus Pedestrian)
12. F (pages 911–912; Car Versus Motorcycle)
13. F (pages 915–918; Blast Injuries)
14. T (page 920; Injuries to the Head)
15. T (page 921; Injuries to the Chest)

Fill-in-the-Blank

1. doubles, quadruples (page 902; Energy and Trauma)
2. Penetrating trauma (page 904; Blunt and Penetrating Trauma)
3. coup-contrecoup (page 905; Vehicular Crashes)
4. KE = ½ m × V² (page 902; Energy and Trauma)
5. rear-end (page 909; Rear-End Crashes)
6. deceleration (page 907; Frontal Crashes)
7. Multisystem (pages 918–919; Multisystem Trauma)
8. lateral (page 910; Lateral Crashes)
9. ejection (page 910; Rollover Crashes)
10. solid (page 921; Injuries to the Abdomen)
11. Glasgow Coma (page 926; Table 25-3 Glasgow Coma Scale)
12. pneumothorax (page 921; Injuries to the Chest)
13. Platinum 10 (page 922; Scene Time)
14. Newton's first law (page 903; Words of Wisdom)
15. medical (page 901; Introduction)

Fill-in-the-Table (pages 901–904; Penetrating Trauma)

Table 25-1 Recognizing Developing Problems in Trauma Patients

Mechanism of Injury	Signs and Symptoms	Index of Suspicion
Blunt or penetrating trauma to the neck	• **Noisy or labored breathing** • **Increased respiratory rate** • **Swelling of the face or neck** • **Altered gag reflex** • **Decreasing/low Glasgow Coma Scale (GCS); <9 in severe** • **Decreasing/low SpO$_2$** • **Rapid, weak pulse** • **Decreasing/low blood pressure**	• Significant bleeding or foreign bodies in the upper or lower airway, causing obstruction • Be alert for airway compromise.
Significant chest wall trauma from motor vehicle, car-versus-pedestrian, and other crashes; penetrating trauma to the chest wall	• **Significant chest pain** • **Shortness of breath** • **Increased respiratory rate** • **Asymmetrical chest wall movement** • **Subcutaneous emphysema** • **Decreasing GCS (<9 is severe)** • **Decreasing/low SpO$_2$** • **Presence of jugular venous distention** • **Rapid, weak pulse** • **Decreasing/low blood pressure** • **Loss of peripheral pulses during respiration** • **Narrowing pulse pressures**	• Cardiac or pulmonary contusion • Pneumothorax or hemothorax • Broken ribs, causing breathing compromise

Mechanism of Injury	Signs and Symptoms	Index of Suspicion
Any significant blunt force trauma from motor vehicle crashes or penetrating injury	• **Blunt or penetrating trauma to the neck, chest, abdomen, or groin** • **Blows to the head sustained during motor vehicle crashes, falls, or other incidents, producing loss of consciousness, altered mental status, inability to recall events, combativeness, or changes in speech patterns** • **Inability to maintain airway** • **Difficulty moving extremities; headache, especially with nausea and vomiting** • **Decreasing GCS (<9 is severe)** • **Decreasing/low SpO$_2$** • **Rapid, weak pulse** • **Decreasing/low blood pressure or increasing blood pressure with slow pulse**	• Injuries in these regions may tear and cause damage to the large blood vessels located in these body areas, resulting in significant internal and external bleeding. • Be alert to the possibility of bruising to the brain and bleeding in and around the brain tissue, which may cause the development of excess pressure inside the skull around the brain.
Any significant blunt force trauma, falls from a significant height, or penetrating trauma	• **Severe back and/or neck pain, history of difficulty moving extremities, loss of sensation or tingling in the extremities** • **Decreasing GCS (<9 is severe)** • **Rapid, weak pulse or slow pulse**	• Injuries to the bones of the spinal column or to the spinal cord

Critical Thinking

Short Answer

1. Potential energy is the product of mass (weight), force of gravity, and height and is mostly associated with the energy of falling objects. (pages 901–904; Energy and Trauma)

2. **1.** Collision of the car against another car or other object

   2. Collision of the passenger against the interior of the car

   3. Collision of the passenger's internal organs against the solid structures of the body (pages 904–911; Vehicular Crashes)

3. **1.** The height of the fall

   2. The surface struck

   3. The part of the body that hit first, followed by the path of energy displacement (page 910; Falls)

4. A bullet, because of its speed, creates pressure waves that emanate from its path, causing distant damage. (pages 913–915; Penetrating Trauma)

5. The size (mass) and speed (velocity) of the projectile affect the potential damage. If the mass is doubled, the potential energy is doubled. If the velocity is doubled, the potential energy is quadrupled. (pages 901–904; Penetrating Trauma)

6. Lateral chest and abdominal/internal organ injuries on the side of impact; fractures of the lower extremities, pelvis, and ribs; and injuries to the aorta (pages 912–913; Lateral Crashes)

7. The deformity of the motorcycle, the side of most damage, the distance of skid in the road, the deformity of stationary objects or other vehicles, and the extent and location of deformity in the helmet (pages 911–912; Car Versus Motorcycle)

8. A comprehensive regional resource that is a tertiary care facility; capable of providing total care for every aspect of injury, from prevention through rehabilitation (page 923; Table 25-2 Key Elements for Trauma Centers)

Ambulance Calls

1. Given the highway speeds and lack of a shoulder belt and airbag, along with his complaints of head and neck pain, your index of suspicion for head and spinal injuries is very high. It is a positive sign that he is awake and able to communicate; however, this should not encourage you to spend any more time on scene than is necessary to extricate this patient and place him in full spinal precautions. His condition could change at any time, and his inability to remember the details of the event likely indicate the presence of a closed head injury. Provide high-flow oxygen (if appropriate) and prompt transport.

2. Each story is 10 feet (3 m), so this patient fell approximately 20 feet (6 m) from the ladder to the hard ground. He is now unconscious. Assume he has significant head and spinal injuries; determine if he is responsive and manage his airway because he will be unable to protect it. Provide high-flow oxygen and prompt transport to the nearest appropriate facility, taking care not to waste time in determining other injuries.

3. 1. Apply high-flow oxygen.
   2. Stabilize the object in place with bulky dressings.
   3. Monitor his vital signs.
   4. Transport the patient in a supine position. Provide rapid transport due to abdominal penetration.

4. 1. Estimate the speed of the vehicle that struck the patient.
   2. Determine whether the patient was thrown through the air and at what distance.
   3. Determine if the patient was struck and pulled under the vehicle.
   4. Evaluate the vehicle for structural damage that might indicate contact points with the patient and alert you to potential injuries.

CHAPTER

26 | Bleeding

General Knowledge

Matching

1. J   (page 935; Figure 26-2)
2. E   (page 935; The Heart)
3. K   (page 935; The Heart)
4. F   (pages 935–937; Blood Vessels and Blood)
5. C   (page 935; The Heart)
6. H   (page 935; Figure 26-2)
7. B   (pages 938–941; Characteristics of External Bleeding)
8. I   (page 940; Internal Bleeding)

9. M   (pages 951–954; Bleeding From the Nose, Ears, and Mouth)
10. A   (pages 935–937; Signs and Symptoms of Internal Bleeding)
11. D   (pages 938–941; Characteristics of External Bleeding)
12. L   (page 938; External Bleeding)
13. G   (page 938; The Significance of External Bleeding)

Multiple Choice

1. B   (pages 935–937; Blood Vessels and Blood)
2. D   (page 934; Anatomy and Physiology of the Cardiovascular System)
3. C   (page 935; The Heart)
4. C   (page 935; Figure 26-2)
5. B   (page 935; Figure 26-2)
6. A   (pages 935–937; Blood Vessels and Blood)
7. B   (pages 935–937; Blood Vessels and Blood)
8. D   (pages 935–937; Blood Vessels and Blood)
9. C   (pages 935–937; Blood Vessels and Blood)
10. B   (page 937; Pathophysiology and Perfusion)
11. C   (page 937; Pathophysiology and Perfusion)
12. C   (pages 935–937; Blood Vessels and Blood)
13. A   (pages 935–937; Blood Vessels and Blood)
14. D   (page 937; Pathophysiology and Perfusion)
15. A   (page 955; Emergency Medical Care for Internal Bleeding, page 946; Emergency Medical Care for External Bleeding)
16. B   (page 938; The Significance of External Bleeding)
17. B   (page 938; The Significance of External Bleeding)
18. A   (page 938; The Significance of External Bleeding)

19. C   (page 938; The Significance of External Bleeding)
20. C   (pages 938–941; Characteristics of External Bleeding)
21. A   (pages 942–943; History Taking)
22. B   (pages 938–941; Characteristics of External Bleeding)
23. C   (pages 944–946; Emergency Medical Care for External Bleeding)
24. A   (pages 944–946; Emergency Medical Care for External Bleeding)
25. A   (pages 944–946; Emergency Medical Care for External Bleeding)
26. C   (page 951; Splints, page 951; Pelvic Binder)
27. B   (page 940; Internal Bleeding)
28. D   (page 940; Nature of Illness for Internal Bleeding)
29. D   (pages 940–941; Signs and Symptoms of Internal Bleeding)
30. A   (pages 935–937; Signs and Symptoms of Internal Bleeding)
31. C   (pages 935–937; Signs and Symptoms of Internal Bleeding)

True/False

1. F (pages 938–941; Characteristics of External Bleeding)
2. F (page 938; The Significance of External Bleeding)
3. F (page 947; Skill Drill 26-1 Controlling External Bleeding)
4. T (page 947; Skill Drill 26-1 Controlling External Bleeding)
5. F (pages 949–951; Tourniquets)
6. T (pages 949–951; Tourniquets)
7. F (pages 944–946; Emergency Medical Care for External Bleeding)
8. F (pages 949–951; Tourniquets)
9. T (page 944; Reassessment)

Fill-in-the-Blank

1. right (page 935; Figure 26-2)
2. Perfusion (page 937; Pathophysiology and Perfusion)
3. bruise (page 940; Internal Bleeding)
4. Internal (page 940; Internal Bleeding)
5. 100 (page 944; Secondary Assessment)
6. Hematemesis (page 941; Signs and Symptoms of Internal Bleeding)
7. Capillary (page 939; Characteristics of External Bleeding)
8. autonomic nervous (page 936; Blood Vessels and Blood)
9. Capillaries (page 935; Blood Vessels and Blood)
10. heart (page 935; The Heart)

Labeling

1. The Left and Right Sides of the Heart (page 935; Figure 26-2 A and B)

   A. Left pulmonary artery
   B. Aorta
   C. Superior vena cava
   D. Right pulmonary artery
   E. Right atrium
   F. Inferior vena cava
   G. Right ventricle
   H. Right pulmonary veins
   I. Oxygen-rich blood to head and upper body
   J. Aorta
   K. Left pulmonary veins
   L. Left atrium
   M. Left ventricle
   N. Oxygen-rich blood to lower body

2. Perfusion (page 937; Figure 26-5)

   A. Artery
   B. Arterioles
   C. Capillaries
   D. Organ or tissue
   E. Capillaries
   F. Venules
   G. Vein

Critical Thinking

Multiple Choice

1. C (pages 949–951; Tourniquets)
2. D (pages 949–951; Tourniquets)
3. D (pages 951–954; Bleeding From the Nose, Ears, and Mouth)
4. B (pages 951–954; Bleeding From the Nose, Ears, and Mouth)
5. B (pages 938–941; Characteristics of External Bleeding)

Short Answer

1. It redirects blood away from nonessential organs to the heart, brain, lungs, and kidneys. (pages 935–937; Blood Vessels and Blood)

2. **Artery:** Bright red, spurting

   Vein: Dark color with steady flow

   Capillary: Darker color, oozes (pages 938–941; Characteristics of External Bleeding)

3. 1. Direct pressure and elevation

   2. Pressure dressings

   3. Tourniquets

   4. Hemostatic agent/splints (page 945; Figure 26-8)

4. 1. Tachycardia

   2. Weakness, fainting, or dizziness on standing or at rest

   3. Thirst

   4. Nausea and vomiting

   5. Cold, moist (clammy) skin

   6. Shallow, rapid breathing

   7. Dull eyes

   8. Slightly dilated pupils, slow to respond to light

   9. Capillary refill in infants and children of more than 2 seconds

   10. Weak, rapid (thready) pulse

   11. Decreasing blood pressure

   12. Altered level of consciousness (pages 935–937; Signs and Symptoms of Internal Bleeding)

5. 1. Follow standard precautions.

   2. Maintain the airway with cervical spine immobilization (if needed).

   3. Administer high-flow oxygen and provide artificial ventilation as necessary.

   4. Control all obvious external bleeding.

   5. Treat suspected internal bleeding in an extremity by applying a splint.

   6. Depending on local protocols, use a pelvic compression device or splint to control suspected internal bleeding from the pelvic area.

   7. Monitor and record the patient's vital signs at least every 5 minutes.

   8. Keep the patient warm.

   9. Give nothing by mouth, not even small sips of water.

   10. Provide prompt transport for all patients with signs and symptoms of hypoperfusion. Report changes in condition to the emergency department. (page 955; Emergency Medical Care for Internal Bleeding)

Ambulance Calls

1. Control bleeding with direct pressure, a pressure dressing, and a tourniquet if the previous steps are not effective. Consider applying oxygen (if needed), and place the patient in a position of comfort. Monitor the patient's vital signs, and provide rapid transport.

2. You must control bleeding through direct pressure, pressure dressings, and a tourniquet, as needed. You must also transport the amputated portion of the limb with the patient to the hospital. Quickly attempt to determine how much blood has been lost and assess his skin and vital signs because

these will provide accurate indicators of the significance of blood loss. Place the patient in a position of comfort, consider applying oxygen as necessary, and provide prompt transport.

3. This is an isolated injury that, depending on the severity of the injury to the antecubital vein, can result in significant blood loss. Attempt to control the bleeding through direct pressure, pressure dressings, and a tourniquet, as needed. Something as benign as a pen can cause significant damage in the hands of a determined person.

Fill-in-the-Patient Care Report

EMS Patient Care Report (PCR)					
Date: Today's date	**Incident No.:** 2010-123	**Nature of Call:** Laceration		**Location:** 1467 Abner Lane	
Dispatched: 1653	**En Route:** 1653	**At Scene:** 1658	**Transport:** 1710	**At Hospital:** 1715	**In Service:** 1735

Patient Information	
Age: 42 years **Sex:** Male **Weight (in kg [lb]):** 77 kg (170 lb)	**Allergies:** Amoxicillin **Medications:** Crestor **Past Medical History:** TIA—1 year ago **Chief Complaint:** Laceration to lower left leg

Vital Signs				
Time: 1704	**BP:** 136/86	**Pulse:** 88 strong/regular	**Respirations:** 16 GTV	**SpO$_2$:** 97%
Time: 1710	**BP:** 122/76	**Pulse:** 102 weak/regular	**Respirations:** 20 shallow	**SpO$_2$:** 94%

EMS Treatment (circle all that apply)				
Oxygen @ ___ L/min via (circle one): NC NRM BVM		**Assisted Ventilation**	**Airway Adjunct**	**CPR**
Defibrillation	⟨Bleeding Control⟩	⟨Bandaging⟩	Splinting	⟨Other: Shock treatment⟩

Narrative
Dispatched for a leg laceration. Arrived on scene to find the patient, a 42-year-old man, on the back deck of his home. He was conscious and alert, had a patent airway, and was breathing with good tidal volume. The patient was holding a blood-soaked shirt on his lower leg and was sitting in a large pool of blood. Patient stated that he had been chopping wood when the axe blade bounced off the wood and struck his leg. I immediately applied direct pressure using a large sterile dressing and manually elevated the patient's leg. I then applied a pressure dressing to maintain bleeding control. We obtained the patient's vitals. The patient's skin was found to be pale, cool, and diaphoretic. The patient's wife disclosed the patient history of TIA (1 year ago), amoxicillin allergy, and current Crestor use. We placed the patient onto the gurney, covered him with a blanket, placed him in a position of comfort, and moved him into the ambulance. I continued to monitor the patient's condition while en route. He remained conscious and alert, but vital sign trending indicated possible hypoperfusion. I checked the pressure dressing and found that bleeding was still controlled. Called in report to receiving facility and subsequently delivered the patient without incident. Gave verbal report to the ED charge nurse.**End of Report**

Skills

Skill Drills

Skill Drill 26-1: Controlling External Bleeding (page 947)

1. Take standard **precautions**. Apply **direct pressure** over the wound with a dry, sterile dressing.

2. Apply a **pressure dressing**.

3. If direct pressure with a **pressure dressing** does not control the bleeding, apply a **tourniquet** above the level of the **bleeding**.

4. Tighten the **tourniquet** until bleeding is controlled and **pulses** are no longer palpable **distal** to the tourniquet. Properly position the **patient**. Apply **high-flow oxygen** as necessary. Keep the patient **warm**. Transport promptly.

Skill Drill 26-3: Applying a MAT Commercial Tourniquet (page 950)

1. Apply **pressure** over the bleeding site and place the tourniquet **proximal** to the injury (in the axillary region for upper extremity injuries and at the groin for lower extremity injuries).

2. Click the buckle into place, pull the strap tight, and turn the tightening dial **clockwise** until pulses are no longer palpable **distal** to the tourniquet or until bleeding has been **controlled**.

Assessment Review

1. C (pages 944–946; Emergency Medical Care for External Bleeding)

2. A (page 942; Primary Assessment)

3. B (pages 943–944; Secondary Assessment)

4. D (pages 943–944; Secondary Assessment)

5. C (pages 943–944; Secondary Assessment)

Soft-Tissue Injuries

General Knowledge

Matching

1. G (pagess 963–964; Anatomy)
2. B (pages 963–964; Anatomy)
3. D (pages 963–964; Anatomy)
4. F (pages 963–964; Anatomy)
5. H (pages 963–964; Anatomy)

6. J (pages 966–967; Open Injuries)
7. E (pages 966–967; Open Injuries)
8. A (pages 966–967; Open Injuries)
9. C (pages 966–968; Open Injuries)
10. I (page 977; Abdominal Wounds)

Multiple Choice

1. C (pages 962–964; Anatomy and Physiology of the Skin)
2. B (pages 962–964; Anatomy and Physiology of the Skin)
3. B (pages 963–964; Anatomy)
4. A (pages 963–964; Anatomy)
5. B (page 964; Physiology)
6. C (pages 965–966; Closed Injuries)
7. B (pages 965–966; Closed Injuries)
8. B (pages 965–966; Closed Injuries)
9. C (pages 965–966; Closed Injuries)
10. C (pages 965–966; Closed Injuries)
11. A (page 976; Emergency Medical Care for Closed Injuries)
12. B (pages 966–967; Open Injuries)
13. D (pages 966–967; Open Injuries)
14. C (page 969; Open Injuries)

15. A (pages 966–967; Open Injuries)
16. A (pages 970–971; Scene Size-up)
17. A (page 975; Reassessment)
18. C (page 978; Abdominal Wounds)
19. C (pages 978–979; Neck Injuries)
20. D (page 982; Pathophysiology of Burns)
21. B (pages 983–984; Burn Severity)
22. C (pages 984–985; Depth)
23. B (pages 984–985; Depth)
24. C (pages 984–985; Depth)
25. D (pages 988–989; Burns Secondary Assessment)
26. B (page 986; Burns Scene Size-up)
27. D (pages 994–996; Electrical Burns)
28. A (page 998; Sterile Dressings)
29. A (page 998; Bandages)
30. B (page 982; Pathophysiology of Burns)
31. B (pages 980–981; Small Animal Bites and Rabies)

True/False

1. T (pages 984–985; Depth)
2. F (pages 984–985; Depth)
3. T (pages 984–985; Depth)
4. T (pages 985–986; Extent)
5. T (pages 983–984; Burn Severity)
6. F (pages 987–988; Burns History Taking)
7. F (pages 989–991; Emergency Medical Care for Burns)

8. T (pages 994–996; Electrical Burns)
9. F (pages 965–966; Closed Injuries)
10. T (page 998; Bandages)
11. F (page 998; Bandages)
12. F (page 998; Bandages)
13. T (page 998; Bandages)
14. F (pages 965–966; Closed Injuries)
15. F (page 967; Open Injuries)

Fill-in-the-Blank

1. alpha, beta, gamma (page 996; Radiation Burns)
2. cool (page 964; Physiology)
3. dermis (pages 963–964; Anatomy)
4. crush syndrome (pages 965–966; Closed Injuries)
5. constrict (page 964; Physiology)
6. cheek, chest (page 978; Impaled Objects)
7. Thermal, 111 (page 982; Pathophysiology of Burns)
8. amputation (page 968; Open Injuries)
9. epidermis, dermis (pages 963–964; Anatomy)
10. radiated (page 964; Physiology)

Labeling

1. Skin (page 963; Figure 27-1)

   A. Hair
   B. Pore
   C. Epidermis
   D. Germinal layer of epidermis
   E. Sebaceous gland
   F. Arrector pilli muscle
   G. Dermis
   H. Nerve (sensory)
   I. Sweat gland
   J. Hair follicle
   K. Blood vessel
   L. Subcutaneous fat
   M. Fascia
   N. Subcutaneous tissue
   O. Muscle

2. Rule of Nines (page 985; Figure 27-19)

   A. 9
   B. 18
   C. 9
   D. 18
   E. 9
   F. 12
   G. 18
   H. 18
   I. 1
   J. 9
   K. 18
   L. 18
   M. 18
   N. 9
   O. 18
   P. 9
   Q. 9
   R. 1
   S. 1
   T. 16.5
   U. 16.5
   V. 13.5
   W. 13.5

Critical Thinking

Multiple Choice

1. D   (pages 984–985; Depth)
2. D   (pages 966–970; Open Injuries)
3. C   (page 976; Emergency Medical Care for Closed Injuries)
4. A   (pages 966–970; Open Injuries)
5. B   (pages 976–977; Emergency Medical Care for Open Injuries)

Short Answer

1. 1. Superficial (first degree)
   2. Partial thickness (second degree)
   3. Full thickness (third degree) (pages 984–985; Burns)

2. 1. Closed injuries
   2. Open injuries
   3. Burns (pages 984–985; Depth)

3. **R:** rest

    I: ice

    C: compression

    E: elevation

    S: splinting (page 976; Emergency Medical Care for Closed Injuries)

4. Any full-thickness burn

    Partial-thickness burns covering more than 20% of the body's total surface area (page 986; Table 27-2 Classification of Burns in Infants and Children)

5. Brush off dry chemicals, and then remove the patient's clothing (including shoes, stockings, gloves, jewelry, and eyeglasses) because there may be small amounts of chemicals in the creases. (pages 993–994; Chemical Burns)

6. First, there may be a deep tissue injury not visible on the outside. Second, there is a danger of cardiac arrest from the electrical shock. (pages 994–996; Electrical Burns)

7. 1. Primary

    2. Secondary

    3. Tertiary (pages 966–970; Open Injuries)

8. 1. To control bleeding

    2. To protect the wound from further damage

    3. To prevent further contamination and infection (page 998; Dressing and Bandaging)

9. 1. Abrasions

    2. Lacerations

    3. Avulsions

    4. Penetrating wounds (pages 966–970; Open Injuries)

10. 1. Depth of the burn

    2. Extent of the burn

    3. Involvement of critical areas (face, upper airway, hands, feet, genitalia)

    4. Preexisting medical conditions or other injuries

    5. Age younger than 5 years or older than 55 years (pages 983–984; Burn Severity)

Ambulance Calls

1. Take standard precautions and apply direct pressure. Elevate the extremity and apply a pressure dressing. If the bleeding is not controlled, move to the use of a tourniquet. Once the bleeding is controlled, splint the arm to decrease movement. Apply high-flow oxygen (if appropriate), and transport the patient in a position of comfort. Monitor her vital signs en route to the hospital.

2. Unfortunately, this scenario has occurred in households throughout the country. This is why it is so important to "turn pot handles in" when cooking in the home of a small, inquisitive child. You must evaluate the child quickly to determine the extent and severity of the burns. Assess airway, breathing, and circulation, and quickly apply sterile dressings and high-flow oxygen. Promptly transport the patient according to local protocols.

3. Apply direct pressure to control any bleeding using sterile dressings. Have the patient lie down because this injury will be quite painful. Even the toughest person can suddenly feel faint, especially if he or she looks at the injury. Find the piece of avulsed tissue, wrap it in sterile dressings, and transport it with you to the hospital. Oxygen via a nasal cannula can assist with any nausea that the patient may experience.

Fill-in-the-Patient Care Report

EMS Patient Care Report (PCR)			
Date: Today's date	**Incident No.:** 2011-2222	**Nature of Call:** Gunshot wound	**Location:** 14th and Berry
Dispatched: 1321	**En Route:** 1321	**At Scene:** 1329	**Transport:** 1334	**At Hospital:** 1341	**In Service:** 1411

Patient Information	
Age: 24 years **Sex:** Male **Weight (in kg [lb]):** 73 kg (161 lb)	**Allergies:** Unknown **Medications:** Unknown **Past Medical History:** Unknown **Chief Complaint:** Gunshot wound to neck

Vital Signs

Time: 1334	BP: 92/60	Pulse: 120	Respirations: 20 Shallow	SpO$_2$: 92%
Time: 1337	BP: 92/58	Pulse: 124	Respirations: 20 Shallow	SpO$_2$: 94%

EMS Treatment
(circle all that apply)

Oxygen @ 15 L/min via (circle one): NC (NRM) BVM	Assisted Ventilation	Airway Adjunct	CPR
Defibrillation	(Bleeding Control)	(Bandaging)	(Splinting)	(Other: Shock treatment)

Narrative

Medic 19 dispatched on emergency call for a police officer with a gunshot wound. Arrived on scene and was led to 24-year-old patient with a gunshot wound on left lateral neck. Bleeding was manually controlled, but evidence of severe blood loss was present. The patient was conscious and alert but subdued. I placed an occlusive dressing and pressure dressing over the wound and initiated high-flow oxygen therapy. The patient was secured to a long backboard due to MOI, and immediate transport was initiated; no other wounds present. Baseline vital signs indicated that the patient was hypoperfusing, so we transported rapidly and covered the patient with blankets to retain body heat. Called in report to the receiving trauma center and provided ETA. Subsequent vital signs showed no improvement of the shock condition but also no further deterioration. Remainder of transport was without incident, and we then delivered the patient to the emergency department and gave a verbal report to the attending physician and charge nurse. Medic 19 returned to service at 1411.**End of Report**

Skills

Skill Drills

Skill Drill 27-1: Stabilizing an Impaled Object

1. Do not attempt to **move** or remove the object. **Stabilize** the impaled body part.

2. Control **bleeding**, and stabilize the object in place using **soft dressings**, gauze, and/or tape.

3. Tape a **rigid** item over the stabilized object to prevent it from **moving** during transport. (page 921; Emergency Medical Care for Open Injuries)

Skill Drill 27-2: Caring for Burns

1. Follow **standard** precautions to help prevent **infection**. If safe to do so, remove the **patient** from the burning area; extinguish or **remove** hot clothing and jewelry as necessary. If the wound is still burning or hot, **immerse** the hot area in **cool**, sterile **water**, or cover with a wet, cool **dressing**.

2. Provide **high-flow oxygen**, and continue to assess the **airway**.

3. Estimate the **severity** of the burn, and then cover the area with a **dry**, sterile dressing or clean **sheet**. Assess and treat the patient for any other **injuries**.

4. Prepare for transport. Treat for **shock**. Cover the patient with **blankets** to prevent loss of **body heat**. Transport promptly. (page 990; Emergency Medical Care for Burns)

Assessment Review

1. C (page 986; Burns Scene Size-up)
2. B (pages 988–989; Burns Secondary Assessment)
3. D (page 989; Burns Reassessment)
4. A (page 989; Emergency Medical Care for Burns)
5. D (page 969; Words of Wisdom)

CHAPTER

28 Face and Neck Injuries

General Knowledge

Matching

1. G (pages 1008–1009; The Eye)
2. H (pages 1008–1009; The Eye)
3. L (pages 1028–1030; Injuries of the Ear)
4. C (pages 1008–1009; The Eye)
5. J (pages 1008–1009; The Eye)
6. K (pages 1008–1009; The Eye)
7. I (pages 1006–1008; Anatomy and Physiology)
8. E (pages 1006–1008; Anatomy and Physiology)
9. O (pages 1008–1009; The Eye)
10. B (pages 1008–1009; The Eye)
11. F (pages 1008–1009; The Eye)
12. M (pages 1006–1008; Anatomy and Physiology)
13. A (pages 1027–1028; Injuries of the Nose)
14. D (pages 1028–1030; Injuries of the Ear)
15. N (pages 1008–1009; The Eye)

Multiple Choice

1. D (page 1006; Introduction)
2. B (pages 1006–1008; Anatomy and Physiology)
3. C (pagses 1006–1008; Anatomy and Physiology)
4. D (pages 1006–1008; Anatomy and Physiology)
5. A (pages 1006–1008; Anatomy and Physiology)
6. D (pages 1006–1008; Anatomy and Physiology)
7. C (pages 1006–1008; Anatomy and Physiology)
8. D (pages 1009–1011; Injuries of the Face and Neck)
9. A (pages 1015–1016; Emergency Medical Care)
10. D (pages 1027–1028; Injuries of the Nose)
11. B (pages 1027–1028; Injuries of the Nose)
12. C (pages 1028–1030; Injuries of the Ear)
13. D (page 1033; Laryngeal Injuries)
14. C (page 1030; Facial Fractures)
15. D (page 1032; Blunt Injuries)
16. A (page 1032; Injuries of the Neck)
17. A (pages 1008–1009; The Eye)
18. C (pages 1016–1019; Foreign Objects)
19. B (pages 1016–1019; Injuries of the Eyes: Foreign Objects)
20. C (page 1021; Burns of the Eye)

True/False

1. T (pages 1009–1011; Injuries of the Face and Neck)
2. T (pages 1015–1016; Emergency Medical Care)
3. F (pages 1015–1016; Emergency Medical Care)
4. F (pages 1028–1030; Injuries of the Ear)
5. T (page 1031; Injuries of the Neck: Blunt Injuries)
6. T (page 1006; Introduction)
7. F (pages 1006–1008; Anatomy and Physiology)
8. F (pages 1006–1008; Anatomy and Physiology)
9. T (page 1011; Patient Assessment)
10. T (pages 1011–1012; Primary Assessment)
11. T (pages 1008–1009; The Eye)
12. F (pages 1016–1019; Injuries of the Eyes: Foreign Objects)
13. T (page 1023; Light Burns)
14. T (page 1023; Injuries of the Eyes: Lacerations)
15. F (pages 1024–1025; Injuries of the Eyes: Blunt Trauma)
16. F (pages 1026–1027; Contact Lenses and Artificial Eyes)
17. T (page 1033; Laryngeal Injuries)
18. F (pages 1015–1016; Emergency Medical Care)
19. T (pages 1015–1016; Emergency Medical Care)

Fill-in-the-Blank

1. carotid (page 1008; Anatomy and Physiology)
2. cervical (page 1007; Anatomy and Physiology)
3. temporal (page 1006; Anatomy and Physiology)
4. trachea (pages 1006–1008; Anatomy and Physiology)
5. cartilage (pages 1006–1008; Anatomy and Physiology)
6. men, women (pages 1006–1008; Anatomy and Physiology)
7. foramen magnum (page 1006; Anatomy and Physiology)
8. blowout fracture (page 1025; Injuries of the Eyes: Blunt Trauma)
9. basilar skull fracture (page 1027; Injuries of the Nose)
10. crown, root (page 1031; Dental Injuries)
11. air embolism (page 1032; Injuries of the Neck: Penetrating Injuries)

Labeling

1. The Face (page 1007; Figure 28-1)

    A. Nasal bone

    B. Zygoma

    C. Maxilla

    D. Mandible

2. The Larynx (page 1008; Figure 28-4)

    A. Laryngeal prominence (Adam's apple)

    B. Thyroid cartilage

    C. Cricothyroid membrane

    D. Cricoid cartilage

    E. Trachea

3. The Eye (page 1008; Figure 28-5)

    A. Anterior compartment filled with aqueous humor

    B. Posterior compartment filled with vitreous humor

    C. Anterior chamber

    D. Posterior chamber

    E. Vein

    F. Iris

    G. Cornea

    H. Pupil

    I. Artery

    J. Lens

    K. Optic nerve

    L. Retina

    M. Choroid

    N. Sclera

4. The Ear (page 1029; Figure 28-29)

    A. Pinna

    B. External auditory canal

    C. Tympanic membrane

    D. Cochlea

    E. Hammer

    F. Anvil

    G. Stirrup

Critical Thinking

Short Answer

1. Apply direct manual pressure with a dry dressing. Use roller gauze around the circumference of the head to hold the pressure dressing in place. Make sure you do not apply excessive pressure if there is a possibility of an underlying skull fracture. (page 1015; Emergency Medical Care)

2. **1.** Apply direct pressure to the bleeding site using a gloved fingertip if necessary to control bleeding.

   2. Apply a sterile occlusive dressing to ensure that air does not enter a vein or artery.

   3. Secure the dressing in place with roller gauze, adding more dressings if needed.

   4. Wrap the gauze around and under the patient's shoulder. To avoid possible airway and circulation problems, do not wrap the gauze around the neck. (page 1032; Injuries of the Neck: Penetrating Injuries)

3. Start on the outer aspect of the eye and work your way in toward the pupil. Examine the eye for any obvious foreign matter. Observe for discoloration of the eye. Evaluate the clarity of the patient's vision. Assess for redness of or bleeding into the iris. Look for symmetry between the two eyes. Assess the pupils for equal size and reaction to light. Determine if unequal pupils are caused by physiologic or pathologic issues. Determine if the patient is able to follow your finger with his or her eyes. Assess visual acuity by having the patient read normal print. Question about blurry vision or sensitivity to light. (page 1013; Secondary Assessment)

4. **1.** Never exert pressure on or manipulate the injured eye (globe) in any way.

   2. If part of the eyeball is exposed, gently apply a moist, sterile dressing to prevent drying.

   3. Cover the injured eye with a protective metal eye shield, cup, or sterile dressing. Apply soft dressings to both eyes, and provide prompt transport to the hospital. (page 1023; Injuries of the Eyes: Lacerations)

5. **1.** One pupil larger than the other

   2. The eyes not moving together or pointing in different directions

   3. Failure of the eyes to follow the movement of your finger as instructed

   4. Bleeding under the conjunctiva, which obscures the sclera of the eye

   5. Protrusion or bulging of one eye (pages 1025–1026; Eye Injuries Following Head Injury)

Ambulance Calls

1. Depending on where the dog's teeth have punctured the skin, you may have a variety of soft-tissue injuries and swelling. If you notice the presence of subcutaneous emphysema, the dog punctured or perforated the child's trachea. You must also assume the presence of cervical spine injuries and take appropriate precautions. Assess his level of consciousness, airway, breathing, and circulation. Control any bleeding and apply other dressings, as needed, after airway management is accomplished and while en route to the hospital. Always follow local protocols.

2. Apply direct pressure to the bleeding site using gloved fingertips and a sterile occlusive dressing. Secure the dressing in place and apply pressure, if necessary. You may need to treat for shock. Provide prompt transport with the patient immobilized to a long backboard, and apply high-flow oxygen en route.

3. You should determine what objects were used to cause injury to this man's face. Baseball bats would be readily available and would increase your index of suspicion. You should determine the presence of head and neck pain. If the area of injury is limited to his nose, and the need for spinal precautions is not indicated, you can instruct the patient in controlling his bleeding by ensuring that he pushes on the cartilage of his nose and does not lean his head backward. Swallowing blood will cause nausea. Do not allow the patient to blow his nose, and consider using ice, as needed, to reduce swelling and pain. Transport according to local protocols.

Skills

Skill Drills

Skill Drill 28-1: Removing a Foreign Object From Under the Upper Eyelid

1. Have the patient look **down**, grasp the upper **lashes**, and gently pull the **lid** away from the eye.

2. Place a cotton-tipped applicator on the **outer** surface of the **upper** lid.

3. Pull the lid **forward** and **up**, folding it back over the applicator.

4. Gently remove the foreign object from the eyelid with a moistened, **sterile**, cotton-tipped applicator. (page 1018; Emergency Medical Care for Specific Injuries)

Skill Drill 28-2: Stabilizing a Foreign Object Impaled in the Eye

1. To prepare a doughnut ring, wrap a 2-inch roll around your fingers and thumb seven or eight times. Adjust the diameter by spreading your fingers or squeezing them together.

2. Remove the gauze from your hand and wrap the remainder of the gauze roll radially around the ring that you have created.

3. Work around the entire ring to form a doughnut.

4. Place the dressing over the eye and impaled object to hold the impaled object in place, and then secure it with a roller bandage. (page 1020; Emergency Medical Care for Specific Injuries)

Assessment Review

1. D   (page 1011; Scene Size-up)
2. B   (pages 1014–1015; Reassessment)
3. D   (pages 1027–1028; Injuries of the Nose)
4. A   (page 1031; Dental Injuries)
5. C   (page 1028; Injuries of the Ear)

CHAPTER

29 Head and Spine Injuries

General Knowledge

Matching

1. D (page 1049; Epidural Hematoma)
2. E (page 1063; Cushing Triad)
3. H (page 1050; Subdural Hematoma)
4. G (page 1051; Concussion)
5. A (page 1051; Concussion)
6. C (page 1051; Concussion)
7. B (page 1049; Traumatic Brain Injuries)
8. I (pages 1042–1043; Peripheral Nervous System)
9. J (page 1045; Spinal Column)
10. F (page 1042; Protective Coverings)

Multiple Choice

1. D (pages 1041–1042; Central Nervous System)
2. B (page 1040; Anatomy and Physiology: Nervous System)
3. C (pages 1041–1042; Central Nervous System)
4. C (page 1046; Head Injuries)
5. A (page 1042; Protective Coverings)
6. B (page 1044; Figure 29-6)
7. D (pages 1042–1043; Peripheral Nervous System)
8. D (page 1042; Protective Coverings)
9. C (pages 1043–1044; How the Nervous System Works)
10. A (page 1045; Spinal Column)
11. D (page 1055; Assessing for Signs and Symptoms of a Head or Spine Injury)
12. D (page 1053; Scene Size-up)
13. B (page 1045; Spinal Column)
14. D (page 1070; Preparation for Transport)
15. B (page 1067; Cervical Collars)
16. A (pages 1067–1075; Preparation for Transport: Supine Patients)
17. A (page 1062; Circulation)
18. B (pages 1075–1077; Sitting Patients)
19. D (page 1050; Subarachnoid Hemorrhage)
20. B (page 1051; Concussion)
21. C (page 1051; Concussion)
22. D (page 1049; Epidural Hematoma)
23. C (page 1078; Short Backboards)
24. B (page 1058; Physical Examination)
25. B (page 1056; Airway, Breathing, and Circulation Considerations)
26. C (page 1053; Patient Assessment)
27. C (page 1055; Assessing for Signs and Symptoms of a Head or Spine Injury)
28. A (page 1046; Table 29-1 General Signs and Symptoms of a Head Injury)
29. C (page 1063; Cushing Triad)
30. D (pages 1054–1055; Spinal Motion Restriction Considerations)
31. C (page 1080; Helmet Removal)
32. D (pages 1067–1075; Preparation for Transport: Supine Patients)

True/False

1. F (page 1050; Intracerebral Hematoma)
2. T (pages 1043–1044; How the Nervous System Works)
3. F (pages 1043–1044; How the Nervous System Works)
4. T (pages 1043–1044; How the Nervous System Works)
5. F (pages 1043–1044; How the Nervous System Works)
6. F (pages 1054–1055; Spinal Motion Restriction Considerations)
7. F (page 1055; Assessing for Signs and Symptoms of a Head or Spine Injury)
8. T (page 1067; Preparation for Transport)
9. T (page 1075; Sitting Patients)
10. T (page 1066; Cervical Collars)

Fill-in-the-Blank

1. motor (pages 1042–1043; Peripheral Nervous System)
2. meninges (page 1042; Protective Coverings)
3. central (pages 1041–1042; Central Nervous System)
4. 31 (pages 1042–1043; Peripheral Nervous System)
5. cranial (pages 1042–1043; Peripheral Nervous System)
6. intervertebral disks (page 1045; Spinal Column)
7. cranium, facial (pages 1044–1045; Skull)
8. arachnoid, pia mater (page 1042; Protective Coverings)
9. sympathetic (page 1044; How the Nervous System Works)
10. parasympathetic (page 1044; How the Nervous System Works)
11. intracerebral hematoma (page 1050; Intracerebral Hematoma)
12. contusion (page 1051; Contusion)
13. padding (page 1083; Alternative Method)
14. pulse, motor, sensory (page 1070; Supine Patients)
15. jaw-thrust (page 1055; Airway, Breathing, and Circulation Considerations)

Labeling

1. Brain (page 1041; Figure 29-2)

   A. Cerebrum
   B. Parietal lobe
   C. Frontal lobe
   D. Occipital lobe
   E. Temporal lobe
   F. Brainstem
   G. Cerebellum
   H. Spinal cord
   I. Foramen magnum

2. Connecting Nerves in the Spinal Cord (page 1043; Figure 29-5)

   A. Motor nerve
   B. Sensory nerve
   C. Connecting nerve cell
   D. Spinal cord

3. Spinal Column (page 1045; Figure 29-7)

   A. Cervical (7)
   B. Thoracic (12)
   C. Lumbar (5)
   D. Sacrum (5)
   E. Coccyx (4)

Critical Thinking

Short Answer

1. 1. Motor vehicle collision (including motorcycles, snowmobiles, and all-terrain vehicles)
   2. Pedestrian–motor vehicle collision
   3. Falls >20 feet (>6 m) (adult)
   4. Falls >10 feet (>3 m) (pediatric)
   5. Blunt trauma
   6. Penetrating trauma to the head, neck, back, or torso
   7. Rapid deceleration injuries
   8. Hangings
   9. Axial loading injuries
   10. Diving accidents (page 1053; Patient Assessment)

2. • Muscle spasms in the neck
   • Substantial increased pain
   • Numbness, tingling, or weakness in the arms or legs
   • Compromised airway or ventilations (page 1065; Spinal Motion Restriction of the Cervical Spine)

3. Primary brain injury is injury to the brain and its associated structures that results instantaneously from impact to the head. Secondary brain injury refers to a multitude of processes that increase the severity of a primary brain injury and therefore negatively affect the outcome. Secondary brain injuries result from cerebral edema, intracranial hemorrhage, increased intracranial pressure, cerebral ischemia, and infection. Hypoxia and hypotension are the two most common causes of secondary brain injuries. (page 1048; Traumatic Brain Injuries)

4. • Lacerations, contusions, or hematomas to the scalp
   • Soft area or depression on palpation
   • Visible fractures or deformities of the skull
   • Decreased mentation, irregular breathing pattern, widening pulse pressure, slow pulse rate
   • Ecchymosis about the eyes or behind the ear over the mastoid process
   • Clear or pink cerebrospinal fluid leakage from a scalp wound, the nose, or the ear
   • Failure of the pupils to respond to light
   • Unequal pupil size
   • Loss of sensation and/or motor function
   • A period of unconsciousness
   • Amnesia
   • Seizures
   • Numbness or tingling in the extremities
   • Irregular respirations
   • Dizziness

- Visual complaints
- Combative or other abnormal behavior
- Nausea or vomiting
- Posturing (decorticate or decerebrate) (page 1046; Table 29-1 General Signs and Symptoms of a Head Injury)

5. **1.** Establish an adequate airway.

2. Control bleeding.

3. Assess the patient's baseline level of consciousness. (page 1061; Emergency Medical Care of Head Injuries)

6. **1.** Is the patient's airway clear?

2. Is the patient breathing adequately?

3. Can you maintain the airway and assist ventilations if the helmet remains in place?

4. Can the face guard be easily removed to allow access to the airway without removing the helmet?

5. How well does the helmet fit?

6. Can the patient move within the helmet?

7. Can the spine be immobilized in a neutral position with the helmet on? (page 1079; Helmet Removal)

Ambulance Calls

1. This incident involves a significant mechanism of injury. The impact with the car, the lack of a helmet, the obvious head trauma, and the patient's decreased level of consciousness all indicate significant life-threatening injuries. You must quickly apply full spinal precautions and manage her airway. Provide prompt transport and high-flow oxygen, and perform reassessment while en route to the nearest appropriate medical facility.

2. This child landed facedown on a concrete surface, with significant force. She is now unconscious, with a partially obstructed airway. You must move her to a supine position to manage her airway. Take note of any apparent injuries to her back as you reposition her. Ideally, you will have the appropriate equipment and adequate staffing to quickly and safely move her to a long backboard immediately. However, do not delay appropriately

moving her to a supine position because you must do this to assess and manage her airway. This may be difficult because she likely has facial fractures and possibly broken teeth, blood, and secretions in her airway. Be prepared to suction her airway and apply positive pressure ventilations (this may be especially challenging in the presence of significant facial fractures). Use high-flow oxygen and promptly transport her to the nearest appropriate facility according to your local protocols.

3. Leave the patient in his car seat. Pad appropriately to immobilize the patient. Use blow-by oxygen if the patient will tolerate it. Monitor vital signs. Continue assessment. Provide rapid transport due to mechanism of injury and death in the vehicle.

Skills

Skill Drills

Skill Drill 29-1: Performing Manual In-Line Stabilization (page 1065)

1. Take standard precautions. Kneel behind the patient and firmly place your hands around the **base** of the **skull** on either **side**.

2. Support the lower jaw with your **index** and **long** fingers, and support the head with your **palms**. Gently lift the head into a **neutral, eyes-forward** position, aligned with the torso. Do not move the head or neck excessively, forcefully, or rapidly.

3. Continue to manually **support** the head while your partner places a rigid **cervical collar** around the neck. Maintain **manual support** until you have completely secured the patient to a backboard.

Skill Drill 29-3: Securing a Patient to a Long Backboard (pages 1068–1069)

1. Apply and maintain cervical stabilization. Assess distal functions in all extremities.

2. Apply a cervical collar.

3. Rescuers kneel on one side of the patient and place hands on the far side of the patient.

4. On command, rescuers roll the patient toward themselves, quickly examine the back, slide the backboard under the patient, and roll the patient onto the backboard.

5. Center the patient on the backboard.

6. Secure the upper torso first.

7. Secure the pelvis and upper legs.

8. Begin to secure the patient's head using a commercial immobilization device or rolled towels.

9. Place tape across the patient's forehead to secure the immobilization device.

10. Check all straps and readjust as needed. Reassess distal functions in all extremities.

Skill Drill 29-5: Securing a Patient Found in a Sitting Position (pages 1075–1077)

1. Take standard precautions. Stabilize the head and neck in a **neutral, in-line** position. Assess pulse, motor, and sensory function in each extremity. Apply a **cervical collar**.

2. Insert an immobilization device between the patient's **upper back** and the seat.

3. Open the side flaps, and position them around the patient's **torso**, snug around the armpits.

4. Secure the upper torso flaps, then the mid-torso flaps.

5. Secure the **groin** (leg) straps. Check and adjust the **torso** straps.

6. **Pad** between the head and the device as needed. Secure the forehead strap and fasten the **lower** head strap around the cervical collar.

7. Place a long backboard next to the patient's buttocks, **perpendicular** to the trunk.

8. Turn and lower the patient onto the backboard. Lift the **patient**, and slip the backboard under the immobilization device.

9. Secure the immobilization device and backboard to each other. **Loosen** or **release** the groin straps. Reassess pulse, motor, and sensory function in each extremity.

Skill Drill 29-2: Application of a Cervical Collar (pages 1066–1067)

1. Apply in-line **stabilization**.

2. Measure the proper **collar size**.

3. Place the **chin support** first.

4. **Wrap** the collar around the neck and **secure** the collar.

5. Ensure proper **fit** and maintain **neutral, in-line** stabilization until the patient is secured to a **backboard**.

Assessment Review

1. D   (pages 1053–1061; Patient Assessment)
2. C   (page 1065; Emergency Medical Care of Spinal Injuries)
3. B   (page 1070; Supine Patients)
4. C   (page 1078; Short Backboards)
5. A   (page 1081; Preferred Method)

Chest Injuries

General Knowledge

Matching

1. B (pages 1092–1093; Anatomy and Physiology)
2. D (pages 1092–1093; Anatomy and Physiology)
3. K (pages 1092–1093; Anatomy and Physiology)
4. A (pages 1092–1093; Anatomy and Physiology)
5. E (pages 1092–1093; Anatomy and Physiology)
6. H (pages 1095–1097; Injuries of the Chest)
7. I (pages 1096–1097; Signs and Symptoms of Chest Injury)
8. J (pages 1105–1106; Cardiac Tamponade)
9. F (pages 1095–1097; Injuries of the Chest)
10. G (pages 1096–1097; Signs and Symptoms of Chest Injury)
11. C (pages 1092–1093; Anatomy and Physiology)

Multiple Choice

1. B (pages 1092–1093; Anatomy and Physiology)
2. A (pages 1092–1093; Anatomy and Physiology)
3. C (pages 1094–1095; Mechanics of Ventilation)
4. D (pages 1095–1097; Injuries of the Chest)
5. D (pages 1096–1097; Signs and Symptoms of Chest Injury)
6. C (pages 1096–1097; Signs and Symptoms of Chest Injury)
7. A (page 1109; Commotio Cordis)
8. B (pages 1098–1099; Primary Assessment)
9. D (pages 1102–1105; Pneumothorax)
10. C (pages 1102–1105; Pneumothorax)
11. A (page 1104; Simple Pneumothorax)
12. B (pages 1105–1106; Cardiac Tamponade)
13. C (page 1105; Tension Pneumothorax)
14. A (page 1105; Hemothorax)
15. C (page 1109; Blunt Myocardial Injury)
16. A (page 1107; Rib Fractures)
17. C (page 1109; Traumatic Asphyxia)
18. D (pages 1094–1095; Mechanics of Ventilation)
19. A (pages 1099–1100; History Taking)
20. B (pages 1092–1093; Anatomy and Physiology)

True/False

1. T (pages 1096–1097; Signs and Symptoms of Chest Injury)
2. F (pages 1096–1097; Signs and Symptoms of Chest Injury)
3. T (page 1105; Tension Pneumothorax)
4. F (page 1102; Special Populations)
5. F (pages 1105–1106; Cardiac Tamponade)
6. F (page 1110; Laceration of the Great Vessels)
7. F (pages 1092–1093; Anatomy and Physiology)
8. T (pages 1094–1095; Mechanics of Ventilation)
9. F (pages 1102–1105; Pneumothorax)
10. T (pages 1095–1097; Injuries of the Chest)
11. T (pages 1098–1099; Primary Assessment)
12. F (pages 1100–1101; Secondary Assessment)
13. T (pages 1098–1099; Primary Assessment)
14. T (pages 1095–1097; Injuries of the Chest)
15. F (pages 1092–1093; Anatomy and Physiology)

Fill-in-the-Blank

1. back (page 1093; Anatomy and Physiology)
2. decreases (page 1094; Mechanics of Ventilation)
3. sternum (page 1093; Anatomy and Physiology)
4. bronchi (page 1093; Anatomy and Physiology)
5. phrenic (page 1094; Mechanics of Ventilation)
6. ribs (page 1093; Anatomy and Physiology)
7. diaphragm (page 1092; Anatomy and Physiology)
8. Pleura (page 1093; Anatomy and Physiology)
9. hypercarbia (page 1095; Injuries of the Chest)
10. contracts (page 1094; Mechanics of Ventilation)
11. Ventilation (page 1092; Anatomy and Physiology)
12. C6, C7 (page 1092; Anatomy and Physiology)
13. Tidal volume (page 1095; Mechanics of Ventilation)
14. respiratory rate (page 1101; Secondary Assessment)
15. traumatic forces (page 1110; Laceration of the Great Vessels)

Labeling

1. Anterior Aspect of the Chest (page 1092; Figure 30-1)

   A. Subclavian artery
   B. Superior vena cava
   C. Heart
   D. Aorta
   E. Pulmonary arteries
   F. Pleural lining
   G. Lungs
   H. Diaphragm

2. Pneumothorax (page 1102; Figure 30-8)

   A. Parietal pleura
   B. Air in the pleural space
   C. Wound site
   D. Lung
   E. Collapsed lung
   F. Heart
   G. Visceral pleura
   H. Diaphragm

Critical Thinking

Short Answer

1. • Pain at the site of injury

   • Pain localized at the site of injury that is aggravated by or increased with breathing

   • Bruising to the chest wall

   • Crepitus with palpation of the chest

   • Any penetrating injury to the chest

   • Dyspnea (difficulty breathing, shortness of breath)

   • Hemoptysis (coughing up blood)

   • Failure of one or both sides of the chest to expand normally with inspiration

   • Rapid, weak pulse and low blood pressure

   • Cyanosis around the lips or fingernails (pages 1096–1097; Signs and Symptoms of Chest Injury)

2. 1. Seal the wound with a large airtight dressing that seals all four sides.

   2. Seal the wound with a dressing that seals three sides, with the fourth side as a flutter valve. Your local protocol will dictate the way that you are to care for this injury. (pages 1102–1105; Pneumothorax)

3. Maintain the airway, provide respiratory support if necessary, and give supplemental oxygen. Perform an ongoing assessment for possible pneumothorax or other respiratory complications. Provide positive pressure ventilation with a bag-mask device as needed. Use PPV in place of splinting with a bulky dressing. (pages 1107–1108; Flail Chest)

4. Sudden severe compression of the chest, causing a rapid increase of pressure within the chest. Characteristic signs include distended neck veins, facial and neck cyanosis, and hemorrhage in the sclera of the eye. (page 1109; Traumatic Asphyxia)

5. 1. Airway obstruction

   2. Bronchial disruption

   3. Diaphragmatic tear

   4. Esophageal injury

   5. Open pneumothorax

   6. Tension pneumothorax

   7. Massive hemothorax

   8. Flail chest

   9. Cardiac tamponade

   10. Thoracic aortic dissection

   11. Myocardial contusion

   12. Pulmonary contusion (page 1099; Table 30-1 Deadly Dozen Chest Injuries)

Ambulance Calls

1. You should be concerned with the presence of rib and sternal fractures as well as pulmonary contusions and pneumothoraces. This patient may require assistance in breathing because it will be extremely painful for him to breathe in. If he requires assistance with a bag-mask device, you must be careful not to become too aggressive in your ventilations. Time your ventilations with the patient's respirations and be gentle. Provide high-flow oxygen and take spinal precautions according to your local protocols.

2. This patient's chest has been crushed with a significant amount of weight. This mechanism of injury indicates the high potential for rib, sternal, and thoracic fractures as well as other soft-tissue injuries. Patients who experience sternal fractures will find it difficult to be placed supine because this will likely increase their pain. There will be little you can do to ease this pain because the patient should be immobilized on a long backboard. Provide prompt transport and high-flow oxygen, and monitor the pulse, motor, and sensations, particularly distal to the suspected spinal injury.

3. Apply high-flow oxygen via a nonrebreathing mask or a bag-mask device. Provide full cervical spine immobilization. Provide rapid transport and monitor vital signs en route.

Skills

Assessment Review

1. B (pages 1102–1105; Pneumothorax)
2. D (pages 1102–1105; Pneumothorax)
3. C (page 1098; Primary Assessment)
4. D (pages 1107–1108; Flail Chest)
5. A (page 1101; Secondary Assessment)

CHAPTER

31 Abdominal and Genitourinary Injuries

General Knowledge

Matching

1. E (pages 1121–1122; Closed Abdominal Injuries)
2. I (pages 1122–1123; Open Abdominal Injuries)
3. F (pages 1127–1128; Secondary Assessment)
4. A (pages 1126–1127; History Taking)
5. H (pages 1119–1121; Hollow and Solid Organs)
6. C (pages 1124–1125; Solid Organ Injuries)
7. D (pages 1122–1123; Open Abdominal Injuries)
8. G (page 1143; Vital Vocabulary)
9. B (pages 1119–1121; Hollow and Solid Organs)

Multiple Choice

1. D (page 1118; Introduction)
2. B (pages 1119–1121; Hollow and Solid Organs)
3. C (pages 1119–1121; Hollow and Solid Organs)
4. D (pages 1119–1121; Hollow and Solid Organs)
5. B (pages 1119–1121; Hollow and Solid Organs)
6. C (pages 1119–1121; Hollow and Solid Organs)
7. A (pages 1119–1121; Hollow and Solid Organs)
8. C (pages 1124–1125; Solid Organ Injuries)
9. B (pages 1123–1124; Hollow Organ Injuries)
10. A (page 1119; Abdominal Quadrants)
11. A (pages 1124–1125; Solid Organ Injuries)
12. C (pages 1122–1123; Open Abdominal Injuries)
13. B (pages 1121–1122; Injuries From Seat Belts and Airbags)
14. A (pages 1119–1121; Hollow and Solid Organs)
15. B (pages 1125–1126; Primary Assessment)
16. B (pages 1125–1126; Primary Assessment)
17. C (pages 1125–1126; Primary Assessment)
18. B (pages 1124–1125; Solid Organ Injuries)
19. D (pages 1126–1127; History Taking)
20. D (pages 1121–1122; Injuries From Seat Belts and Airbags)
21. C (pages 1127–1128; Secondary Assessment)
22. A (pages 1122–1123; Open Abdominal Injuries)
23. D (pages 1122–1123; Open Abdominal Injuries)
24. D (pages 1130–1131; Abdominal Evisceration)
25. A (pages 1119–1121; Hollow and Solid Organs)
26. C (pages 1131–1132; Anatomy of the Genitourinary System)
27. D (page 1133; Injuries of the Genitourinary System)
28. C (page 1133; Injuries of the Kidneys)
29. A (pages 1133–1134; Injuries to the Urinary Bladder)
30. B (pages 1137–1138; External Male Genitalia)
31. B (pages 1134–1135; Injuries of the Female Genitalia)
32. B (pages 1138–1139; Sexual Assault and Rape)

True/False

1. T (pages 1123–1124; Hollow Organ Injuries)
2. T (pages 1125–1126; Primary Assessment)
3. F (pages 1124–1125; Solid Organ Injuries)
4. T (pages 1119–1121; Hollow and Solid Organs)
5. F (pages 1130–1131; Abdominal Evisceration)
6. F (page 1133; Injuries of the Kidneys)
7. T (pages 1119–1121; Hollow and Solid Organs)
8. F (page 1119; Abdominal Quadrants)
9. T (pages 1126–1127; History Taking)

Fill-in-the-Blank

1. solid (page 1120; Hollow and Solid Organs)
2. kidneys, blood (page 1124; Solid Organ Injuries)
3. retroperitoneal (pages 1120–1121; Hollow and Solid Organs)
4. other organs (page 1133; Injuries of the Kidneys)
5. peritonitis (page 1120; Hollow and Solid Organs)
6. peritoneal cavity (page 1120; Hollow and Solid Organs)
7. blunt injuries (page 1129; Closed Abdominal Injuries)
8. penetrating injuries (page 1129; Open Abdominal Injuries)
9. flank (page 1128; Secondary Assessment)
10. evisceration (page 1130; Abdominal Evisceration)

Labeling

1. Hollow Organs (page 1120; Figure 31-2)

   A. Stomach

   B. Gallbladder

   C. Bile duct

   D. Large intestine

   E. Ureter

   F. Small intestine

   G. Fallopian tubes

   H. Rectum

   I. Appendix

   J. Uterus

   K. Urinary bladder

2. Solid Organs (page 1120; Figure 31-3)

   A. Liver

   B. Spleen

   C. Adrenal gland

   D. Adrenal gland

   E. Pancreas

   F. Kidney

   G. Kidney

   H. Ovaries

Critical Thinking

Short Answer

1. Stomach, intestines, ureters, bladder, gallbladder, bile duct, appendix, uterus, fallopian tubes, and rectum (page 1120; Figure 31-2)
2. Liver, spleen, pancreas, adrenal glands, ovaries, and kidneys (page 1120; Figure 31-3)
3. • Pain
   • Guarding
   • Distention
   • Tenderness
   • Bruising and discoloration
   • Abrasions
   • Tachycardia
   • Shock signs
   • Lacerations
   • Bleeding
   • Difficulty with movement because of pain (pages 1127–1128; Secondary Assessment, pages 1126–1127; History Taking)

4. • An abrasion, laceration, or contusion in the flank

   • A penetrating wound in the flank (the region below the rib cage and above the hip) or the upper abdomen

   • Fractures on either side of the lower rib cage or of the lower thoracic or upper lumbar vertebrae

   • A hematoma in the flank region (page 1133; Injuries of the Kidneys)

Ambulance Calls

1. Assess the patient's ABCs and apply high-flow oxygen or a bag-mask device if needed. Control any bleeding. Stabilize the knife in place with bulky dressings—do not remove it. Keep movement of the patient to the bare minimum so as not to create further injury. (Sliding the patient very carefully onto a backboard may help to minimize movement.) Monitor vital signs, and provide rapid transport. Keep patient warm and treat for shock if signs and symptoms present. Bandage minor lacerations en route.

2. Ensure that the scene is safe. Quickly visualize the area to determine how badly he has cut himself and whether he has in fact amputated any portion of his penis. You will need to control bleeding because blood loss in this area can be significant. Use direct pressure and/or pressure dressings to control bleeding. If a portion of the penis is amputated, wrap it in a moist, sterile dressing, place it in a plastic bag, and transport it in a cooled container. Do not allow it to come in direct contact with ice. Provide high-flow oxygen and prompt transport. Also, request the presence of a police officer during transport because this patient will likely need to be restrained and could be unpredictable during transport.

3. Cover the abdomen and the portion of the protruding bowel with a moistened, sterile dressing and/or an occlusive dressing. Secure these dressings with tape. Allow the patient to draw up his knees as needed for comfort. Apply high-flow oxygen, cover the patient to preserve warmth, treat for shock as needed, and promptly transport to the hospital.

Skills

Assessment Review

1. A   (pages 1130–1131; Abdominal Evisceration)
2. A   (pages 1137–1138; External Male Genitalia)
3. D   (page 1133; Injuries of the Kidneys)
4. D   (pages 1137–1138; External Male Genitalia)
5. C   (pages 1138–1139; Sexual Assault and Rape)

CHAPTER

32

Orthopaedic Injuries

General Knowledge

Matching

1. G (pages 1146–1147; Muscles)
2. J (pages 1146–1147; Muscles)
3. D (pages 1146–1147; Muscles)
4. I (pages 1148–1149; The Skeleton)
5. F (pages 1148–1149; The Skeleton)
6. B (pages 1152–1155; Fractures)
7. K (page 1154; Figure 32-17)
8. A (pages 1152–1155; Fractures)
9. C (pages 1148–1149; The Skeleton)
10. E (pages 1152–1155; Fractures)
11. H (page 1181; Traction Splints)

Multiple Choice

1. A (page 1179; Fractures of the Pelvis)
2. B (pages 1146–1147; Muscles)
3. A (pages 1148–1149; The Skeleton)
4. B (pages 1148–1149; The Skeleton)
5. C (pages 1148–1149; The Skeleton)
6. B (page 1155; Dislocations)
7. C (pages 1156–1157; Sprains)
8. A (page 1157; Strain)
9. D (page 1151; Musculoskeletal Injuries)
10. A (pages 1151–1152; Mechanism of Injury)
11. B (pages 1151–1152; Mechanism of Injury)
12. C (pages 1151–1152; Mechanism of Injury)
13. D (pages 1151–1152; Mechanism of Injury)
14. B (pages 1152–1155; Fractures)
15. C (pages 1152–1155; Fractures)
16. D (pages 1152–1155; Fractures)
17. A (page 1153; Figure 32-14)
18. C (page 1154; Tenderness)
19. D (pages 1152–1155; Fractures)
20. A (pages 1152–1155; Fractures)
21. C (pages 1152–1155; Fractures)
22. B (pages 1152–1155; Fractures)
23. A (page 1154; Swelling)
24. C (page 1154; Bruising)
25. D (page 1156; Dislocations)
26. C (page 1157; Sprains)
27. D (pages 1161–1162; Secondary Assessment)
28. B (page 1192; Compartment Syndrome)
29. D (pages 1161–1162; Secondary Assessment)
30. A (page 1164; Splinting)
31. C (pages 1181–1186; Traction Splints)
32. D (page 1165; Types of Splints)
33. B (pages 1181–1186; Traction Splints)
34. A (page 1169; Hazards of Improper Splinting)
35. B (pages 1169–1171; Injuries of the Clavicle and Scapula)
36. B (pages 1169–1171; Injuries of the Clavicle and Scapula)
37. D (pages 1179–1180; Dislocation of the Hip)
38. C (pages 1180–1181; Fractures of the Proximal Femur)
39. B (page 1187; Injuries of Knee Ligaments)
40. D (page 1187; Injuries of Knee Ligaments)
41. C (pages 1187–1188; Dislocation of the Knee)
42. B (page 1188; Fractures About the Knee)
43. A (page 1189; Injuries of the Tibia and Fibula)
44. C (pages 1189–1190; Ankle Injuries)

True/False

1. T   (pages 1164–1165; Splinting)
2. T   (pages 1164–1165; Splinting)
3. F   (pages 1181–1186; Traction Splints)
4. T   (pages 1181–1186; Traction Splints)
5. T   (pages 1164–1165; Splinting)
6. F   (pages 1163–1164; Emergency Medical Care)
7. T   (pages 1162–1163; Reassessment)
8. T   (pages 1148–1149; The Skeleton)
9. T   (page 1192; Compartment Syndrome)
10. T   (pages 1175–1176; Fractures of the Forearm)

Fill-in-the-Blank

1. calcaneus (page 1150; The Skeleton)
2. blood cells (page 1148; The Skeleton)
3. hinged (page 1148; The Skeleton)
4. clavicle (page 1148; The Skeleton)
5. mechanism of injury (pages 1151–1152; Mechanism of Injury)
6. open fracture (page 1153; Fractures)
7. sciatic nerve (page 1179; Dislocation of the Hip)
8. Pelvic binders (page 1168; Pelvic Binders)
9. crepitus (page 1155; Crepitus)
10. reduce (page 1155; Dislocations)
11. neurovascular status (page 1192; Compartment Syndrome)

Labeling

1. Pectoral Girdle (page 1149; Figure 32-5)

   A. Sternoclavicular joint
   B. Clavicle
   C. Acromioclavicular joint
   D. Manubrium
   E. Acromion process
   F. Humerus
   G. Sternum
   H. Glenohumeral (shoulder) joint
   I. Acromion process
   J. Glenoid fossa
   K. Humerus
   L. Scapula

2. Anatomy of the Wrist and Hand (page 1149; Figure 32-7)

   A. Index
   B. Long
   C. Ring
   D. Little
   E. Phalanges
   F. Thumb
   G. Metacarpals
   H. Scaphoid
   I. Carpals
   J. Radius
   K. Ulna

3. Bones of the Thigh, Leg, and Foot (page 1150; Figure 32-8)

   A. Pelvis (hip bone)
   B. Hip
   C. Femur
   D. Thigh
   E. Patella (kneecap)
   F. Knee
   G. Fibula
   H. Leg
   I. Tibia (shin bone)
   J. Ankle
   K. Tarsals (ankle)
   L. Foot
   M. Metatarsals
   N. Phalanges

Critical Thinking

Short Answer

1. **1.** Direct blows

   2. Indirect forces

   3. Twisting forces

   4. High-energy injuries (pages 1151–1152; Mechanism of Injury)

2. • Deformity

   • Tenderness (point)

   • Guarding

   • Swelling

   • Bruising

   • Crepitus

   • False motion

   • Exposed fragments

   • Pain

   • Locked joint (pages 1152–1155; Fractures)

3. **1.** Pain

   2. Paralysis

   3. Paresthesia (numbness or tingling)

   4. Pulselessness

   5. Pallor

   6. Pressure (pages 1161–1162; Secondary Assessment)

4. **1.** Remove clothing from the area.

   2. Note and record the patient's neurovascular status distal to the site of the injury.

   3. Cover all wounds with a dry, sterile dressing before splinting.

   4. Do not move the patient before splinting.

   5. For a suspected fracture of the shaft of any bone, immobilize the joints above and below the fracture.

   6. For a joint injury, immobilize the bones above and below the injured joint.

   7. Pad all rigid splints.

   8. Maintain manual immobilization to minimize movement of the limb and to support the injury site.

   9. If a fracture of a long-bone shaft has resulted in severe deformity, use a constant, gentle manual traction to align the limb.

   10. If you encounter resistance to limb alignment, splint the limb in its deformed position.

   11. Stabilize all suspected spinal injuries in a neutral in-line position on a backboard.

   12. If the patient has signs of shock, align the limb in the normal anatomic position, and provide transport.

   13. When in doubt, splint. (page 1165; General Principles of Splinting)

5. **1.** Stabilize the fracture fragments to prevent excessive movement.

   2. Align the limb sufficiently to allow it to be placed in a splint.

   3. Avoid potential neurovascular compromise. (pages 1181–1186; Traction Splints)

Ambulance Calls

1. This patient likely has a compression injury to his lumbar spine. The force exerted on his body from the landing will be transferred up from his feet through his legs to his pelvis and spine. You must take all spinal precautions, apply high-flow oxygen, and provide prompt transport to the nearest appropriate facility. Continue to monitor any changes in the pulse, motor, and sensation, specifically in his lower body.

2. Because circulation is intact, splint the arm in the position found. Use a board splint for support with a sling and swathe. Immobilize the hand in the position of function. Apply oxygen as needed and transport the patient in a position of comfort.

Provide normal transport and monitor vital signs and neurovascular function.

3. This patient presents with signs of an anterior hip dislocation. Do not attempt to reduce the dislocation. It is preferable to use a scoop stretcher to move the patient to avoid any further injury. Manage her ABCs and give oxygen as needed. Assess for a pulse in the right foot before and after moving. Splint the dislocation in the position found, and place the patient supine on the backboard using a scoop stretcher to lift her. Support her right leg with pillows and rolled blankets, then secure the entire limb to the backboard with long straps so that the hip region will not move. Provide prompt transport and reassess frequently.

Skills

Skill Drills

Skill Drill 32-1: Caring for Musculoskeletal Injuries (page 1163)

1. Cover open wounds with a **dry**, **sterile** dressing and apply pressure to control **bleeding**. Assess distal pulse and motor and sensory function. If bleeding cannot be controlled, quickly apply a tourniquet.

2. Apply a **splint**, and elevate the extremity about 6 inches (15 cm) (slightly above the level of the heart). Assess distal pulse and motor and sensory function.

3. Apply cold packs if there is **swelling**, but do not place them directly on the skin.

4. Position the patient for transport, and secure the **injured area**.

Skill Drill 32-2: Applying a Rigid Splint (page 1166)

1. Provide gentle **support** and **in-line traction** for the limb. Assess distal pulse and motor and sensory function.

2. Place the splint **alongside** or **under** the limb. **Pad** between the limb and the splint as needed to ensure even pressure and contact.

3. Secure the splint to the limb with **bindings**.

4. Assess and record **distal neurovascular** function.

Skill Drill 32-3: Applying a Vacuum Splint (page 1168)

1. Assess distal pulse and motor and sensory function. Your partner **stabilizes** and **supports** the injury.

2. Place the splint, and **wrap** it around the limb.

3. **Draw** the air out of the splint through the **suction valve**, and then **seal** the valve. Assess distal pulse and motor and sensory function.

Skill Drill 32-5: Applying a Hare Traction Splint (page 1177)

1. Expose the injured limb and check pulse and motor and sensory function. Place the splint beside the uninjured limb, adjust the splint to proper length, and prepare the straps.

2. Support the injured limb as your partner fastens the ankle hitch about the foot and ankle.

3. Continue to support the limb as your partner applies gentle in-line traction to the ankle hitch and foot.

4. Slide the splint into position under the injured limb.

5. Pad the groin and fasten the ischial strap.

6. Connect the loops of the ankle hitch to the end of the splint as your partner continues to maintain traction. Carefully tighten the ratchet to the point that the splint holds adequate traction.

7. Secure and check support straps. Assess pulse and motor and sensory functions.

8. Secure the patient and splint to the backboard in a way that will prevent movement of the splint during patient movement and transport.

Skill Drill 32-4: Splinting the Hand and Wrist (page 1183)

1. Support the injured limb and move the hand into the **position** of **function**. Place a soft **roller bandage** in the palm.

2. Apply a **padded board** splint on the **palmar** side with fingers **exposed**.

3. Secure the splint with a **roller bandage**.

Assessment Review

1. A   (pages 1159–1160; Primary Assessment)
2. B   (pages 1162–1163; Reassessment)
3. B   (pages 1176–1177; Injuries of the Wrist and Hand)
4. D   (pages 1181–1186; Traction Splints)

CHAPTER

33 Environmental Emergencies

General Knowledge

Matching

1. J (page 1202; Cold Exposure)
2. H (page 1222; Air Embolism)
3. K (page 1202; Cold Exposure)
4. O (page 1211; Heat Exposure)
5. A (page 1220; Resuscitation Efforts)
6. N (page 1203; Hypothermia)
7. I (page 1202; Cold Exposure)
8. C (pages 1218–1220; Drowning)
9. B (page 1214; Secondary Assessment)
10. E (page 1202; Cold Exposure)
11. G (page 1203; Hypothermia)
12. M (page 1202; Cold Exposure)
13. L (page 1211; Heat Cramps)
14. D (pages 1218–1220; Drowning)
15. F (pages 1229–1230; Hymenoptera Stings)

Multiple Choice

1. D (page 1202; Cold Exposure)
2. A (page 1202; Cold Exposure)
3. D (pages 1202–1203; Cold Exposure)
4. C (page 1203; Hypothermia)
5. C (pages 1203–1205; Hypothermia: Signs and Symptoms)
6. B (page 1203; Hypothermia)
7. A (page 1204; Figure 33-1)
8. C (pages 1203–1205; Hypothermia: Signs and Symptoms)
9. D (pages 1209–1210; General Management of Cold Emergencies)
10. D (page 1205; Local Cold Injuries)
11. A (page 1211; Heat Exposure)
12. D (page 1211; Heat Exposure)
13. D (page 1224; Diving Emergencies: History Taking)
14. A (page 1211; Heat Cramps)
15. D (pages 1211–1212; Heat Exhaustion)
16. A (page 1218; Spinal Injuries in Submersion Incidents)
17. A (pages 1212–1213; Heatstroke)
18. D (pages 1212–1213; Heatstroke)
19. B (pages 1218–1220; Drowning)
20. D (page 1223; Assessment of Drowning and Diving Emergencies: Scene Size-up)
21. B (pages 1222–1223; Decompression Sickness)
22. A (pages 1218–1220; Drowning)
23. B (page 1220; Resuscitation Efforts)
24. B (page 1220; Diving Emergencies)
25. A (page 1220; Descent Emergencies)
26. D (page 1222; Air Embolism)
27. A (page 1222; Air Embolism)
28. D (pages 1228–1229; Black Widow Spider)
29. A (pages 1232–1233; Coral Snakes)
30. A (page 1234; Tick Bites)
31. B (pages 1231–1232; Pit Vipers)
32. C (page 1234; Tick Bites)
33. A (page 1229; Brown Recluse Spider)
34. D (pages 1231–1232; Pit Vipers)
35. B (pages 1211–1212; Heat Exhaustion)
36. D (page 1217; Heatstroke)
37. B (page 1202; Cold Exposure)
38. D (page 1217; Management of Heat Emergencies: Heatstroke)
39. C (pages 1201–1202; Factors Affecting Exposure)
40. A (pages 1201–1202; Factors Affecting Exposure)
41. A (page 1217; Heatstroke)

True/False

1. T   (page 1202; Cold Exposure)
2. T   (page 1203; Hypothermia: Signs and Symptoms)
3. F   (page 1203; Hypothermia: Signs and Symptoms)
4. T   (pages 1210–1211; Heat Exposure)
5. T   (pages 1210–1211; Heat Exposure)
6. F   (page 1226; Other Water Hazards)
7. T   (page 1220; Resuscitation Efforts)
8. F   (pages 1231–1232; Pit Vipers)
9. F   (pages 1231–1232; Pit Vipers)
10. T   (pages 1231–1232; Pit Vipers)
11. F   (page 1234; Tick Bites)
12. F   (page 1235; Injuries From Marine Animals)
13. F   (page 1207; Assessment of Cold Injuries: Primary Assessment)
14. T   (pages 1209–1210; General Management of Cold Emergencies)
15. T   (pages 1227–1228; Lightning: Emergency Medical Care)
16. F   (pages 1201–1202; Factors Affecting Exposure)
17. F   (page 1223; Assessment of Drowning and Diving Emergencies: Scene Size-up)
18. T   (pages 1206–1207; Assessment of Cold Injuries: Scene Size-up)
19. F   (page 1213; Assessment of Heat Emergencies: Scene Size-up)

Fill-in-the-Blank

1. moderate, severe (page 1209; General Management of Cold Emergencies)
2. ascent (page 1222; Ascent Emergencies)
3. rewarming (page 1210; Emergency Care of Local Cold Injuries)
4. high-altitude pulmonary edema (page 1226; High Altitude)
5. Shivering (page 1203; Hypothermia: Signs and Symptoms)
6. diving reflex (page 1220; Resuscitation Efforts)
7. Radiation (page 1202; Cold Exposure)
8. 93.2°F (34°C), 98°F (36.7°C) (page 1203; Hypothermia: Signs and Symptoms)
9. cardiovascular, nervous (page 1227; Lightning)
10. Lightning (page 1227; Lightning)
11. Antivenin (pages 1228–1229; Black Widow Spider)
12. Hymenoptera (page 1229; Hymenoptera Stings)
13. April, October (page 1230; Snake Bites)
14. rattlesnake (page 1231; Pit Vipers)
15. Scorpions (page 1233; Scorpion Stings)
16. summer (page 1234; Tick Bites)
17. bull's-eye (page 1234; Tick Bites)
18. vinegar (page 1235; Injuries From Marine Animals)
19. envenomations (page 1235; Injuries From Marine Animals)
20. heat sensitive (page 1235; Injuries From Marine Animals)

Critical Thinking

Short Answer

1. 1. Increase or decrease heat production: shiver, jump, walk around, etc.
   2. Move to an area where heat loss is decreased or increased: out of wind, into sun, etc.
   3. Wear insulated clothing, which helps decrease heat loss in several ways: layer with wool, down, synthetics, etc. (page 1203; Cold Exposure)

2. 1. Move the patient out of the hot environment and into the ambulance.
   2. Set the air conditioning to maximum cooling.
   3. Remove the patient's clothing.
   4. Administer high-flow oxygen if indicated. If needed, assist the patient's ventilations with a bag-mask device and appropriate airway adjuncts as per your protocol.
   5. Provide cold-water immersion in an ice bath, if possible.
   6. Cover the patient with wet towels or sheets, or spray the patient with cool water and fan him or her to quickly evaporate the moisture on the skin.

7. Aggressively and repeatedly fan the patient with or without dampening the skin.

8. Exclude other causes of altered mental status and check blood glucose level, if possible.

9. Provide rapid transport to the hospital.

10. Notify the hospital as soon as possible so that staff can prepare to treat the patient immediately on arrival.

11. Do not overcool the patient. Call for ALS assistance if the patient begins to shiver. (page 1217; Management of Heat Emergencies: Heatstroke)

3. An air embolism is a bubble of air in the blood vessels caused by breath-holding during rapid ascent. The air pressure in the lungs remains at a high level while the external pressure on the chest decreases. As a result, the air inside the lungs expands rapidly, causing the alveoli in the lungs to rupture. (page 1222; Air Embolism)

4. Treatment of air embolism and decompression sickness. The recompression treatment allows the bubbles of gas to dissolve into the blood and equalize the pressures inside and outside the lungs. (pages 1222–1223; Decompression Sickness)

5. **1.** Remove the patient from further exposure to the cold.

2. Handle the injured part gently, and protect it from further injury.

3. Remove any wet or restricting clothing from the patient, especially over the injured part.

4. Remove any jewelry from the injured part and cover the injury loosely with a dry, sterile dressing.

5. Splinting a frostbitten extremity may also help prevent secondary injury by limiting use.

6. Evaluate the patient's general condition for the signs or symptoms of systemic hypothermia.

7. Support the vital functions as necessary, and provide rapid transport to the hospital. (page 1210; Emergency Care of Local Cold Injuries)

6. **1.** Do not break blisters.

2. Do not rub or massage area.

3. Do not apply heat or rewarm unless instructed by medical control.

4. Do not allow patient to stand or walk on a frostbitten foot.

5. Do not reexpose the injury to cold. (page 1210; Emergency Care of Local Cold Injuries)

7. **1.** Have the patient lie flat and stay quiet.

2. Wash the bite area with soapy water; consider a constricting band for hypotensive patients.

3. Splint the extremity.

4. Mark the skin with a pen to monitor advancing swelling. (pages 1231–1232; Pit Vipers)

8. **1.** Black widow: Bite has a systemic effect (venom is neurotoxic).

2. Brown recluse: Bite destroys tissue locally (venom is cytotoxic). (page 1229; Spider Bites)

Ambulance Calls

1. Provide BLS. Administer oxygen. Transport the patient in the left lateral recumbent position with the head down. Transport to a facility with hyperbaric chamber access.

2. Your main concern for this patient is hypothermia. Although this patient could also likely have localized cold injuries such as frostbite or frostnip, hypothermia can be fatal. You must handle this patient carefully, remove any wet clothing, and prevent further heat loss. Assessing the extent of the hypothermia through mentation will be difficult in this case because your patient is likely confused. Take note of the presence of shivering (this protective mechanism stops at core temperatures >90°F or 32°C), and if possible, take his temperature (rectally). Assess airway, breathing, and circulation. Provide warm, humidified oxygen (if possible) and passive rewarming measures, such as increasing the heat in the patient compartment. Promptly transport.

3. This patient is suffering from heat exhaustion. The hot environment coupled with the strenuous activity and poor hydration has overwhelmed his ability to thermoregulate. Promptly move him to the back of the ambulance with the air conditioner on high. Remove any excessive clothing. Administer high-flow oxygen, and assess his glucose level because his mental status is altered. Cover the

patient with cool, wet towels and place ice packs on the trunk of the body—groin, axillae, neck. Because he is already nauseated, transport as left lateral recumbent. Assess his skin turgor, and call for ALS rendezvous for more aggressive treatment if his symptoms do not clear up promptly.

Skills

Skill Drills

Skill Drill 33-1: Treating for Heat Exhaustion (page 1216)

1. Move the patient to a **cooler environment**. Remove extra **clothing**.

2. Give **oxygen** if indicated. Check the patient's blood glucose level if indicated. Perform cold-water immersion or other cooling measures as available. Place the patient in a **supine** position and fan the patient.

3. If the patient is fully alert, give **water** by mouth.

4. If **nausea** develops, secure and transport the patient on his or her left side.

Skill Drill 33-2: Stabilizing a Suspected Spinal Injury in the Water (page 1221)

1. Turn the patient to a supine position by rotating the entire upper half of the body as a single unit.

2. As soon as the patient is turned, begin artificial ventilation using the mouth-to-mouth method or a pocket mask.

3. Float a buoyant backboard under the patient.

4. Secure the patient to the backboard.

5. Remove the patient from the water.

6. Maintain the body's normal temperature and apply oxygen if the patient is breathing. Begin CPR if breathing and pulse are absent.

Assessment Review

1. B (page 1206; Figure 33-4)
2. A (page 1203; Cold Exposure)
3. B (page 1211; Heat Exposure)
4. B (pages 1227–1228; Lightning)
5. C (page 1235; Injuries From Marine Animals)

CHAPTER

34 Obstetrics and Neonatal Care

General Knowledge

Matching

1. D (page 1244; Anatomy and Physiology of the Female Reproductive System)
2. C (pages 1255–1256; Stages of Labor)
3. L (page 1245; Anatomy and Physiology of the Female Reproductive System)
4. B (page 1245; Anatomy and Physiology of the Female Reproductive System)
5. N (page 1244; Anatomy and Physiology of the Female Reproductive System)
6. H (page 1245; Anatomy and Physiology of the Female Reproductive System)
7. M (pages 1278–1279; Vital Vocabulary)
8. E (page 1245; Anatomy and Physiology of the Female Reproductive System)
9. F (pages 1255–1256; Stages of Labor)
10. O (pages 1270–1271; Breech Delivery)
11. K (pages 1271–1272; Presentation Complications)
12. I (pages 1278–1279; Vital Vocabulary)
13. A (page 1263; Umbilical Cord Around the Neck)
14. G (pages 1270–1271; Breech Delivery)
15. J (page 1250; Abortion)

Multiple Choice

1. C (page 1263; Umbilical Cord Around the Neck)
2. B (page 1254; History Taking)
3. B (pages 1266–1269; Additional Resuscitation Efforts)
4. B (pages 1264–1265; Delivery of the Placenta)
5. A (pages 1269–1270; The Apgar Score)
6. C (page 1267; Figure 34-10 Basic Neonatal Resuscitation Algorithm)
7. D (pages 1269–1270; The Apgar Score)
8. D (pages 1266–1269; Additional Resuscitation Efforts)
9. A (pages 1271–1272; Presentation Complications)
10. A (pages 1271–1272; Presentation Complications)
11. B (pages 1250–1251; Substance Abuse)
12. A (pages 1255–1256; Stages of Labor)
13. B (pages 1255–1256; Stages of Labor)
14. C (pages 1255–1256; Stages of Labor)
15. A (pages 1255–1256; Stages of Labor)
16. C (pages 1255–1256; Stages of Labor)
17. B (pages 1247–1248; Hypertension in Pregnancy)
18. B (pages 1248–1250; Bleeding)
19. D (pages 1256–1258; Preparing for Delivery)
20. C (pages 1246–1247; Normal Changes in Pregnancy)
21. D (page 1248; Hypertension in Pregnancy)
22. D (pages 1271–1272; Presentation Complications)
23. C (pages 1248–1250; Bleeding)
24. B (pages 1248–1250; Bleeding)
25. A (pages 1247–1248; Hypertension in Pregnancy)
26. B (pages 1250–1251; Substance Abuse)
27. D (page 1260; Skill Drill 34-1 Delivering the Newborn: Step 1)
28. D (page 1263; Unruptured Amniotic Sac)
29. C (pages 1255–1256; Stages of Labor)
30. D (page 1274; Postpartum Complications)
31. D (pages 1264–1265; Delivery of the Placenta)
32. B (page 1244; Anatomy and Physiology of the Female Reproductive System)
33. C (page 1244; Anatomy and Physiology of the Female Reproductive System)
34. B (pages 1248–1250; Bleeding)
35. B (pages 1269–1270; The Apgar Score)
36. C (pages 1272–1273; Multiple Gestation)
37. A (page 1273; Premature Birth)
38. D (page 1273; Postterm Pregnancy)
39. C (page 1274; Postpartum Complications)
40. C (pages 1265–1266; Neonatal Assessment and Resuscitation)

True/False

1. T (page 1244; Anatomy and Physiology of the Female Reproductive System)
2. F (pages 1255–1256; Stages of Labor)
3. F (pages 1255–1256; Stages of Labor)
4. F (pages 1278–1279; Vital Vocabulary)
5. F (pages 1256–1258; Preparing for Delivery)
6. T (pages 1270–1271; Breech Delivery)
7. T (pages 1264–1265; Delivery of the Placenta)
8. F (pages 1264–1265; Delivery of the Placenta)
9. F (pages 1264–1265; Delivery of the Placenta)
10. T (pages 1271–1272; Presentation Complications)
11. T (pages 1272–1273; Multiple Gestation)
12. T (page 1253; Teenage Pregnancy)
13. T (pages 1254–1255; Secondary Assessment)
14. T (page 1250; Abuse)
15. T (pages 1273–1274; Fetal Death)
16. F (page 1273; Premature Birth)
17. T (page 1274; Postpartum Complications)

Fill-in-the-Blank

1. placenta (pages 1264–1265; Delivery of the Placenta)
2. arteries, vein (page 1245; Anatomy and Physiology of the Female Reproductive System)
3. 500, 1,000 (page 1245; Anatomy and Physiology of the Female Reproductive System)
4. 39, 40, 6 (page 1245; Anatomy and Physiology of the Female Reproductive System)
5. 20 (pages 1246–1247; Normal Changes in Pregnancy)
6. 50% (pages 1246–1247; Normal Changes in Pregnancy)
7. ectopic pregnancy (pages 1248–1250; Bleeding)
8. 10 (pages 1270–1271; Breech Delivery)
9. fontanelles (page 1260; The Delivery: Step 2)
10. Spina bifida (page 1272; Spina Bifida)
11. spontaneous abortion (page 1250; Abortion)
12. Braxton-Hicks (pages 1255–1256; Stages of Labor)
13. umbilical vein (page 1245; Anatomy and Physiology of the Female Reproductive System)
14. perineum (page 1244; Anatomy and Physiology of the Female Reproductive System)
15. falls (pages 1251–1252; Special Considerations for Trauma and Pregnancy)

Fill-in-the-Table (page 1269; Table 34-4 Apgar Scoring System)

Area of Activity	Score		
	2	**1**	**0**
Appearance	**Entire newborn is pink.**	**Body is pink, but hands and feet remain blue.**	**Entire newborn is blue or pale.**
Pulse	**More than 100 beats/min.**	**Fewer than 100 beats/min.**	**Absent pulse.**
Grimace or irritability	**Newborn cries and tries to move foot away from finger snapped against sole of foot.**	**Newborn gives a weak cry in response to stimulus.**	**Newborn does not cry or react to stimulus.**
Activity or muscle tone	**Newborn resists attempts to straighten hips and knees.**	**Newborn makes weak attempts to resist straightening.**	**Newborn is completely limp, with no muscle tone.**
Respiration	**Rapid respirations.**	**Slow respirations.**	**Absent respirations.**

Labeling

1. Anatomic Structures of the Pregnant Woman (page 1244; Figure 34-1)

   A. Placenta

   B. Uterus

   C. Cervix

   D. Amniotic fluid

   E. Sacrum

   F. Rectum

   G. Bladder

   H. Vagina

   I. Pubic symphysis

Critical Thinking

Multiple Choice

1. C   (pages 1269–1270; The Apgar Score)

2. A   (pages 1269–1270; The Apgar Score)

3. B   (pages 1269–1270; The Apgar Score)

Short Answer

1. Early: spontaneous abortion (miscarriage) or ectopic pregnancy

   Late: Placenta previa or abruptio placentae (pages 1248–1250; Bleeding, page 1250; Abortion)

2. On the left side, to prevent supine hypotensive syndrome (low blood pressure occurring from the weight of the fetus compressing the inferior vena cava) (pages 1247–1248; Hypertension in Pregnancy)

3. **1.** Uterine contractions

   2. Bloody show

   3. Rupture of amniotic sac (pages 1255–1256; Stages of Labor)

4. **1.** How long have you been pregnant?

   2. When are you due?

   3. Is this your first baby?

   4. Are you having contractions? If so, how far apart are the contractions? How long do the contractions last?

   5. Do you feel as though you will have a bowel movement?

   6. Have you had any spotting or bleeding?

   7. Has your water broken?

   8. Do you feel the need to push?

   9. Were any of your previous children delivered by cesarean section?

   10. Did you have any problems in this or any previous pregnancy?

   11. Do you use drugs, drink alcohol, or take any medications?

   12. Is there a chance you will have multiple deliveries (having more than one baby)?

   13. Does your physician expect any other complications? (page 1257; Preparing for Delivery)

5. Place your sterile gloved hand over the emerging bony parts of the head, avoid the eyes and fontanelles, and by exerting minimal pressure, control the delivery of the head. (page 1263; Delivering the Head)

6. The brain is only covered by skin and membrane at the fontanelles. (page 1263; Delivering the Head)

7. Apply gentle pressure across the perineum with a sterile gauze pad. (page 1263; Delivering the Head)

8. **1.** During a breech delivery to protect the infant's airway

 2. When the umbilical cord is prolapsed (pages 1270–1271; Breech Delivery, pages 1271–1272; Presentation Complications)

9. **1.** Prematurity

 2. Low birth weight

 3. Severe respiratory depression (pages 1250–1251; Substance Abuse)

10. **1.** Severe or persistent headache

 2. Visual abnormalities such as seeing spots, blurred vision, or sensitivity to light

 3. Swelling in the hands and feet (edema)

 4. Anxiety

 5. Severe hypertension (pages 1247–1248; Hypertension in Pregnancy)

Ambulance Calls

1. This patient has classic signs of preeclampsia. If she does not receive medical care soon to control her hypertension, she will likely experience a seizure. Provide high-flow oxygen, obtain a set of vital signs (especially blood pressure), and provide prompt transport with the patient on her left side. Consider ALS intercept, if available.

2. Position the mother for delivery and apply high-flow oxygen. As crowning occurs, use a clamp to puncture the sac or tear it by twisting it between your fingers, away from the baby's face. Push the ruptured sac away from the infant's face as the head is delivered. Clear the newborn's mouth and nose, using the bulb syringe if required by your protocols, and wipe the mouth and nose with gauze. Continue with the delivery as normal.

Skills

Skill Drill

Skill Drill 34-1: Delivering the Newborn (pages 1260–1262)

1. Crowning is the definitive sign that delivery is imminent, and transport should be delayed until after the child has been born.

2. Use your hands to support the bony parts of the head as it emerges. The child's body will naturally rotate to the right or left at this point in the delivery. Continue to support the head to allow it to turn in the same direction.

3. As the upper shoulder appears, guide the head down slightly by applying gentle downward traction to deliver the shoulder.

4. Support the head and upper body as the lower shoulder delivers; guide the head up if needed.

5. Handle the newborn firmly but gently, support the head, and keep the neck in a neutral position to maintain the airway. Consider placing the newborn on the mother's abdomen with the umbilical cord still intact; allow skin-to-skin contact to warm the newborn. Otherwise, keep the newborn approximately at the level of the vagina until the cord has been cut.

6. After delivery and prior to cutting the cord, if the child is gurgling or shows other signs of respiratory distress, suction the mouth and oropharynx to clear any amniotic fluid and ease the infant's initiation of air exchange.

7. Wait for the umbilical cord to stop pulsing. Place a clamp on the cord. Milk the blood from a small section of the cord on the placental side of the clamp. Place a second clamp 2 inches to 3 inches away from the first.

8. Cut between the clamps.

9. Allow the placenta to deliver itself. Do not pull on the cord to speed delivery.

Assessment Review

1. A (page 1263; The Delivery)

2. A (pages 1266–1269; Additional Resuscitation Efforts)

3. A (page 1254; History Taking)

4. D (page 1264; The Delivery)

5. B (page 1264; Postdelivery Care)

CHAPTER

35 | Pediatric Emergencies

General Knowledge

Matching

1. C (page 1289; Adolescents)
2. I (page 1311; Croup)
3. F (page 1285; The Infant)
4. A (page 1299; Table 35-5 Abnormal Breath Sounds)
5. D (page 1338; Neglect)
6. G (page 1284; Introduction)
7. J (page 1312; Pertussis)
8. H (page 1287; The Preschool-Age Child)
9. B (pages 1297–1302; Hands-On XABCs)
10. E (page 1286; The Toddler)

Multiple Choice

1. B (page 1285; The Infant: 2 to 6 Months)
2. C (page 1285; The Infant: 6 to 12 Months)
3. D (page 1286; The Toddler: 12 to 18 Months)
4. C (page 1287; The Preschool-Age Child)
5. A (pages 1290–1292; The Respiratory System)
6. A (pages 1290–1292; The Respiratory System)
7. D (page 1292; The Circulatory System)
8. B (page 1322; Altered Mental Status)
9. C (page 1329; Pediatric Trauma Emergencies and Management)
10. C (pages 1297–1302; Hands-On XABCs)
11. A (pages 1297–1302; Hands-On XABCs)
12. B (pages 1297–1302; Hands-On XABCs)
13. A (pages 1297–1302; Hands-On XABCs)
14. D (page 1303; History Taking)
15. C (pages 1292–1293; The Musculoskeletal System)
16. D (page 1308; Respiratory Emergencies and Management)
17. C (pages 1295–1296; Pediatric Assessment Triangle)
18. B (pages 1310–1311; Asthma)
19. D (pages 1308–1310; Airway Obstruction)
20. B (pages 1310–1311; Asthma)
21. A (pages 1310–1311; Asthma)
22. A (page 1311; Pneumonia)
23. A (page 1312; Bronchiolitis)
24. D (pages 1320–1322; Shock)
25. C (pages 1328–1329; Shock)
26. D (pages 1321–1322; Anaphylaxis, pages 1308–1310; Airway Obstruction)
27. D (pages 1322–1323; Seizures)
28. B (pages 1323–1324; Meningitis)
29. C (pages 1324–1325; Gastrointestinal Emergencies and Management)
30. A (page 1325; Poisoning Emergencies and Management)
31. D (page 1325; Poisoning Emergencies and Management)
32. A (page 1327; Table 35-14 Vital Signs and Symptoms of Dehydration)
33. B (page 1326; Dehydration Emergencies and Management)
34. D (page 1327; Fever Emergencies and Management)
35. C (pages 1328–1329; Drowning Emergencies and Management)
36. D (page 1330; Sports Activities)
37. B (page 1333; Abdominal Injuries)
38. B (pages 1333–1335; Burns)
39. B (pages 1335–1336; Disaster Management)
40. C (page 1339; Sudden Unexplained Infant Death and Sudden Infant Death Syndrome)
41. D (page 1339; Sudden Unexplained Infant Death and Sudden Infant Death Syndrome)
42. A (page 1342; Communication and Support of the Family After the Death of a Child)

True/False

1. F (page 1285; 6 to 12 months)
2. T (pages 1286–1287; The Toddler: Assessment)
3. F (pages 1286–1287; The Toddler: Assessment)
4. T (page 1289; Adolescents)
5. T (page 1289; Adolescents)
6. F (page 1308; Respiratory Emergencies and Management)
7. T (page 1329; Pediatric Trauma Emergencies and Management)
8. T (page 1301; Words of Wisdom)
9. F (pages 1297–1302; Hands-On XABCs)
10. T (pages 1302–1303; Transport Decision)
11. F (pages 1304–1306; Secondary Assessment)
12. T (pages 1310–1311; Asthma)
13. T (page 1313; Oropharyngeal Airway)
14. F (page 1316; Oxygen Delivery Devices)
15. T (page 1327; Fever Emergencies and Management)
16. T (pages 1330–1333; Immobilization)
17. F (page 1335; Injuries of the Extremities)
18. T (page 1336; Child Abuse and Neglect)
19. T (pages 1338–1339; Sexual Abuse)
20. F (page 1340; Communication and Support of the Family After the Death of a Child)

Fill-in-the-Blank

1. oxygen demand (pages 1290–1292; The Respiratory System)
2. chest (pages 1290–1292; The Respiratory System)
3. respiratory failure (pages 1290–1292; The Respiratory System)
4. fontanelles (pages 1292–1293; The Musculoskeletal System)
5. pediatric assessment triangle (pages 1295–1296; Pediatric Assessment Triangle)
6. sniffing position (pages 1297–1302; Hands-On XABCs)
7. forward-facing, rear-facing (pages 1302–1303; Transport Decision)
8. oxygen (page 1308; Respiratory Emergencies and Management)
9. Epiglottitis (pages 1311–1312; Epiglottitis)
10. Chest compressions (pages 1308–1310; Airway Obstruction)
11. status asthmaticus (pages 1310–1311; Asthma)
12. nasopharyngeal airway (pages 1314–1316; Nasopharyngeal Airway)
13. Hemophilia (page 1322; Bleeding Disorders)
14. Appendicitis (pages 1324–1325; Gastrointestinal Emergencies and Management)
15. Drowning (pages 1328–1329; Drowning Emergencies and Management)
16. blunt trauma (page 1333; Chest Injuries)
17. infection (page 1338; Burns)
18. Neglect (page 1338; Neglect)

Short Answer

1. **T**—Tone

   I—Interactiveness

   C—Consolability

   L—Look or gaze

   S—Speech or cry (page 1295; Table 35-4 Characteristics of Appearance: The TICLS Mnemonic)

2. **Abnormal airway noise:** Grunting or wheezing

   Accessory muscle use: Contractions of the muscles above the clavicles (supraclavicular)

   Retractions: Drawing in of the muscles between the ribs (intercostal retractions) or of the sternum (substernal retractions) during inspiration

   Head bobbing: The head lifts and tilts back during inspiration, then moves forward during expiration

   Nasal flaring: The nares (the external openings of the nose) widen; usually seen during inspiration

   Tachypnea: Increased respiratory rate

   Tripod position: In older children, this position will maximize the effectiveness of the airway (pages 1295–1296; Pediatric Assessment Triangle)

3. Significant MOI—same MOIs as adults, with the addition of:
   - Any fall from a height equal to or greater than a pediatric patient's height, especially with a headfirst landing
   - Bicycle crash (when not wearing a helmet)

   A history compatible with a serious illness

   A physical abnormality noted during the primary assessment

   A potentially serious anatomic abnormality

   Significant pain

   Abnormal level of consciousness, altered mental status, or signs and/or symptoms of shock (pages 1302–1303; Transport Decision)

4. 70 + (2 × child's age in years) = systolic blood pressure (pages 1304–1306; Secondary Assessment)

5. **Pulse:** Assess both the rate and quality of the pulse. A weak, "thready" pulse is a sign that there is a problem. The appropriate rate depends on the patient's age; generally, except in the case of a newborn, anything over 160 beats/min suggests shock.

   Skin signs: Assess the temperature and moisture of the hands and feet. How does this compare with the temperature of the skin on the trunk of the body? Is the skin dry and warm or cold and clammy?

   Capillary refill time: Squeeze a finger or toe for several seconds until the skin blanches, and then release it. Does the fingertip return to its normal color within 2 seconds, or is it delayed?

   Color: Assess the patient's skin color. Is it pink, pale, ashen, or blue?

   Changes: Changes in pulse rate, color, skin signs, and capillary refill time are all important clues suggesting shock. (pages 1320–1322; Shock)

Ambulance Calls

1. Young children typically experience febrile seizures when their temperature rises rapidly. As with any call, you should assess the airway, breathing, and circulation of this 2-year-old patient. Ensure that his airway is patent; assist him with breathing using a bag-mask device and airway adjunct, as necessary; apply high-flow oxygen; and remove excessive clothing. The child's level of consciousness should improve. If the child's level of consciousness doesn't improve or if the child experiences additional seizure activity, then this is a very serious sign that should be relayed to the receiving emergency department.

2. Immediately open and suction the airway. Assess breathing and apply high-flow oxygen via a nonrebreathing mask or bag-mask device. Assess the patient further en route during rapid transport. Obtain the history from the grandmother en route. Reassess the patient's airway and vital signs en route as well.

3. Allow the mother to ride in the patient compartment of the ambulance to comfort the child. Provide rapid transport in a position of comfort, with as much oxygen as she will tolerate. Continually assess the patient for signs of altered mental status and decreasing tidal volume; be prepared to assist ventilations. Obtain further history en route.

4. This infant is deceased, possibly as a result of SIDS. After you have quickly assessed the infant and made this determination, you must communicate the condition of the baby to the mother and family. This may be difficult, and they will possibly request resuscitation attempts regardless of your findings. This becomes a judgment call, which can be clarified by utilizing online medical direction and/or standing orders. You should survey the scene and document any history of recent illness, congenital conditions, and so forth. Be supportive of family members and assist them as appropriate. Calls involving infants and children can be traumatic experiences for emergency medical providers as well. Request debriefing as necessary and follow local protocols.

Skills

Skill Drills

Skill Drill 35-1: Positioning the Airway in a Pediatric Patient (page 1298)

1. Position the pediatric patient on a **firm** surface.

2. Place a **folded** towel about 1 inch (2.5 cm) thick under the **shoulders** and **back**.

3. **Stabilize** the forehead to limit **movement**, and use the head tilt–chin lift maneuver to open the airway.

Skill Drill 35-2: Inserting an Oropharyngeal Airway in a Pediatric Patient (page 1314)

1. Determine the appropriately **sized** airway. Confirm the correct size **visually** by placing it next to the pediatric patient's **face**.

2. Position the pediatric patient's **airway** with the appropriate method.

3. Open the mouth. Insert the airway until the **flange** rests against the **lips**. **Reassess** the airway.

Skill Drill 35-3: Inserting a Nasopharyngeal Airway in a Pediatric Patient (page 1315)

1. Determine the correct airway size by comparing its **diameter** to the opening of the **nostril** (nare). Place the airway next to the pediatric patient's **face** to confirm correct **length**. **Position** the airway.

2. **Lubricate** the airway. Insert the **tip** into the right naris, with the bevel pointing toward the **septum**.

3. Carefully move the tip forward until the **flange** rests against the **outside** of the nostril. Reassess the **airway**.

Skill Drill 35-4: One-Person Bag-Mask Ventilation on a Pediatric Patient (page 1319)

1. Open the airway and insert the appropriate airway adjunct.

2. Hold the mask on the patient's face with a one-handed head tilt–chin lift technique (EC clamp method). Ensure a good mask–face seal while maintaining the airway.

3. Squeeze the bag using the correct ventilation rate of 1 breath every 3 to 5 seconds or 12 to 20 breaths/min. Allow adequate time for exhalation.

4. Assess effectiveness of ventilation by watching bilateral rise and fall of the chest.

Skill Drill 35-6: Immobilizing a Patient in a Car Seat (page 1332)

1. **Stabilize** the head in a **neutral** position.

2. Place a **short backboard** or pediatric **immobilization device** between the patient and the surface he or she is resting on.

3. Slide the patient onto the **short backboard** or pediatric **immobilization device**.

4. Place a **towel** under the back, from the **shoulders** to the **hips**, to ensure **neutral** head position.

5. Secure the **torso** first; pad any **voids**.

6. Secure the head to the short backboard or pediatric **immobilization device**.

CHAPTER

36 Geriatric Emergencies

General Knowledge

Matching

1. E (pages 1354–1357; Changes in the Cardiovascular System: Pathophysiology)
2. C (pages 1357–1358; Changes in the Nervous System: Vision)
3. G (pages 1359–1360; Delirium)
4. I (pages 1358–1359; Dementia)
5. J (page 1360; Syncope)
6. F (pages 1353–1354; Pulmonary Embolism)
7. D (pages 1364–1365; Changes in the Musculoskeletal System: Pathophysiology)
8. H (pages 1365–1367; Toxicology)
9. A (pages 1364–1365; Changes in the Musculoskeletal System: Pathophysiology)
10. B (page 1356; Heart Failure)

Multiple Choice

1. C (page 1352; Table 36-1 Common Conditions and the Leading Causes of Death in Geriatric Patients)
2. A (page 1350; Introduction)
3. D (pages 1350–1351; Generational Considerations)
4. C (pages 1350–1351; Generational Considerations)
5. A (page 1351; Communication and Older Adults)
6. C (page 1352; Table 36-1 Common Conditions and the Leading Causes of Death in Geriatric Patients)
7. D (page 1369; Scene Size-up)
8. C (page 1379; Response to Nursing and Skilled Care Facilities)
9. A (page 1353; Changes in the Respiratory System: Anatomy and Physiology)
10. A (page 1371; History Taking)
11. D (page 1371; History Taking)
12. B (page 1377; Secondary Assessment)
13. C (pages 1374–1375; Trauma and Geriatric Patients: Anatomic Changes and Fractures)
14. A (page 1368; The GEMS Diamond)
15. D (page 1353; Changes in the Respiratory System: Anatomy and Physiology)
16. B (page 1353; Pneumonia)
17. A (pages 1353–1354; Pulmonary Embolism)
18. C (pages 1354–1357; Changes in the Cardiovascular System: Pathophysiology)
19. A (pages 1354–1357; Changes in the Cardiovascular System: Pathophysiology)
20. D (pages 1353–1354; Pulmonary Embolism)
21. C (pages 1359–1360; Delirium)
22. B (pages 1356–1357; Stroke)
23. D (pages 1357–1358; Changes in the Nervous System: Anatomy and Physiology)
24. D (pages 1357–1358; Vision)
25. A (page 1358; Hearing)
26. D (pages 1358–1359; Dementia)
27. B (page 1360; Changes in the Gastrointestinal System: Anatomy and Physiology)
28. A (pages 1360–1362; Changes in the Gastrointestinal System: Pathophysiology)
29. C (page 1362; The Acute Abdomen: Nongastrointestinal Complaints)
30. C (pages 1362–1363; Changes in the Renal System)
31. D (page 1363; Changes in the Endocrine System: Anatomy and Physiology)
32. A (pages 1364–1365; Changes in the Musculoskeletal System: Pathophysiology)
33. C (pages 1364–1365; Changes in the Musculoskeletal System: Pathophysiology)
34. B (pages 1365–1367; Toxicology)
35. D (page 1367; Depression)
36. C (page 1374; Trauma and Geriatric Patients)
37. B (pages 1367–1368; Suicide)

38. D (page 1374; Trauma and Geriatric Patients)
39. B (page 1382; Assessment of Elder Abuse)
40. D (pages 1374–1375; Trauma and Geriatric Patients: Anatomic Changes and Fractures)
41. C (page 1379; Response to Nursing and Skilled Care Facilities)
42. D (page 1379; Response to Nursing and Skilled Care Facilities)
43. D (page 1380; Advance Directives)
44. D (page 1383; Signs of Physical Abuse)
45. B (page 1383; Signs of Physical Abuse)

True/False

1. T (pages 1350–1351; Generational Considerations)
2. T (page 1351; Communication and Older Adults)
3. F (page 1352; Common Complaints and the Leading Causes of Death in Older People)
4. T (page 1354; Changes in the Cardiovascular System: Anatomy and Physiology)
5. T (page 1371; Primary Assessment)
6. T (page 1371; History Taking)
7. T (page 1368; The GEMS Diamond)
8. F (page 1353; Changes in the Respiratory System: Anatomy and Physiology)
9. F (page 1354; Changes in the Cardiovascular System: Anatomy and Physiology)
10. F (pages 1355–1356; Myocardial Infarction (Heart Attack))
11. T (pages 1356–1357; Stroke)
12. T (pages 1357–1358; Vision)
13. T (page 1358; Taste)
14. F (page 1360; Neuropathy)
15. T (pages 1360–1362; Changes in the Gastrointestinal System: Pathophysiology)
16. F (pages 1360–1362; Changes in the Gastrointestinal System: Pathophysiology)
17. F (page 1363; Changes in the Endocrine System: Pathophysiology)
18. T (page 1363; Changes in the Immune System)
19. F (page 1360; Changes in the Gastrointestinal System: Anatomy and Physiology)
20. T (pages 1367–1368; Suicide)
21. F (page 1374; Trauma and Geriatric Patients)
22. F (page 1375; Special Considerations in Assessing Geriatric Trauma Patients)
23. T (page 1377; Reassessment)
24. T (page 1375; Environmental Injury)
25. T (page 1380; Advance Directives)

Fill-in-the-Blank

1. name (page 1351; Communication and Older Adults)
2. osteoporosis (pages 1374–1375; Anatomic Changes and Fractures)
3. Oxygen (page 1372; Reassessment)
4. Pneumonia (page 1353; Pneumonia)
5. mucus production (page 1353; Pneumonia)
6. Arteriosclerosis (page 1354; Changes in the Cardiovascular System: Anatomy and Physiology)
7. aneurysm (pages 1354–1357; Changes in the Cardiovascular System: Pathophysiology)
8. left-sided (page 1356; Heart Failure)
9. Presbycusis (page 1358; Hearing)
10. touch, pain (page 1358; Touch)
11. Diverticulosis (pages 1360–1362; Changes in the Gastrointestinal System: Pathophysiology)
12. Pressure ulcers (page 1365; Changes in Skin)
13. head injuries (pages 1374–1375; Anatomic Changes and Fractures)
14. Bystander information (pages 1375–1376; Special Considerations in Assessing Geriatric Trauma Patients: Scene Size-up)
15. airway obstruction (pages 1370–1371; Special Considerations in Assessing a Geriatric Medical Patient: Primary Assessment)
16. flaccid abdominal wall (page 1377; Special Considerations in Assessing Geriatric Trauma Patients: Secondary Assessment)
17. kyphosis (pages 1377–1378; Special Considerations in Assessing Geriatric Trauma Patients: Reassessment)
18. pelvic (pages 1374–1375; Anatomic Changes and Fractures)
19. Nursing homes (page 1379; Response to Nursing and Skilled Care Facilities)
20. Advance directives (page 1380; Advance Directives)

Fill-in-the-Table (page 1383; Table 36-5)

Fill in the missing parts of the table.

Categories of Elder Abuse	
Physical	• **Assault** • **Neglect or abandonment** • **Dietary (malnutrition)** • **Poor maintenance of home** • **Poor personal hygiene** • **Sexual assault**
Psychological	• **Benign neglect** • **Verbal** • **Treating the person as an infant** • **Deprivation of sensory stimulation**
Financial	• **Theft of valuables** • **Embezzlement**

Critical Thinking

Short Answer

1. 1. Hypertension

   2. Arthritis

   3. Heart disease

   4. Cancer

   5. Diabetes mellitus

   6. Asthma

   7. Chronic bronchitis or emphysema

   8. Stroke (page 1352; Table 36-1 Common Conditions and the Leading Causes of Death in Geriatric Patients)

2. **Motor nerves:** muscle weakness, cramps, spasms, loss of balance, and loss of coordination

   Sensory nerves: tingling, numbness, itching, and pain; burning, freezing, or extreme sensitivity to touch

   Autonomic nerves: affected involuntary functions that could include changes in blood pressure and heart rate, constipation, bladder and sexual dysfunction (page 1360; Neuropathy)

3. HHNS is a type 2 diabetic complication. It does not cause ketosis; instead, it leads to osmotic diuresis and a shift of fluid to the intravascular space that results in dehydration. HHNS does not present with Kussmaul respirations.

   DKA is a type 1 diabetic complication. It causes ketosis as a result of the hyperglycemia. The blood glucose is typically over 600 mg/dL in DKA, and patients tend to present with Kussmaul respirations. (page 1363; Changes in the Endocrine System: Pathophysiology)

4. • Caregiver apathy about the patient's condition

   • Overly defensive reaction by caregiver to your questions

   • Caregiver does not allow patient to answer questions

- Repeated visits to the emergency department or clinic
- A history of being accident-prone
- Soft-tissue injuries
- Unbelievable, vague, or inconsistent explanations of injuries
- Psychosomatic complaints
- Chronic pain without medical explanation
- Self-destructive behavior
- Eating and sleep disorders
- Depression or lack of energy
- A history of substance and/or sexual abuse (page 1382; Assessment of Elder Abuse)

5. 1. Dysrhythmias and heart attack: The heart is beating too fast or too slowly, the cardiac output drops, and blood flow to the brain is interrupted. A heart attack can also cause syncope.

2. Vascular and volume changes: Medication interactions can cause venous pooling and vasodilation, the widening of a blood vessel that results in a drop in blood pressure and inadequate blood flow to the brain. Another cause of syncope can be a drop in blood volume because of hidden bleeding (such as an aneurysm).

3. Neurologic cause: Syncope can be a sign of transient ischemic attack or stroke. (page 1360; Table 36-2 Possible Causes of Syncope in Geriatric Patients)

Ambulance Calls

1. This situation appears to be one of neglect and possible elder abuse. Perform a thorough assessment, especially if the patient is confused or is otherwise unable to express how or why she ended up on the floor. Ask for the patient's medical chart to obtain accurate information regarding her medical condition(s) and current medications. Immobilize her affected leg (and spine if needed) using the most comfortable methods possible. Geriatric patients need gentle care and many cannot tolerate conventional methods of splinting and immobilizing. Mechanisms of injury not viewed as significant in young, healthy patients can prove quite devastating or result in serious injury in older patients with frail skin and brittle bones.

2. Osteoporosis can be quite insidious in its onset. Individuals who were once relatively strong and healthy can suddenly find themselves with a fracture from something they may have done many times in the past. Postmenopausal, thin, Caucasian women are at higher risk of developing osteoporosis, and a spinal fracture in this scenario should be suspected. Perform an assessment to determine the presence of other injuries, provide full spinal immobilization, apply oxygen, and promptly transport this patient to the nearest appropriate facility. Always follow local protocols.

3. Hip fractures are a misnomer because true "hip fractures" are in fact fractures of the femur. You should determine if the mechanism of injury or

suspicion exists for possible spinal fractures. Survey the scene to determine if there was a reason for the fall or if the break was spontaneous, giving the patient the impression of "tripping" on an object. If you believe that it was a spontaneous fracture, this patient suffers from extreme osteoporosis and likely sustained other fractures during the fall. If no spinal immobilization is deemed necessary, isolated hip fracture care requires an assessment of the patient's pulse, motor, and sensation of both lower extremities. You should also determine if the affected extremity is the same length or shorter than the uninjured side. It is also helpful to note if the leg is rotated inward, outward, or not at all. Immobilize the injured leg using blankets, pillows, and cravats or straps after placing the patient on a long backboard or scoop stretcher. After immobilization has occurred, reassess the pulse and motor and sensory functions of the injured extremity. Provide reassurance for the patient because many feel that hip fractures signal the loss of their independence. Always follow local protocols.

4. Patients with kyphosis are extremely uncomfortable when immobilized on long backboards. You should pad all voids using pillows, blankets, towels, or other appropriate forms of padding. Failure to adequately pad a patient's spine can result in increased pain and the inability of the patient to remain still. This can result in exacerbated injuries, as well as a very unhappy patient. Thoracic spine injuries and injuries to the ribs can make it difficult for patients to breathe without pain. Determine whether her shortness of breath is related to pain during inspiration and/or whether she has a history of respiratory disease, such as emphysema, chronic bronchitis, or asthma. Local weather conditions have likely contributed to her fall. Depending on the length of exposure to the elements, she could be suffering from hypothermia as well. Geriatric patients generally do not tolerate extremes in weather; avoiding extended periods of time in cold temperatures will minimize the likelihood for hypothermia.

Fill-in-the-Patient Care Report

EMS Patient Care Report (PCR)			
Date: Today's date	**Incident No.:** 011727	**Nature of Call:** Unknown medical emergency	**Location:** 222 Orchard Lane
Dispatched: 0843	**En Route:** 0843	**At Scene:** 0849	**Transport:** 0902	**At Hospital:** 0908	**In Service:** 0915

Patient Information	
Age: 78 years **Sex:** Male **Weight (in kg [lb]):** Unknown	**Allergies:** Aspirin
	Medications: Metoprolol, Lisinopril, Actos, metformin, Zocor, Celebrex, allopurinol, Lasix, K-dur, Plavix, and multivitamin
	Past Medical History: MI, CHF, hypertension, diabetes, arthritis, gout, high cholesterol
	Chief Complaint: Head pain

Vital Signs				
Time: 0853	**BP:** 110/68	**Pulse:** 86	**Respirations:** 20	**SpO$_2$:** 98%
Time: 0902	**BP:** 116/76	**Pulse:** 84	**Respirations:** 18	**SpO$_2$:** 100%

EMS Treatment (circle all that apply)				
Oxygen @ _15_ L/min via (circle one): NC (NRM) BVM		Assisted Ventilation	Airway Adjunct	CPR
Defibrillation	(Bleeding Control)	(Bandaging)	(Splinting: Full body/ cervical immobilization)	Other:

Narrative
9-1-1 dispatch for 78-year-old man with an unknown medical problem. Local fire department was also dispatched for an assist per the dispatcher. We arrived on scene and were met by the patient's wife at the front door, who stated that the patient was lying on the bathroom floor and she was unable to help him up. We were directed to the bathroom, where we found our patient lying supine on the floor in no obvious distress, with a hematoma and laceration noted to his right forehead. The patient stated that he was on the toilet and must have fallen but cannot completely remember the incident. The patient denied any chest pain, dyspnea, N/V, dizziness, or sweating. The patient complained of "head pain," which he rated as a 4/10. The patient denied radiation of pain or neck pain. Cervical immobilization was manually maintained while immobilization supplies were gathered. The patient was fully immobilized onto a backboard to include cervical collar, longboard, and head immobilization device. Immobilization was assisted by fire personnel. Oxygen was applied at 15 L/min via a nonrebreathing mask. Primary and secondary assessment were performed, along with vital signs. The patient was secured to a litter and taken to a unit. The patient was transported to Mercy Hospital per his request. Reassessment of the patient indicated his pain continued to be a 4/10. On arrival at the facility, the patient was stable. Care was transferred to ED staff. A verbal report was given to staff. Room 4. No further incidents. Unit cleaned and restocked. Crew went available and returned to station.**End of Report**

Patients With Special Challenges

General Knowledge

Matching

1. C (pages 1400–1401; Cerebral Palsy)
2. H (page 1410; Colostomies, Ileostomies, and Urostomies)
3. F (pages 1393–1394; Developmental Disability)
4. J (pages 1394–1395; Down Syndrome)
5. A (page 1410; Colostomies, Ileostomies, and Urostomies)
6. D (page 1402; Bariatric Patients)
7. G (pages 1397–1398; Hearing Impairment)
8. I (page 1410; Shunts)
9. B (pages 1401–1402; Spina Bifida)
10. E (pages 1403–1405; Tracheostomy Tubes)

Multiple Choice

1. C (pages 1393–1394; Developmental Disability)
2. B (page 1394; Autism Spectrum Disorder)
3. D (pages 1394–1395; Down Syndrome)
4. A (pages 1394–1395; Down Syndrome)
5. A (pages 1394–1395; Down Syndrome)
6. C (pages 1395–1396; Brain Injury)
7. D (pages 1396–1397; Visual Impairment)
8. B (pages 1396–1397; Visual Impairment)
9. D (pages 1397–1398; Hearing Impairment)
10. A (pages 1397–1398; Hearing Impairment)
11. D (pages 1400–1401; Cerebral Palsy)
12. B (pages 1400–1401; Cerebral Palsy)
13. C (pages 1400–1401; Cerebral Palsy)
14. A (pages 1401–1402; Spina Bifida)
15. B (pages 1403–1405; Tracheostomy Tubes)
16. C (pages 1405–1407; Mechanical Ventilators)
17. D (pages 1407–1408; Apnea Monitors)
18. C (page 1408; Ventricular Assist Devices)
19. B (page 1409; Central Venous Catheter)
20. B (pages 1409–1410; Gastronomy Tubes)
21. A (page 1410; Shunts)
22. C (page 1411; Home Care)
23. D (pages 1411–1412; Hospice Care and Terminally Ill Patients)
24. B (page 1402; Bariatric Patients)

True/False

1. T (page 1395; Patient Interaction)
2. F (pages 1396–1397; Visual Impairment)
3. T (page 1402; Paralysis)
4. F (page 1402; Bariatric Patients)
5. T (pages 1403–1405; Tracheostomy Tubes)
6. T (pages 1403–1405; Tracheostomy Tubes)
7. F (pages 1403–1405; Tracheostomy Tubes)
8. T (page 1408; Internal Cardiac Pacemakers)
9. T (pages 1409–1410; Gastronomy Tubes)
10. T (page 1411; Patient Assessment Guidelines)

Fill-in-the-Blank

1. Autism (page 1394; Autism Spectrum Disorder)
2. shoulder (pages 1396–1397; Visual Impairment)
3. Hearing aids (pages 1397–1398; Hearing Impairment)
4. sensorineural, conductive (pages 1397–1398; Hearing Impairment)
5. Cerebral palsy (pages 1400–1401; Cerebral Palsy)
6. vitamin B9 (folic acid) (pages 1401–1402; Spina Bifida)
7. ventricular assist device (page 1408; Ventricular Assist Devices)
8. Shunts (page 1410; Shunts)
9. dehydration (page 1410; Colostomies, Ileostomies, and Urostomies)
10. palliative care (pages 1411–1412; Hospice Care and Terminally Ill Patients)

Fill-in-the-Table (page 1404; Table 37-1)

Complete the missing information to the right of the mnemonic.

DOPE Mnemonic	
D	Displaced, dislodged, or damaged tube
O	Obstruction of the tube (secretions, blood, mucus, vomitus)
P	Pneumothorax, pulmonary problems
E	Equipment failure (kinked tubing, ventilator malfunction, empty oxygen supply)

Critical Thinking

Short Answer

1. 1. Speak slowly and distinctly into a less-impaired ear, or position yourself on that **side**.
   2. Change speakers. Look for a team member with a low-pitched voice if you think pitch is the issue.
   3. Provide paper and a pencil so that you may write your questions and the patient may write responses.
   4. Only one person should ask interview questions to avoid confusing the patient.
   5. Try the "reverse stethoscope" technique: Put the earpieces of your stethoscope in the patient's ears and speak softly into the diaphragm of the stethoscope. (pages 1397–1398; Hearing Impairment)

2. 1. Make sure the hearing aid is turned on.
   2. Try a fresh battery, and check the tubing to make sure it is not twisted or bent. Ensure that the switch is set on M (microphone), not T (telephone).
   3. Try a spare cord for a conventional body-type aid; the old one may be broken or shorted. Make sure the ear mold is not plugged with wax. (pages 1398–1400; Hearing Aids)

3. 1. Behind-the-ear type
   2. Conventional body type
   3. In-the-canal and completely in-the-canal type
   4. In-the-ear type (pages 1398–1400; Hearing Aids)

4. 1. Treat the patient with dignity and respect.
   2. Ask your patient how it is the best to move him or her before attempting to do so.
   3. Avoid trying to lift the patient by only one limb, which would risk injury to overtaxed joints.
   4. Coordinate and communicate all moves to all team members prior to starting to lift.
   5. If the move becomes uncontrolled at any point, stop, reposition, and resume.

6. Look for pinch or pressure points from equipment because they could cause a deep venous thrombosis.

7. Very large patients may have difficulty breathing if you lay the patient in a supine position.

8. Many manufacturers make specialized equipment for morbidly obese patients, and some areas have specially equipped bariatric ambulances for such patients.

9. Plan egress routes to accommodate large patients, equipment, and the lifting crew members.

10. Notify the receiving facility early to allow special arrangements to be made prior to your arrival to accommodate the patient's needs. (pages 1402–1403; Interactions With Patients With Morbid Obesity)

5. 1. What type of heart disorder does the patient have?

2. How long has this device been implanted?

3. What is the patient's normal baseline rhythm and pulse rate?

4. Is the patient's heart completely dependent on the pacemaker device?

5. At what pulse rate will the defibrillator fire?

6. How many times has the defibrillator shocked the patient? (page 1408; Table 37-2 Questions for Patients With Pacemakers)

Ambulance Calls

1. An internal cardiac pacemaker is implanted under the patient's skin to regulate the pulse rate and rhythm. You should provide oxygen and airway management for this patient. Because the automated implanted cardioverter defibrillator is firing, it is likely that the patient has an underlying dysrhythmia. ALS should be contacted for a rendezvous. In addition, you should be prepared for this patient to go into cardiac arrest. Remember not to place AED pads directly over the implanted device. Transport immediately, maintain ABCs, and rendezvous with ALS.

2. Many patients with Down syndrome have epilepsy. Most of the seizures are tonic-clonic. Patient management is the same as with other patients with seizures. Because the patient has had two witnessed seizures, consider requesting ALS. It is likely the patient will seize again. In addition, use the parents and family as a resource for information; they are likely to be very familiar with the patient's medical history and complications. Maintain ABCs, apply oxygen, and assess for any potential injuries that may have occurred during the seizure. Be aware of the potential airway complications faced in patients with Down syndrome, such as a large tongue and smaller oral and nasal cavities.

Skills

Assessment Review

1. C (page 1394; Autism Spectrum Disorder)
2. D (pages 1396–1397; Visual Impairment)
3. D (pages 1403–1405; Tracheostomy Tubes)
4. B (page 1410; Colostomies, Ileostomies, and Urostomies)

CHAPTER

38 Transport Operations

General Knowledge

Matching

1. D (page 1453; Air Medical Operations)

2. A (page 1426; Table 38-1 Basic Ambulance Designs)

3. E (pages 1446–1448; The Cushion of Safety)

4. G (pages 1442–1443; The Postrun Phase)

5. F (pages 1424–1426; Emergency Vehicle Design)

6. C (pages 1442–1443; The Postrun Phase)

7. B (pages 1442–1443; The Postrun Phase)

Multiple Choice

1. C (pages 1424–1426; Emergency Vehicle Design)

2. A (pages 1424–1426; Emergency Vehicle Design)

3. A (pages 1426–1427; The Preparation Phase)

4. B (page 1426; Table 38-1 Basic Ambulance Designs)

5. C (pages 1427–1430; Airway and Ventilation Equipment)

6. D (pages 1427–1430; Airway and Ventilation Equipment)

7. A (pages 1427–1430; Airway and Ventilation Equipment)

8. D (page 1434; Table 38-5 Extrication Equipment)

9. B (page 1428; Table 38-3 Ambulance Equipment Checklist)

10. D (pages 1432–1433; The Jump Kit)

11. A (page 1432; Patient Transfer Equipment)

12. D (page 1435; Daily Inspections)

13. D (pages 1426–1427; The Preparation Phase)

14. C (page 1436; The Dispatch Phase)

15. C (page 1437; En Route to the Scene)

16. D (page 1443; Driver Characteristics)

17. B (page 1437; En Route to the Scene)

18. D (page 1444; Safe Driving Practices)

19. B (page 1446; Table 38-6 Guidelines for Safe Ambulance Driving)

20. A (pages 1450–1451; Use of Warning Lights and Siren)

21. C (page 1448; Vehicle Size and Distance Judgment)

22. D (page 1450; Laws and Regulations)

23. D (page 1444; Safe Driving Practices)

24. C (pages 1450–1451; Use of Warning Lights and Siren)

25. C (page 1451; Right-of-Way Privileges)

26. B (page 1452; Intersection Hazards)

27. D (pages 1437–1438; Arrival at the Scene)

28. D (page 1440; Traffic Control)

29. C (page 1441; The Delivery Phase)

30. D (pages 1450–1451; Use of Warning Lights and Siren)

31. D (page 1455; Establishing a Landing Zone)

True/False

1. T (pages 1426–1427; The Preparation Phase)

2. F (page 1430; CPR Equipment)

3. T (page 1453; Air Medical Operations)

4. F (page 1437; En Route to the Scene)

5. F (pages 1451–1452; Use of Escorts)

6. F (page 1446; Table 38-6 Guidelines for Safe Ambulance Driving)

7. T (page 1456; Landing Zone Safety and Patient Transfer)

8. F (page 1453; Air Medical Operations)

9. F (page 1455; Establishing a Landing Zone)

Fill-in-the-Blank

1. jump kit (pages 1432–1433; The Jump Kit)
2. Star of Life (pages 1424–1426; Emergency Vehicle Design)
3. hearse (pages 1424–1426; Emergency Vehicle Design)
4. First-responder vehicles (pages 1424–1426; Emergency Vehicle Design)
5. nine (page 1426; Phases of an Ambulance Call)
6. with due regard (pages 1450–1451; Use of Warning Lights and Siren)
7. airway (pages 1427–1430; Airway and Ventilation Equipment)
8. CPR board (page 1430; CPR Equipment)

Labeling

1. Helicopter Hand Signals (page 1457; Figure 38-32)

   A. Move right

   B. Move forward

   C. Move rearward

   D. Move upward

   E. Move downward

   F. Move left

Critical Thinking

Multiple Choice

1. A   (pages 1437–1438; Arrival at the Scene)
2. B   (page 1426; Phases of an Ambulance Call)
3. D   (page 1426; Phases of an Ambulance Call)
4. C   (page 1440; Traffic Control)
5. A   (pages 1440–1441; The Transport Phase)

Short Answer

1. **Type I:** Conventional, truck cab-chassis with modular ambulance body that can be transferred to a newer chassis as needed

   Type II: Standard van, forward-control integral cab-body ambulance

   Type III: Specialty van cab with a modular ambulance body that is mounted on a cutaway van chassis (page 1426; Table 38-1)

2. 1. Preparation for the call

   2. Dispatch

   3. En route to scene

   4. Arrival at scene

   5. Transfer of patient to the ambulance

   6. En route to the receiving facility (transport)

   7. At the receiving facility (delivery)

   8. En route to station

   9. Postrun (page 1426; Phases of an Ambulance Call)

3. *Siren syndrome* is the term for the increase in anxiety of other drivers that commonly causes them to drive faster in the presence of sirens. (page 1448; Recognition of Siren Syndrome)

4. **1.** To the best of your knowledge, the unit must be on a true emergency call.

　2. Both audible and visual warning devices must be used simultaneously.

　3. The unit must be operated with due regard for the safety of all others, both on and off the roadway. (pages 1450–1451; Use of Warning Lights and Siren)

5. **1.** At the time of dispatch, select the shortest and least congested route to the scene.

　2. Avoid routes with heavy traffic congestion; know alternative routes to each hospital during rush hours.

　3. Avoid one-way streets. Do not go against the flow of traffic on a one-way street, unless absolutely necessary.

　4. Watch carefully for bystanders as you approach the scene.

　5. Once you arrive at the scene, park the ambulance in a safe place. If you park facing into traffic, turn off your headlights so that they do not blind oncoming drivers, unless they are needed to illuminate the scene. If the vehicle is blocking part of the road, keep your warning lights on to alert oncoming motorists; otherwise, turn them off.

　6. Drive within the speed limit while transporting patients, except in the rare extreme emergency.

　7. Go with the flow of the traffic.

　8. Always drive defensively.

　9. Always maintain a safe following distance. Use the "4-second rule."

　10. Try to maintain an open space or cushion in the lane next to you as an escape route in case the vehicle in front of you stops suddenly.

　11. Use your siren if you turn on the emergency lights, except when you are on a freeway.

　12. Always assume that other drivers will not hear the siren or see your emergency lights. (page 1446; Table 38-6)

6. A hard, level surface a minimum of 100 feet by 100 feet (30 m by 30 m)

A clear site that is free of loose debris, electric or telephone poles and wires, or any other hazards that might interfere with the safe operation of the helicopter (page 1455; Establishing a Landing Zone)

Ambulance Calls

1. Fire departments have a distinct chain of command. You should obtain permission to place yourself en route to this medical emergency from your shift captain or appropriate fire officer. Just because a call is dispatched does not mean you should automatically place yourself en route to that location. The incident commander of the confirmed structure fire may need your immediate assistance on the scene. Because you do not know the nature of the medical emergency at this point, it would be prudent to place that decision in appropriate hands. Always follow local protocols and chain of command.

2. Ideally, you should be very familiar with your response area, and you should take time every shift to study local roads. This can be done individually or as a group shift activity. The larger your coverage area, the more difficult it becomes to memorize addresses, especially if you are not native to the area. Regardless, you should be able to read maps quickly, and you should not rely on your memory to assist in locating a new address. To attempt to memorize all local streets is a good goal, but failing to consult with a map before leaving the station for reasons of pride is downright foolish. Ensure that each and every agency vehicle used in response to emergencies is equipped with local maps and other resources to ensure that you arrive promptly at emergency scenes. Utilize your local dispatch center for directions, if necessary.

3. Park your ambulance in a safe area and ensure your personal safety. Either you or your partner should handle traffic control until the police arrive. The person not handling traffic control should assess the patient. Provide patient care while ensuring personal safety and patient safety.

Fill-in-the-Patient Care Report

EMS Patient Care Report (PCR)			
Date: Today's date	**Incident No.:** 2011-8999	**Nature of Call:** MVC	**Location:** Hwy 12 and Nest Creek Rd.

Dispatched: 0512	**En Route:** 0513	**At Scene:** 0523	**Transport:** 0532	**At Hospital:** 0546	**In Service:** 0557

Patient Information

Age: 41 years **Sex:** Female **Weight (in kg [lb]):** 90 kg (198 lb)	**Allergies:** None **Medications:** Lisinopril **Past Medical History:** TIA at age 36 **Chief Complaint:** Facial pain following MVC

Vital Signs

Time: 0532	**BP:** 142/100	**Pulse:** 100	**Respirations:** 16 Unlabored	**SpO$_2$:** 98%
Time: 0543	**BP:** 142/100	**Pulse:** 100	**Respirations:** 14 Unlabored	**SpO$_2$:** 98%

EMS Treatment
(circle all that apply)

Oxygen @ _15_ L/min via (circle one): NC **(NRM)** BVM	Assisted Ventilation	Airway Adjunct	CPR
Defibrillation	Bleeding Control	Bandaging	**(Splinting)**	Other:

Narrative

Dispatched on an emergency call to a motor vehicle collision on Hwy 12. Arrived on scene to find two vehicles involved and one injured driver (other driver denied any injury). The patient, a 41-year-old woman with a swollen and bleeding nose, was contacted while still belted into the driver's seat of her damaged car. She was conscious and alert and followed directions appropriately. C-spine precautions were taken. The patient was properly secured to a long backboard, removed from the vehicle, and given high-concentration oxygen via a nonrebreathing mask. The patient was loaded into the ambulance and was found to have no other obvious or stated injuries. Initial vital signs indicated elevated blood pressure, which the patient stated was normal; all other observations indicated that the patient was stable. While en route, I contacted the receiving facility to provide a report and completed a second set of vital signs to compare to the first and found no change other than a slightly lower respiratory rate. Transport was completed without incident. Once at the County Medical Center, the patient was transferred appropriately to the staff's care. I provided a full verbal report to the accepting nurse. Ambulance was then cleaned and restocked, and we returned to service without delay.**End of Report**

CHAPTER

39 Vehicle Extrication and Special Rescue

General Knowledge

Matching

1. E (pages 1465–1466; Fundamentals of Extrication)
2. A (page 1472; Simple Access)
3. L (pages 1467–1469; Arrival and Scene Size-up)
4. F (pages 1465–1466; Fundamentals of Extrication)
5. B (pages 1475–1476; Technical Rescue Situations)
6. J (page 1477; Tactical Emergency Medical Support)
7. D (page 1472; Complex Access)
8. H (pages 1476–1477; Search and Rescue)
9. I (pages 1475–1476; Technical Rescue Situations)
10. G (page 1479; Structure Fires)
11. K (page 1479; Structure Fires)
12. C (pages 1469–1470; Hazard Control)

Multiple Choice

1. B (pages 1465–1466; Fundamentals of Extrication)
2. D (pages 1467–1469; Arrival and Scene Size-up)
3. A (page 1468; Words of Wisdom)
4. B (pages 1465–1466; Fundamentals of Extrication)
5. D (pages 1467–1469; Arrival and Scene Size-up)
6. C (pages 1467–1469; Arrival and Scene Size-up)
7. D (pages 1469–1470; Hazard Control)
8. B (pages 1465–1466; Fundamentals of Extrication)
9. B (pages 1469–1470; Hazard Control)
10. C (page 1470; Support Operations)
11. A (pages 1473–1474; Removal of the Patient)
12. B (page 1472; Simple Access)
13. C (page 1475; Specialized Rescue Situations)
14. D (page 1477; Trench Rescue)
15. B (page 1477; Tactical Emergency Medical Support)

True/False

1. T (page 1479; Structure Fires)
2. F (pages 1476–1477; Search and Rescue)
3. T (pages 1475–1476; Technical Rescue Situations)
4. T (page 1475; Termination)
5. T (page 1475; Specialized Rescue Situations)
6. T (pages 1467–1469; Arrival and Scene Size-up)
7. T (pages 1473–1474; Removal of the Patient)
8. T (pages 1473–1474; Removal of the Patient)
9. T (pages 1467–1469; Arrival and Scene Size-up)
10. T (page 1470; Alternative Fuel Vehicles)
11. F (pages 1473–1474; Removal of the Patient)
12. T (pages 1472–1473; Emergency Care)
13. F (page 1472; Simple Access)
14. T (pages 1470–1472; Gaining Access)
15. F (pages 1469–1470; Hazard Control)
16. T (pages 1464–1465; Vehicle Safety Systems)
17. F (page 1466; Table 39-1 Ten Phases of Extrication)

Fill-in-the-Blank

1. hazardous materials (page 1479; Structure Fires)
2. rapid extrication (pages 1470–1472; Gaining Access)
3. Entrapment (pages 1465–1466; Fundamentals of Extrication)
4. primary assessment (pages 1472–1473; Emergency Care)
5. Size-up (pages 1467–1469; Arrival and Scene Size-up)

6. hearing protection (pages 1473–1474; Removal of the Patient)

7. EMS providers (pages 1465–1466; Fundamentals of Extrication)

8. firefighters (pages 1465–1466; Fundamentals of Extrication)

9. danger zone (pages 1469–1470; Hazard Control)

10. battery (pages 1469–1470; Hazard Control)

11. stabilized (pages 1469–1470; Hazard Control)

12. protective gear (pages 1467–1469; Arrival and Scene Size-up)

13. rescue team (pages 1465–1466; Fundamentals of Extrication)

14. Communication (pages 1465–1466; Fundamentals of Extrication)

15. leadership (pages 1475–1476; Technical Rescue Situations)

16. fire-resistant blanket, backboard (pages 1470–1472; Gaining Access)

17. specialized rescue (page 1475; Specialized Rescue Situations)

18. air transport (pages 1475–1476; Technical Rescue Situations)

19. incident commander (pages 1476–1477; Search and Rescue)

20. Vibration (page 1477; Trench Rescue)

21. 4 feet (page 1477; Trench Rescue)

22. structure fire (page 1479; Structure Fires)

Critical Thinking

Short Answer

1. **EMS personnel:** Responsible for assessing and providing immediate medical care, performing triage and assigning priority to patients, packaging the patient, providing additional assessment and care as needed once the patient has been removed, and providing transport to the emergency department.

   Firefighters: Responsible for extinguishing any fire, preventing additional ignition, ensuring that the scene is safe, and washing down spilled fuel.

   Law enforcement: Responsible for traffic control and direction, maintaining order at the scene, investigating the crash or crime scene, and establishing and maintaining a perimeter so that bystanders are kept at a safe distance and out of the way of rescuers.

   Rescue team: Responsible for properly securing and stabilizing the vehicle, providing safe entrance and access to patients, safely extricating any patients, ensuring that patients are properly protected during extrication or other rescue activities, and providing adequate room so that patients can be removed properly. (pages 1465–1466; Fundamentals of Extrication)

2. 1. Is the patient in a vehicle or in some other structure?

   2. Is the vehicle or structure severely damaged?

   3. What hazards exist that pose a risk to the patient and rescuers?

   4. In what position is the vehicle? On what type of surface? Is the vehicle stable, or is it likely to roll over? (pages 1470–1472; Gaining Access)

3. 1. Address any exsanguinating hemorrhage with direct pressure or a tourniquet if appropriate.

   2. Provide manual stabilization to protect the cervical spine, as needed.

   3. Open the airway.

   4. Provide high-flow oxygen.

   5. Assist or provide for adequate ventilation.

   6. Control any significant external bleeding.

   7. Treat all critical injuries. (pages 1472–1473; Emergency Care)

4. **1.** Preparation

    2. En route to the scene

    3. Arrival and scene size-up

    4. Hazard control

    5. Support operations

    6. Gaining access

    7. Emergency care

    8. Removal of the patient

    9. Transfer of the patient

    10. Termination (page 1466; Table 39-1)

5. **F**—Failure to understand the environment or underestimating it

    A—Additional medical problems not considered

    I—Inadequate rescue skills

    L—Lack of teamwork or experience

    U—Underestimating the logistics of the incident

    R—Rescue versus recovery mode not considered

    E—Equipment not mastered (page 1479; Words of Wisdom)

Ambulance Calls

1. Unless there is an immediate threat of fire, explosion, or other danger, once entrance and access to the patient have been provided and the scene is safe, you should perform a primary assessment and provide care before further extrication begins. She is obviously alert, and her airway is open. The first concern is to address the arterial bleeding, which is best managed with a tourniquet in this situation. You should direct your partner to take cervical spine control, and you should attempt to calm the patient and assess her mental status as you control the bleeding. Explain to her what you are doing, and offer encouragement. Provide oxygen as needed, and look for other life threats. Once these have been addressed, the extrication can continue, and you should participate in the preparation for patient removal.

2. Entering the water could be a death sentence for you both. If you have a cell phone and/or department radio with you, your best course of action would be to inform incoming units of the boy's location and situation. It would be advisable to direct some responding units downstream so that if the boy should lose his grasp on the log, other responders will be available to retrieve him. If your department has areas that contain the possibility of swift-water rescue (even if only seasonal), training should be conducted, and appropriate helmets, throw bags, and life jackets should be made available for safe response. You must assess the scene before trying to effect immediate rescue operations. Many responders have been killed by "jumping into" all types of rescues without performing a scene size-up or using the proper gear. Don't become a victim. Doing so will only make you part of the problem.

3. Try to learn as much about the chemical as possible by having the dispatcher contact CHEMTREC or another agency to find out about possible effects to the patient. Prepare necessary equipment to manage the airway and ventilation. Be prepared to do CPR, if necessary. Have all equipment within reach. Once the patient is brought to you, rapidly begin to manage the ABCs and prepare for rapid transport.

CHAPTER

Incident Management

40

General Knowledge

Matching

1. H (pages 1507–1508; Carboys)
2. N (pages 1514–1515; Establishing Control Zones)
3. B (pages 1514–1515; Establishing Control Zones)
4. J (pages 1487–1490; Incident Command System)
5. E (pages 1514–1515; Establishing Control Zones)
6. O (pages 1488–1489; Command)
7. L (page 1502; Disaster Management)
8. I (pages 1514–1515; Establishing Control Zones)

9. A (pages 1506–1508; Container Volume)
10. G (pages 1508–1509; The Department of Transportation Marking System)
11. C (pages 1497–1498; Triage)
12. F (pages 1506–1508; Container Volume)
13. D (pages 1497–1498; Triage)
14. M (pages 1487–1490; Incident Command System)
15. K (pages 1514–1515; Establishing Control Zones)

Multiple Choice

1. B (pages 1486–1487; National Incident Management System)
2. D (pages 1486–1487; National Incident Management System)
3. A (pages 1487–1490; Incident Command System)
4. D (page 1489; Finance/Administration)
5. A (page 1490; Command Staff)
6. C (page 1492; EMS Response Within the ICS: Scene Size-up)
7. B (page 1493; EMS Response Within the ICS: What Do I Need to Do?)
8. C (page 1493; Establishing Command)
9. D (page 1493; Triage Supervisor)
10. B (page 1494; Transportation Supervisor)
11. B (page 1495; Rehabilitation Supervisor)
12. A (page 1486; Introduction)
13. B (pages 1498–1499; Triage Categories)
14. C (pages 1514–1515; Table 40-1 Triage Priorities)
15. B (page 1498; Table 40-1 Triage Priorities)

16. D (pages 1514–1515; Table 40-1 Triage Priorities)
17. A (pages 1514–1515; Table 40-1 Triage Priorities)
18. C (pages 1489–1490; Logistics)
19. A (pages 1499–1500; START Triage)
20. C (pages 1499–1500; START Triage)
21. A (pages 1500–1501; JumpSTART Triage for Pediatric Patients)
22. C (pages 1499–1500; START Triage)
23. B (pages 1503–1504; Recognizing a Hazardous Material)
24. D (pages 1506–1508; Container Volume)
25. C (page 1507; Drums)
26. C (pages 1508–1509; The Department of Transportation Marking System)
27. B (page 1510; Other Considerations)
28. A (pages 1510–1511; Material Safety Data Sheets)
29. D (pages 1514–1515; Establishing Control Zones)
30. B (pages 1516–1517; Personal Protective Equipment Level)

True/False

1. T (page 1486; Introduction)
2. T (pages 1487–1490; Incident Command System)
3. F (pages 1487–1490; Incident Command System)

4. F (page 1493; What Do I Need to Do?)
5. T (page 1494; Transportation Supervisor)
6. F (page 1494; Staging Supervisor)

7. T   (page 1495; Morgue Supervisor)

8. T   (page 1499; Triage Tags)

9. T   (pages 1500–1501; JumpSTART Triage for Pediatric Patients)

10. F   (pages 1503–1504; Recognizing a Hazardous Material)

11. T   (pages 1504–1505; Senses)

12. T   (page 1507; Drums)

13. F   (pages 1508–1509; The Department of Transportation Marking System)

14. T   (pages 1513–1514; Identification)

15. F   (page 1518; Special Care)

Fill-in-the-Blank

1. flexibility, standardization (pages 1486–1487; National Incident Management System)

2. span of control (pages 1487–1490; Incident Command System)

3. single (pages 1488–1489; Command)

4. planning (page 1490; Planning)

5. Preparedness (pages 1491–1492; Preparedness)

6. triage supervisor (page 1493; Triage Supervisor)

7. Treatment supervisors (pages 1493–1494; Treatment Supervisor)

8. number, category (pages 1497–1498; Triage)

9. location, building (page 1504; Occupancy and Location)

10. bulk, nonbulk (page 1505; Containers)

11. Storage bags (page 1507; Bags)

12. Control zones (pages 1514–1515; Establishing Control Zones)

13. warm zone (pages 1514–1515; Establishing Control Zones)

14. decontamination (pages 1514–1515; Establishing Control Zones)

15. intermodal tank (pages 1506–1508; Container Volume)

Fill-in-the-Table (page 1498; Table 40-1)

Triage Priorities	
Triage Category	**Typical Injuries**
Red tag: first priority (immediate) Patients who need immediate care and transport Treat these patients first and transport as soon as possible	• **Airway and breathing compromise** • **Uncontrolled or severe bleeding** • **Severe medical problems** • **Signs of shock (hypoperfusion)** • **Severe burns** • **Open chest or abdominal injuries**
Yellow tag: second priority (delayed) Patients whose treatment and transport can be temporarily delayed	• **Burns without airway compromise** • **Major or multiple bone or joint injuries** • **Back injuries with or without spinal cord damage**
Green tag: third priority, minimal (walking wounded) Patients who require minimal or no treatment and whose transport can be delayed until last	• **Minor fractures** • **Minor soft-tissue injuries**
Black tag: fourth priority (expectant) Patients who are already dead or have little chance for survival; treat salvageable patients before treating these patients	• **Obvious death** • **Obviously nonsurvivable injury, such as major open brain trauma** • **Respiratory arrest (if limited resources)** • **Cardiac arrest**

Critical Thinking

Short Answer

1. • Command and management
   • Preparedness
   • Resource management
   • Communications and information management
   • Supporting technologies
   • Ongoing management and maintenance (pages 1486–1487; National Incident Management System)

2. 1. Check-in at the incident
   2. Initial incident briefing
   3. Incident record keeping
   4. Accountability
   5. Incident demobilization (page 1591; Mobilization and Deployment)

3. • The total number of patients
   • The number of patients in each of the triage categories
   • Recommendations for extrication and movement of patients to the treatment area
   • Resources needed to complete triage and begin movement of patients (pages 1497–1498; Triage)

4. • An understanding of what hazardous substances are and the risks associated with them
   • An understanding of the potential outcomes of an incident
   • The ability to recognize the presence of hazardous substances
   • The ability to identify the hazardous substances, if possible
   • An understanding of the role of the first responder awareness individual in the emergency response plan
   • The ability to determine the need for additional resources and to notify the communication center (page 1503; Introduction to Hazardous Materials)

5. • The name of the chemical, including any synonyms for it
   • Physical and chemical characteristics of the material
   • Physical hazards of the material
   • Health hazards of the material
   • Signs and symptoms of exposure
   • Routes of entry
   • Permissible exposure limits
   • Response-party contact
   • Precautions for safe handling (including hygiene practices, protective measures, and procedures for cleaning up spills or leaks)
   • Applicable control measures, including personal protective equipment
   • Emergency and first-aid procedures
   • Appropriate waste disposal (pages 1510–1511; Safety Data Sheets)

Ambulance Calls

1. The 4-year-old should be triaged as first priority (red). The 27-year-old should be triaged as third priority (green). The 42-year-old should be triaged as fourth priority (black). (pages 1497–1498; Triage)

2. It is fortunate that this is occurring on shift change because members from two shifts are available to respond to this mass-casualty incident. Because this is a remote area, which implies extended response times, you should use this time to gather information from the crop-duster pilot/responsible parties regarding the substance and to notify all local hospitals. Area HazMat team members should be requested, and once the chemicals have been identified, appropriate first aid and other instructions should be relayed to the affected patients on-scene through the dispatch center. Law enforcement should be requested to cordon off the area to prevent more individuals, such as coworkers and family members, from entering the contaminated area. Consult HazMat team members and/or CHEMTREC for appropriate information, including medical treatment, PPE, and minimum distances that are required to avoid exposure to the identified substance. Do not enter the area unless you have been trained and have the proper equipment to do so.

3. The good news is that you are uphill from the possible hazardous materials. You should be uphill and upwind from contaminated areas (especially when dealing with an unidentified substance). Each chemical reacts differently to outside air, temperature, and other ambient conditions. You should immediately instruct all civilians along the road to move out of the immediate area and/or instruct them to wait in a specific location if you feel that they have already been contaminated by the substance. Do not allow the driver to contaminate the passersby. Immediately notify law enforcement, as well as the local HazMat team. Attempt to gain information regarding the shipment, keeping a safe distance (using binoculars, PA system to relay instructions, etc). Look for placards or other markings, and use the *Emergency Response Guidebook* in an attempt to ascertain what the truck is carrying. Prevent exposure to yourself and your crew and the members of the public. Always follow local protocols.

Skills

Assessment Review

1. C   (pages 1499–1500; START Triage)
2. B   (pages 1499–1500; START Triage)
3. A   (pages 1499–1500; START Triage)
4. B   (pages 1499–1500; START Triage)

CHAPTER

41

Terrorism Response and Disaster Management

General Knowledge

Matching

1. L (page 1535; Vesicants (Blister Agents))
2. O (page 1535; Vesicants (Blister Agents))
3. E (page 1542; Biologic Agents)
4. N (pages 1536–1537; Pulmonary Agents (Choking Agents))
5. J (page 1545; Neurotoxins)
6. K (page 1544; Bacteria)
7. B (page 1535; Chemical Agents)
8. F (page 1540; Metabolic Agents (Cyanides))
9. D (page 1535; Chemical Agents)
10. M (page 1545; Plague (Bubonic/Pneumonic))
11. C (page 1542; Biologic Agents)
12. I (pages 1546–1548; Ricin)
13. H (page 1542; Biologic Agents)
14. A (page 1549; What Is Radiation?)
15. G (page 1532; Biologic Terrorism/Warfare)

Multiple Choice

1. D (pages 1528–1529; What Is Terrorism?)
2. A (pages 1528–1529; What Is Terrorism?)
3. B (page 1531; Chemical Terrorism/Warfare)
4. B (page 1532; Nuclear/Radiologic Terrorism)
5. A (page 1533; Scene Safety)
6. A (page 1534; Notification Procedures)
7. B (page 1535; Chemical Agents)
8. C (page 1535; Vesicants (Blister Agents))
9. A (pages 1536–1537; Pulmonary Agents (Choking Agents))
10. A (page 1539; Table 41-1)
11. A (pages 1539–1540; Nerve Agent Treatment)
12. B (page 1539; Safety Tips)
13. A (page 1540; Metabolic Agents (Cyanides))
14. B (page 1542; Biologic Agents)
15. D (pages 1543–1544; Viral Hemorrhagic Fevers)
16. D (page 1545; Inhalation and Cutaneous Anthrax)
17. C (page 1545; Plague (Bubonic/Pneumonic))
18. A (pages 1537–1540; Nerve Agents)
19. A (pages 1546–1548; Ricin)
20. B (page 1549; Syndromic Surveillance)
21. B (page 1549; What Is Radiation?)
22. D (page 1552; Radiologic/Nuclear Devices: Protective Measure)
23. B (page 1553; Tissues at Risk)

True/False

1. F (pages 1528–1529; What Is Terrorism?)
2. T (page 1531; Weapons of Mass Destruction)
3. F (pages 1532–1533; Recognizing a Terrorist Event (Indicators))
4. T (pages 1532–1533; Recognizing a Terrorist Event (Indicators))
5. T (page 1533; Scene Safety)
6. F (page 1534; Notification Procedures)
7. F (page 1535; Chemical Agents)
8. F (page 1535; Vesicants (Blister Agents))
9. T (pages 1536–1537; Pulmonary Agents (Choking Agents))
10. F (pages 1537–1540; Nerve Agents)
11. F (pages 1537–1540; Nerve Agents)
12. T (page 1539; Safety Tips)
13. T (page 1540; Metabolic Agents (Cyanides))
14. F (page 1543; Smallpox)

15. F   (pages 1543–1544; Viral Hemorrhagic Fevers)

16. T   (page 1545; Inhalation and Cutaneous Anthrax)

17. T   (page 1545; Plague (Bubonic/Pneumonic))

18. F   (pages 1546–1548; Ricin)

19. F   (pages 1546–1548; Ricin)

20. T   (pages 1550–1551; Radiologic Dispersal Devices)

21. T   (pages 1551–1552; Radiologic/Nuclear Devices: Medical Management)

22. T   (pages 1552–1553; Incendiary and Explosive Devices)

Fill-in-the-Blank

1. domestic terrorism (page 1528; What Is Terrorism?)
2. weapon of mass destruction (page 1531; Weapons of Mass Destruction)
3. State-sponsored terrorism (page 1532; Nuclear/ Radiologic Terrorism)
4. secondary infection (page 1535; Vesicants (Blister Agents))
5. Cross-contamination (page 1534; Responder Safety (Personnel Protection))
6. Route of exposure (page 1535; Chemical Agents)
7. contact hazard (page 1535; Chemical Agents)
8. Nerve agents (pages 1537–1540; Nerve Agents)
9. Off-gassing (pages 1537–1540; Nerve Agents)
10. Dissemination (page 1542; Biologic Agents)
11. Virus (page 1543; Viruses)
12. viral hemorrhagic fevers (pages 1543–1544; Viral Hemorrhagic Fevers)
13. Anthrax (page 1545; Inhalation and Cutaneous Anthrax)
14. lymph nodes (page 1545; Plague (Bubonic/Pneumonic))
15. botulinum (page 1546; Botulinum Toxin)
16. Points of distribution (page 1549; Points of Distribution (Strategic National Stockpile))
17. radiologic dispersal device (pages 1550–1551; Radiologic Dispersal Devices)
18. secondary blast injury (pages 1552–1553; Incendiary and Explosive Devices: Mechanism of Injury)

Critical Thinking

Short Answer

1. 1. What are your initial actions?
   2. Whom should you notify, and what should you tell them?
   3. What type of additional resources might you require?
   4. How should you proceed to address the needs of the victims?
   5. How do you ensure your own and your partner's safety, as well as the safety of the victims?
   6. What is the clinical presentation of a victim exposed to a WMD?
   7. How are WMD patients to be assessed and treated?
   8. How do you avoid becoming contaminated or cross-contaminated with a WMD agent? (page 1528; Introduction)
2. 1. Vesicants (blister agents)
   2. Respiratory agents (choking agents)
   3. Nerve agents
   4. Metabolic agents (cyanides) (page 1531; Chemical Terrorism/Warfare)
3. 1. Type of location
   2. Type of call
   3. Number of patients
   4. Victims' statements
   5. Preincident indicators (pages 1532–1533; Recognizing a Terrorist Event (Indicators))

4. 1. Skin irritation, burning, and reddening

  2. Immediate, intense skin pain

  3. Formation of large blisters

  4. Gray discoloration of skin

  5. Swollen and closed or irritated eyes

  6. Permanent eye injury

  7. If vapors inhaled:

     a. Hoarseness and stridor

     b. Severe cough

     c. Hemoptysis

     d. Severe dyspnea (page 1535; Vesicants (Blister Agents))

5. 1. Shortness of breath

  2. Chest tightness

  3. Hoarseness and stridor due to upper airway constriction

  4. Gasping and coughing (pages 1536–1537; Pulmonary Agents (Choking Agents))

6. 1. Salivation, sweating

  2. Lacrimation

  3. Urination

  4. Defecation, drooling, diarrhea

  5. Gastric upset and cramps

  6. Emesis

  7. Muscle twitching, miosis (page 1539; Table 41-1)

7. 1. Shortness of breath and gasping respirations

  2. Tachypnea

  3. Flushed skin

  4. Tachycardia

  5. Altered mental status

  6. Seizures

  7. Coma

  8. Apnea

  9. Cardiac arrest (page 1540; Metabolic Agents (Cyanides))

8. 1. Fever

  2. Chills

  3. Headache

  4. Muscle aches

  5. Nausea

  6. Vomiting

  7. Diarrhea

8. Severe abdominal cramping

9. Dehydration

10. Gastrointestinal bleeding

11. Necrosis of liver, spleen, kidneys, and gastrointestinal tract (pages 1546–1548; Ricin)

9. 1. Hospitals

2. Colleges and universities

3. Chemical and industrial sites (pages 1549–1550; Sources of Radiologic Material)

10. 1. Time

2. Distance

3. Shielding (page 1552; Protective Measure)

Ambulance Calls

1. There is no confirmation regarding the nature of the explosion. It could have been caused by a number of hazards, but precautions should be taken any time there is the chance for a terrorist attack. No one should rush into the scene because terrorists have been known to deliberately target first responders by placing secondary explosive devices. Request all available resources, including local, state, and federal specialized HazMat and law enforcement agencies, to assist in this call. Notify all local and regional hospitals of the situation; assess the scene from a distance. Establish command, and designate a staging area for incoming units. Enter the scene only when it has been determined to be safe. Regularly scheduled mock drills to include expected agencies to respond in this type of situation can greatly improve communications and the overall effectiveness and efficiency of response.

2. The presence of numerous people with the same signs and symptoms, who were in the same location at the same time, should immediately send up red flags. These patients were exposed to contaminated food, air, or water in which they ingested some sort of toxin. Ingestion of ricin can produce these signs and symptoms within 4 to 8 hours after exposure. It can be difficult to initially determine what substances caused these signs and symptoms, but through careful history taking and investigation of the patients' commonalities, the exposure can be found. Unfortunately, there is no vaccination or other specific treatment available for exposure to ricin. Only supportive measures for airway, breathing, and circulation can be applied.

3. Cyanide is colorless and has an odor similar to bitter almonds. It interferes with the body's ability to utilize oxygen and can result in headache, shortness of breath, tachypnea, altered levels of consciousness, apnea, seizures, and even death. Antidotes can be given but are rarely carried on ambulances. Patients' clothing must be removed to avoid exposure to the cyanide because it is released as a gas from the clothing fibers. For most patients, simply removing them from the source of cyanide and providing supportive therapy for their ABCs will be all that is needed. However, those with significant exposure may require aggressive airway intervention.

Skills

Assessment Review

1. C   (page 1543; Smallpox)

2. B   (page 1545; Plague (Bubonic/Pneumonic))

3. D   (page 1545; Inhalation and Cutaneous Anthrax)

4. A   (pages 1543–1544; Viral Hemorrhagic Fevers)